New Feminist Stories of Child Sexual Abuse

Child sexual abuse is a multifaceted event, interpreted in many different ways, in many different contexts. In *New Feminist Stories of Child Sexual Abuse* contributors try to untangle some of the complex ways in which stories of child sexual abuse are translated through and into personal, professional and social practices.

The first section of the book explores the cultural and political landscape of child sexual in Western and non-Western contexts. It examines the ways in which radical aspects of feminism can be undermined in Western cultures and how Westernised ideologies of childhood, sex and gender have been used to structure discussions about child sexual abuse across the world.

The second section traces the effects of these wider cultural and political narratives through the various contexts in which child sexual abuse is theorised and around which interventions in the lives of women are structured. It provides insights into how traditional approaches to understanding harm can be challenged and reworked in practice, using alternative therapeutic models based on feminist post-structuralist agendas.

Reworking earlier feminist analyses, *New Feminist Stories of Child Sexual Abuse* asks pertinent questions about how child sexual abuse is produced, rather than merely represented, in the ways we speak about it.

Paula Reavey is a Senior Lecturer in Psychology at South Bank University. **Sam Warner** is a Consultant Clinical Psychologist and Research Fellow at Manchester Metropolitan University.

New Feminist Stories of Child Sexual Abuse

Sexual scripts and dangerous dialogues

Edited by Paula Reavey and Sam Warner

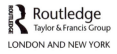
Routledge
Taylor & Francis Group

LONDON AND NEW YORK

First published 2003
by Routledge
11 New Fetter Lane, London EC4P 4EE

Simultaneously published in the USA and Canada
by Routledge
29 West 35th Street, New York, NY 10001

Routledge is an imprint of the Taylor & Francis Group

Typeset in Times by Wearset Ltd, Boldon, Tyne and Wear
Printed and bound in Great Britain by St Edmundsbury Press,
Bury St Edmunds, Suffolk

British Library Cataloguing in Publication Data
A catalogue record for this book is available from the British
Library

Library of Congress Cataloging in Publication Data
A catalog record for this book has been requested

ISBN 0-415-25943-6 (hbk)
ISBN 0-415-25944-4 (pbk)

To my family, Alex and Oskar (PR)
To my mum and dad, Thelma and Geoff Lidster (SW)

Contents

List of contributors   ix
Acknowledgements   xii

1 **Introduction**   I
   PAULA REAVEY AND SAM WARNER

PART I
**Exploring the cultural and political landscape of child
sexual abuse**   13

2 **Feminism's restless undead: the radical/lesbian/victim theorist
   and conflicts over sexual violence against children and women**   15
   CHRIS ATMORE

3 **Childhood, sexual abuse and contemporary political
   subjectivities**   34
   ERICA BURMAN

4 **Problems of cultural imperialism in the study of child sexual
   abuse**   52
   ANN LEVETT

5 **Traumatic revisions: remembering abuse and the politics
   of forgiveness**   77
   JANICE HAAKEN

6 **Creating discourses of 'false memory': media coverage and
   production dynamics**   94
   JENNY KITZINGER

7 The vigilant(e) parent and the paedophile: the *News of the World* campaign 2000 and the contemporary governmentality of child sexual abuse 108
VIKKI BELL

PART II
How we theorise and intervene in the lives of women who have experienced child sexual abuse 129

8 The 'harm' story in childhood sexual abuse: contested understandings, disputed knowledges 131
LINDSAY O'DELL

9 When past meets present to produce a sexual 'other': examining professional and everyday narratives of child sexual abuse and sexuality 148
PAULA REAVEY

10 Diagnosing distress and reproducing disorder: women, child sexual abuse and 'borderline personality disorder' 167
SAM WARNER AND TRACY WILKINS

11 Writing the effects of sexual abuse: interrogating the possibilities and pitfalls of using clinical psychology expertise for a critical justice agenda 187
NICOLA GAVEY

12 Working at being survivors: identity, gender and participation in self-help groups 210
MARCIA WORRELL

13 Disrupting identity through Visible Therapy: a feminist post-structuralist approach to working with women who have experienced child sexual abuse 226
SAM WARNER

Index 248

Contributors

Chris Atmore has been a New Zealand government child abuse researcher and educator; activist against sexual violence; and Australian feminist, media and cultural studies academic. She is presently a freelance writer and researcher in Melbourne. She has contributed to an eclectic range of journals and books, including Sharon Lamb's (New York University Press, 1999) edited book, *New Versions of Victims*.

Vikki Bell is a senior lecturer in sociology at Goldsmiths College, University of London. She is the author of *Interrogating Incest: Feminism, Foucault and the Law* (Routledge, 1993), *Feminist Imagination: Genealogies in Feminist Theory* (Sage, 1999) and editor of *Performativity and Belonging* (Sage, 1999). In addition, she has written many articles on cultural theory and identity, several indebted to the work of Michel Foucault, and published in journals such as *Theory, Culture & Society*, *Cultural Values*, *Feminist Theory* and *New Formations*.

Erica Burman is Professor of Psychology and Women's Studies at the Discourse Unit, Department of Psychology and Speech Pathology, the Manchester Metropolitan University. Her previous publications include: *Feminists and Psychological Practice* (Sage, edited, 1990), *Deconstructing Developmental Psychology* (Routledge, 1994a), *Challenging Women: Psychology's Exclusions, Feminist Possibilities* (Open University, co-authored, 1996), *Psychology, Discourse, Practice: From Regulation to Resistance* (Taylor & Francis, co-authored, 1996) and *Deconstructing Feminist Psychology* (Sage, co-authored, 1998).

Nicola Gavey is a clinical psychologist and lecturer in psychology at the University of Auckland, New Zealand. She has authored a wide variety of texts on sexual violence and child sexual abuse. Her recent publications include: 'Women's desire and sexual violence discourse', in S. Wilkinson (ed.) *Feminist Social Psychologies* (Open University Press, 1995). She was also an author in Sharon Lamb's (New York University Press, 1999) edited book *New Versions of Victims*.

Janice Haaken is a professor of psychology at the Portland State University, USA, and a clinical psychologist in private practice. She has published widely in the areas of gender and psychopathology, psychoanalysis and feminism, and psychology of social movements. Her most recent book is *Pillars of Salt: Gender, Memory, and the Perils of Looking Back* (Free Association Press, 1998). She was also an author in Sharon Lamb's (New York University Press, 1999) edited book *New Versions of Victims*.

Jenny Kitzinger is professor in the School of Journalism, Media and Cultural Studies at Cardiff University, UK. Jenny is co-author of *The Mass Media and Power in Modern Britain* (Oxford University Press, 1997) and *The Circuit of Mass Communication* (Sage, 1998) and co-editor of *Developing Focus Group Research: Politics, Theory and Practice* (Sage, 1999). Her work also appears in journals such as *Media, Culture and Society*, *The European Journal of Communication*, and *Sociology of Health and Illness*. Research interests include: media influence, public understandings, audience reception processes, journalistic production practices and feminism. Her substantive research has focused on the media and health, science and 'risk', and on the media and sexual violence.

Ann Levett was an associate professor and a clinical psychologist at the University of Cape Town until 1996. Her main research interests have been in discourse analysis and other qualitative approaches to gender and power-related issues. She is now a psychotherapist. She has published widely on the areas of child sexual abuse, race and culture. She is co-editor with Amanda Kottler, Erica Burman and Ian Parker of *Culture, Power and Difference* (Zed Books Ltd, 1997).

Lindsay O'Dell is a Senior Lecturer in the Department of Psychology at the University of Luton where she co-ordinates modules on Difference and Diversity in Psychology and The Psychology of Sexuality. Lindsay also teaches on Psychological Aspects of Child Sexual Abuse and Critical Social Psychology. Her research interests include the role of science in the production of knowledge about the effects of child sexual abuse; developmentalism and the construction of the child; gender and sexuality.

Paula Reavey is Senior Lecturer in Psychology at South Bank University where she teaches the psychology of mental health, sexuality and qualitative research. Her PhD thesis was a feminist post-structuralist account of professional/therapeutic, self-help and everyday constructions of the effects of child sexual abuse on women's sexuality and identity. She has written a number of articles and given conference papers on sexuality and the construction of 'surviving' abuse as single author and as co-author with Sam Warner. Her research interests include the therapeutic and clinical construction of the effects of child sexual abuse and sexuality in general.

Sam Warner is a consultant clinical psychologist and part-time research fellow at Manchester Metropolitan University. She specialises in the study of child sexual abuse and works freelance as a consultant, trainer, researcher, expert witness and therapist. Sam has written numerous articles and book chapters and is the author of *Understanding Child Sexual Abuse: Making the Tactics Visible* (Handsell, 2000) and co-editor, with Rebecca Horn, of *Positive Directions for Women in Secure Environments: Issues in Criminological and Legal Psychology* (BPS, 2000). Sam is currently writing a book on child sexual abuse for inclusion in the 'Women and Psychology' series (Routledge).

Tracy Wilkins is a post-graduate student at the Discourse Unit, Manchester Metropolitan University, UK. Her research interests are around women patients in high security mental hospitals, child sexual abuse and the social construction of categories of disorder. Tracy works as a psychiatric nurse within a forensic context.

Marcia Worrell is a Senior Lecturer in the Department of Psychology at the University of Luton, where she co-ordinates and teaches on modules relating to child sexual abuse, critical social psychology, differences and diversity in psychology and the psychology of sexuality. Marcia, as a member of the Beryl Curt Collective, has co-authored *Textuality and Tectonics: Troubling Social and Psychological Science* (OUP, 1994). Marcia's research interests include post-structural theorising on child sexual abuse and sexuality as a form of governmentality.

Acknowledgements

We would like to thank Michelle Bacca, senior editorial assistant and Edwina Welham, publisher at Routledge, for their support and encouragement. We would also like to thank Dave Harper and Alex John for their generosity regarding their time, their thoughtfulness, their humour and their residential and culinary facilities – cheers!

Chapter 1

Introduction

Paula Reavey and Sam Warner

This book is about women and child sexual abuse. It is about the ways in which women and child sexual abuse are talked about, how their relationship is understood and the multiple practices this gives rise to. This book is also about dismantling taken-for-granted truths. It is about daring to ask questions concerning the constructed nature of child sexual abuse; how it is *produced*, rather than merely *represented* in the ways in which we speak about it (Reavey and Warner, 2001). In this book we demonstrate that child sexual abuse is never transparent in terms of what it means: either as an event itself or in the memory of it. It is something that, as survivors, theoreticians or practitioners, we *make sense of* in the re-telling, and how we make sense of it shifts according to the contexts in which we speak, with whom we speak with, and who we speak about. It shapes the ways we see ourselves, the way we view others and it structures what we decide our actions around child sexual abuse should be. As such, we argue that child sexual abuse is a matter of translation, debate and politics, and not simply a taken-for-granted fact. Our aim is to enter the debate in order to untangle some of the complex ways we translate stories of child sexual abuse through, and into, personal and social politics. This book, then, provides a sustained and critical engagement with those stories of child sexual abuse that shape our sense of reality and the actions these give rise to.

Sexual scripts and feminist politics: social economies of women and child sexual abuse

It is self-evident that child sexual abuse takes place in a socio-cultural setting (Hacking, 1995), wherein concepts such as 'truth' (about who is guilty or innocent and the aftermath of abuse) are subject to a wide range of interpretations. As argued, this is dependent on who is doing the speaking and the position she (or he) is speaking from. Is the speaker invested with authority and expertise, and by what means is this authority and expertise warranted? In order to elaborate how authority is conferred, and which understandings are most readily accepted, we need to directly address the socio-cultural settings in which such judgements are made. We do not believe that there is an objective standard, by which all understandings can be judged, because any such standard is subjective to the culture that defines it. Indeed, such culturally sanctioned ways of knowing are themselves part of the mechanisms through which specific cultures can be recognised and their dominance *and* subjugation of other cultures can be sustained.

Hence, we are interested in exploring how particular versions of reality, in respect of child sexual abuse (Warner, 2000a), are maintained through the cultural privileging of particular, yet widely available, sexual scripts that position social actors in familiar ways. Specifically, we are interested in the ways that discourses (ways of speaking) produce particular versions of womanhood/femininity that act to reproduce power relations and sustain social hierarchies.

This involves making visible the often-unacknowledged assumptions about sex, gender and childhood that are drawn on to sustain dominant accounts of child sexual abuse. This means socially situating such narratives in order to ward against the instillation of universal and all-pervasive world-views. When we do this we are able to contextualise the way professional and populist understandings about child sexual abuse impact on how sexual abuse can be recognised, and its effects experienced. It allows us to explore how we hear these experiences and what kind of expert and everyday language is used to reconstruct, not just the past but also the present 'effects' of such abuse. Is the language we use, for example, mindful of not just the 'abusive event' itself but the cultural context in which survivors live their lives? Acknowledging the cultural specificity of language domains promotes an awareness of how categories such as 'woman' are socially produced and culturally bound. When investigating child sexual abuse it is, therefore, important to examine wider sexual scripts that frame the identifications women may make with, not only the original abuse(s), but their identifications *as women* living in a heterosexualised society. Hence, we maintain a clear commitment to an explicitly feminist agenda. In order to situate the sexual scripts that we draw on to explicate our understandings of 'the reality' of child sexual abuse, we locate ourselves in our own histories of feminism.

It is now thirty years since second wave feminists forced the issue of sexual violence onto the political agenda, making clear the connection between *male* privilege and the abuse of women and children. Through the various arenas of consciousness-raising groups and self-help forums, women began to narrate their own lives and to articulate their own experiences of sexual exploitation. Women drew on their own personal experiences of violence in order to illustrate the connection between individual life histories and wider gender inequalities. The fact that sexual abuse was a common feature of women's life stories highlighted the need to view issues of abuse as a political/societal problem rather than a private event confined to a few 'unfortunate' individuals. Feminists argued that the sexual exploitation of children generally, and girls specifically, is endemic to all patriarchal societies that prioritise the needs of men in public as well as private settings. In emphasising the effects of patriarchy on all women and promoting the need to speak with one voice, feminists were able to marshal an attack on a social world that was founded on male privilege and maintained through, amongst other things, (enforced) female silence.

Feminists, therefore, enjoined women to participate in the (organised) Women's Liberation Movement in order to struggle against male oppression and to break the silence around abuse. It is this history of activism and theorisation by women in Western cultures that has shaped current understandings of child sexual abuse and the many practices these give rise to. This is not only in terms of the influence this history has had on women writing in this book (indeed, many of us have been part of this movement), but more generally in terms of the influence this has had on the diverse and dispersed cultures in which we variously reside. These women ensured that sex and gender politics could no longer be entirely marginalised and both self-help and professional services made some moves to take real-life oppression seriously. Yet, the Women's Liberation Movement foundered.

For some women in Western cultures the early gains made by feminists led to a premature belief that gender equality had arrived. For other women, inequality was still all too real. Indeed, whilst the Women's Liberation Movements around the (Westernised) world had found their strength in a shared belief in a common identity and common cause, similarity had become over-determined. Many women within, and outside of, Western cultures felt misunderstood, marginalised and ultimately excluded from the very movement that sought to represent them (see Warner, 2000b). Speaking 'as women' was no longer an easy solution for addressing social inequality, as patriarchy could no longer be considered the primary social oppression and women struggled with their troubled and troubling relationships with each other. It was time to find new ways of speaking about gender and abuse that could still recognise commonality, but that never closes down difference nor predetermines political strategy. It was in this context that some feminists, at the end of the twentieth century, turned to post-structuralism to fashion new ways of theorising difference and commonality.

This book is about these new narratives. They are new in as much as they are intimately tied to our own specific historical and geopolitical moment and so are nascent and evolving. But their newness is also illusionary, as they are rooted in our various, at times conflicting, histories of womanhood. There may no longer be *a* movement of women that can be spoken about, but it is the interventions that women have made in theory and practice that provide the foundation for our current actions. Without reference to our pasts we lose sense of our achievements and lose sight of all that we have learnt (Warner, 2000b). This is why we do not call for a rejection of feminist politics. We still believe that emancipation and equality are useful goals – however variable and socially specific emancipation and equality may be.

Dangerous dialogues: speaking between feminism and post-structuralism

We recognise the role that feminists have played in ensuring that child sexual abuse can be spoken about and its effects addressed. We note that, in Western cultures, 'sex' is now readily acknowledged as a significant context in which children are abused. What was once depicted as a marginal concern to 'feminists' is now a central issue in the mainstream and that professionals have recuperated what was a political social agenda into a more individual, therapeutic one. We do not deny that child sexual abuse is prevalent nor that it can have devastating effects, but we do challenge the too-ready presumption of inevitable harm and the narrowing of concern that this has given rise to. As such, we maintain a (feminist) commitment to ensuring that concerns about 'the personal' effects of child sexual abuse do not restrict our concerns about 'the political' ramifications of it. At the same time, we recognise that feminists have been in danger of replacing one truth totality with another totalising story of patriarchal privilege. We argue that abuse, power, gender and sex are fragmentary and that they exist in a multiple array of knowledges, practices and strategies. There can never be, therefore, a final account of what they are or how they correspond to each other. Rather, as post-structuralism suggests, our concern is with how individuals *come to be known* through discursive practices, rather than claiming to be able to provide an objective account of who these individuals *really* are.

If feminism is to remain relevant then it must engage with the *specific* as the impact of feminist theories and practices will always be socially mediated and historically located. As such, feminism can no longer make claim to being the truth-sayer about child sexual abuse, as what is 'true' can never be absolute. So if we are suggesting that truth is always relative are we then saying that child sexual abuse is a myth or that women's stories of abuse are mere fictions? Is this book then a backlash against previous feminist work or a denial of women's lived experience? The simple answer is 'no'. All of the authors in this book share the conviction that these voices are real, and that child sexual abuse can give rise to distress, both in the short and long term. Yet, what we experience and talk about as 'real abuse' and the forms that our distress may take in relation to it, are already constructed through language. In order to tease apart what we 'know' about child sexual abuse and its 'effects' we need to revisit existing theories of power, experience and identity.

We draw on recent developments in post-structuralist theory to enable a more critical reading of women and child sexual abuse: to do more than simply articulate women's experience but to theorise why particular experiences are raised or ignored and what institutions and institutional practices these invite and sustain (Foucault, 1978). As argued, we need to be mindful of our own desires to circumscribe want counts as the truth. Hence, rather than situating power in a fixed system structured around patriarchy, we view power as a complex of knowledges that, although reified through repetition, ultimately remain unstable. Thus, our concern is with those forms of knowledge (professional and everyday) that claim to be able to speak the truth and consequently fix identities as a result – this does not reside in one place, therefore, but in a multitude of private and public spaces. And such claims to truth are *powerful* precisely because they exhibit 'an ability to hide [their] own mechanism[s]' (Foucault, 1978: 86). This is about making our own ways of understanding and the positions from which we speak explicit.

Our aim in this book, then, is to come together, *as* women, to articulate new feminist stories *about* women and child sexual abuse. We do not presume to speak, with one voice, *for* all women. Rather, our aim is to continue debating and arguing in order to illuminate how women's lives are regulated through the particular ways we are enjoined to theorise child sexual abuse and its effects. Our strategies are local and specific and never final. Hence, whilst all the authors share a feminist orientation and commitment, the forms and application of this commitment are varied. Our interventions into, and our dialogues with, feminist politics, post-structuralist theories, mainstream and everyday practices are dangerous because we are no longer prepared to rely on received wisdom (even when from feminism) to justify our actions.

This book aims to contribute to a continuing critical engagement with academic, professional, activist and everyday practices around, and under-standings of, women and child sexual abuse. We argue that if critique is to be sustained, then political action can nowhere be presumed in advance (see Butler, 1990). We aim to contribute to the ongoing development of critical practices in respect of child sexual abuse. We maintain a commitment to the emancipatory politics that feminism speaks of. However, we note that although 'structural change is important ... it is conceptual change that is revolutionary' (Warner, 2000a: 9). Our introduction of post-structuralist ideas into feminist debates is an act of politics that is about furthering this revolution. Our aim is to disrupt mainstream understand-ings of child sexual abuse that continue to rely on and, thereby, reproduce structural inequalities. We view gender and power as mutable terms rather than concrete and invariant objects. Part of our aim, then, is to deconstruct not only psychological and sociological knowledges about child sexual abuse, but also feminist ones. This reflects a shared commitment to socially situating the issue of child sexual abuse such that issues of gender and power cannot be separated from those of class, race and sexuality.

This book systematically explores the ways in which recent feminist and post-structuralist practices have converged to illuminate the issue of child sexual abuse in a wide variety of theoretical and practical arenas. We draw on our varied experiences, as academics, clinicians and/or activists across (some of) the world, to interrogate child sexual abuse in terms of its representation and understanding within populist, academic, clinical, legal and media contexts. Post-structuralism, like feminism, also takes many forms and it is the sustained and evolving dialogue between these areas of theorising which locate this book and which give rise to its particular contribution regarding the issue of child sexual abuse. We recognise that there are multiple ways in which women and child sexual abuse can be understood and their utility is provisionally located in specific historical and geopolitical contexts. The authors speak from a range of discursive and actual locations around the world and our writing reflects this. This is not a corporate body of work, but a selected sample of the various ways we have taken up ideas from feminism and post-structuralism to fashion our different stories about women and child sexual abuse.

The chapters

The book is organised into two main sections. In Part I we explore the cultural and political landscape of child sexual abuse in both Western and so-called non-Western contexts.

The aim is to examine the multiple ways in which child sexual abuse is spoken about within, and between, different societal and cultural contexts in order to elaborate what is constructed as the relevant field of interest. The authors variously demonstrate the particular formations of authority and authenticity that are implicated in regulating different cultural understandings and practices in respect of child sexual abuse. The chapters move from discussions regarding the ways radical aspects of feminism can be undermined within Westernised cultures to considering the ways dominant Westernised ideologies regarding childhood, sex and gender have been used to structure discussions about child sexual abuse across the world. The authors resist the globalising of theory through specific discussions of child sexual abuse within an African context and with respect to critiquing dominant understandings within Western cultures regarding the nature and status of memories of abuse and populist action around child sexual abuse. Consideration is also given to the potential for non-Western theories and practices to impact on, and to inform, Western approaches to addressing the aftermath of child sexual abuse.

In Part II we trace the discursive effects of these wider cultural and political narratives through the various contexts in which the effects of child sexual abuse are theorised and around which interventions in the lives of women are structured. Central to this analysis is an examination of psychological and (some second wave) feminist constructions of enduring 'harm' which is said to follow episodes of child sexual abuse. The authors map out the various trajectories that narratives of harm can take in shaping lived-experiences of child sexual abuse. Specifically the authors discuss normative assumptions regarding child development, sexuality and mental (dis)order that are implicated in Western narratives of harm. Consideration is then given to how narratives of survival can work to destabilise narratives of harm, but still install naturalised and global representations of womanhood. Finally, the authors provide insight into the ways in which traditional approaches to understanding harm can be disrupted, challenged and reworked *in practice*, using alternative clinical/therapeutic models founded on feminist post-structuralist agendas.

Part I: exploring the cultural and political landscape of child sexual abuse

Chris Atmore opens this section of the book by exploring the ways in which we – as women/feminists engaged in work around sexual abuse are seen and represented in wider culture. By drawing on her own lived experience of recent political, intellectual and geographical migration (from New Zealand to Australia), she explores how changes in feminist theorising and activism around sexual violence have led to a growing reluctance by some to acknowledge the still *radical* potential of feminist politics. She illuminates the ways in which radical feminism has been characterised as being terminally essentialist and, hence, outmoded in our increasingly 'postmodern' world. She argues that this has occasioned a too-ready dismissal of what *was* radical and subversive about feminist work, and which may *still* be relevant today. She concludes that we need to maintain our relationship, however ambivalent, with feminism's 'restless undead' who offer a trope that provides a context in which to verbalise our enduring relationship (and fascination?) with sex and violence.

In the next chapter, Erica Burman elaborates critiques of identity to consider how pervasive Westernised notions of subjectivity mediate the territory of childhood generally and child sexual abuse specifically. Erica explores some of the political consequences that developmental and psychological theories of maturation have for children who have been sexually abused. She examines unacknowledged assumptions in these theories, regarding gender, authenticity and naturalness which sediment childhood as a 'special' state and which are implicated in how child sexual abuse and its effects are understood. She demonstrates that children and childhood are, in fact, socially constituted within multiple institutional relationships (such as those involving the family, school and healthcare) that vary within and between different cultural contexts. She argues that notions of 'development' are prescriptive, rather than descriptive and that they represent moral judgements regarding what an 'ideal' child is, which serve to regulate all 'other' children (whether abused, neglected, or from the so-called Third World). Erica concludes that the political and economic landscape (however fragmented) must be taken into account if the specificities of child sexual abuse are to be understood.

Ann Levett extends this critique to open up for debate the role that Western cultural imperialism plays in regulating how child sexual abuse is spoken about, not only in Western contexts but in African countries as well. She explores how Anglo-American understandings of child sexual abuse and its 'effects' are depicted as being able to speak to 'all' individuals, regardless of cultural context. Ann argues for more culturally specific modes of enquiry and theorisation, and identifies some of the factors implicated in the social production of child sexual abuse in African societies. She critically examines the ways in which childhood, sex, abuse and gender intersect to sometimes raise, and often restrict, concern regarding the sexual exploitation of girls by men in this locale. Ann argues that whilst caution is needed in addressing 'cultural differences' as, too often, 'culture' is negatively associated with being Black, it is necessary to make visible the particular forms that patriarchal power and gendered subjectivities take in different socio-cultural and class contexts. Ann concludes that discursive approaches to research that draw attention to the various social and semiotic codes which relate to different expressions of power, are useful means of enquiry for exploring the geographical and cultural specificities of child sexual abuse.

Jan Haaken demonstrates how formalised Westernised thought does not have to be restrictive, but can be appropriated to vitalise our (feminist) understandings of child sexual abuse and its effects. Jan draws on psychoanalytic theory to consider how socially sanctioned versions of female suffering are translated into individual memories and beliefs. She begins by arguing that both feminist and clinical discourses on female suffering have tended to focus on the presence of abuse, rather than the absence of care. Her contention is that it is not just the presence of abuse in women's lives that constitutes female oppression, but also the pervasive neglect that girls experience. Jan explores how culturally sanctioned forms of remembering fail to invite this recognition of women's more general oppression. She argues that scientific/clinical discourses on storytelling and memory must be 'opened up' to include the social/symbolic threads of women's oppression more generally. This entails a dialogue with the larger cultural context of female suffering rather than representing abuse as *the* site of female grievance. Jan also argues for dialogue across cultures to enable a more detailed explication of women's relationship to recovery. To this end, Jan enlists the insights of African women to unsettle normative feminist concerns regarding the territory of reparation and forgiveness.

Jenny Kitzinger continues to explore the status of women's memories of abuse by interrogating how child sexual abuse is treated in the production of news in the UK. Jenny draws on feminism to elaborate how women are discredited in the British media through the ways in which their memories of child sexual abuse are called into question during debates on false memory syndrome. She analyses data from one year's press and TV coverage, interviews with pressure groups, journalists and so-called 'ordinary people' (including survivors of abuse) to demonstrate that particular versions of reality are sustained in media debates on false memory syndrome that serve to reproduce male privilege and normal gender hierarchies. Jenny critically examines these public portrayals of 'false memory' in order to explicate how the media often functions in a way which marginalises and denies women's voices by too readily accepting the authority of the men they accuse. Jenny demonstrates how the cultural regulation of gender is achieved through the media's unacknowledged (and unknowing?) obfuscation of 'patriarchal privilege' in terms of the use of 'psychological science' to frame the debate.

Vikki Bell continues to trace the impact of the popular press in shaping our understanding of women's actions around child sexual abuse. Vikki provides a Foucauldian analysis of the British media's portrayal of mothers who took to the streets, during the summer of 2000, to mark their protest against the re-housing of 'paedophiles' in local communities. This protest was fuelled by the widespread news coverage of the disappearance (and murder) of the schoolgirl Sarah Payne. The so-called liberal press condemned the action of these 'vigilante' mothers because of concerns that such actions may drive so-called paedophiles underground due to their fear of subsequent attack by members of the public. However, Vikki argues that their actions could be reinterpreted as still politically useful because these women were nevertheless mobilised *as women*. Therefore, she argues for a more complex reading of social action. Vikki does not view this protest as representing a straightforward feminist statement (as many of the women's actions were embedded in reactionary, nationalist and racist discourses). Yet she concludes that their actions have political valance because they represent a particular (working) class *response* to governmental practices which neither offered women adequate information about abusers nor actual protection of their children.

Part II: how we theorise and intervene in the lives of women who have experienced child sexual abuse

Lindsay O'Dell begins this section by examining how the long-term 'effects' of child sexual abuse are constructed in professional and everyday talk. Lindsay provides a macro discourse analysis of transcripts taken from interviews conducted in the UK with survivors of child sexual abuse and the various professionals who work with them. In analysing this data, she details how popular understandings of the 'effects' of child sexual abuse are frequently depicted in terms of formulaic narratives of harm. She argues that these narratives of harm are shot through with developmental-ist assumptions that emphasise a unilateral (bio)logical process from childhood to adulthood. Lindsay elaborates how notions of 'normal' devel-opment are embedded in wider social discourses about sex, gender and race, but that these remain obscured. Furthermore, this analysis explicates how psychological discourses of harm, that individualise pathology through keeping the social foundations of '(ab)normality' hidden, warrant and enforce therapeutic forms of intervention. Lindsay argues that such forms of 'help' not only circumscribe the victim or survivor, but also dictate what families and partners are deemed to 'need' in order to recu-perate them back into normative culture.

Paula Reavey further elaborates how the effects of child sexual abuse are frequently depicted as being inevitably and enduringly harmful. Paula focuses her critique on a discussion of how notions of normal sexual behaviour are drawn on to sustain individual narratives of harm. By tracing discourses of sexuality through narratives of harm, Paula demon-strates how survivors are positioned as 'other' to ideals of normative fem-ininity. Paula bases her analysis on interviews she conducted in the UK with women survivors and therapists, as well as on a selection of popular and readily available 'self-help' books. Her aim was to explore the discur-sive locations in which judgements are made about the effects of abuse on (female) sexuality. Paula argues that 'self-evident' connections, between past abuse and present sexuality, instigate a seemingly straightforward reading of the relationships between (past) abuse and (present) problem-atic sexuality. This narrow understanding of 'cause and effect' renders women's sexual stories and behaviour open to individualistic interpreta-tion that obscures the social foundations of sex/gender relations. Paula argues that causal narratives that locate present problems in terms of past abuse reproduce normative sexual identities and gendered structural hier-archies that are organised around cultural metaphors of male power and female powerlessness.

Sam Warner and Tracy Wilkins continue this detailed exploration of nar-ratives of harm by examining psychiatric classification systems that collapse the 'effects' of child sexual abuse into restrictive categories of (mental) disorder. Drawing on research conducted within a British high security mental hospital, Sam and Tracy challenge current psychiatric understandings of women patients that frequently depict the effects of sexual abuse as resulting in borderline personality disorder. They begin by examining the role of diagnosis in sustaining medical hegemony in psychiatric care. They then explore the ways in which unacknowledged assumptions about gender have given rise to particular understandings of personality disorder. They demonstrate how child sexual abuse is used as a causal explanation for the development of borderline personality disorder, yet is seldom addressed in therapeutic terms. They argue that when the 'effects' of abuse are viewed simply as symptoms of mental categories of disorder, the social foundations of women's distress are paradoxically hidden. They demonstrate that conceptualising the effects of abuse as extant personality disorder obscures the role of others, both in the past and present, who are implicated in the maintenance of disorder. Sam and Tracy conclude that it is through more social understandings of individual distress that women's *actual* experiences of disorder may be situated and addressed.

In the following chapter, Nicola Gavey extends this critique of mainstream depictions of the 'effects' of child sexual abuse to examine the psychological frameworks that are used to theorise the assumed negative effects on adult mental health. Such frameworks often conflate a moral judgement against child sexual abuse with the expectation that it causes particular kinds of psychological harm to those who are abused, and that such understandings are socially prevalent in that they reach wider legal policy and practices regarding compensation for instances of harm. Specifically, she explores the New Zealand Accident Compensation Corporation's past policy of awarding lump sum compensation to victims of child sexual abuse for whom there was expert testimony of 'emotional pain and suffering' and 'loss of amenities or capacity to enjoy life'. Nicola uses a reflexive discourse analytic approach to critically analyse professional psychology documents she wrote for this scheme in the context of her own clinical psychology practice. Using this body of work as an illustrative case study, Nicola identifies and elaborates the tensions between using psychological expertise for 'victim' advocacy and feminist notions of empowerment.

Marcia Worrell's chapter moves away from a focus on inevitable 'harm' to elaborate on contrasting approaches that reconfigure narratives of harm as narratives of survival. Marcia considers how self-help groups utilise narratives of survival to challenge the usual ways women are represented as being essentially damaged by their experiences of child sexual abuse. Drawing on research conducted with a British self-help group for survivors of childhood sexual abuse she explores how survivor identities are 'created', and sustained, in this context through regulating the kinds of subject positions available to women in the group. Marcia examines the ways in which survivors come to know themselves and each other by sharing narratives on abuse. She demonstrates that these group narratives are informed and fashioned by wider discourses on gender and survival (in respect to child sexual abuse). Marcia argues that survivor identity cannot, in itself, act as a panacea for all women who have experienced child sexual abuse (or as a trope of social change). This is because such narratives of survival are sedimented in global representations of womanhood that fail to recognise or elaborate difference between women.

In the final chapter, Sam Warner moves beyond and between narratives of harm and survival to develop a theoretical framework for explicating therapeutic practices with women who have experienced child sexual abuse. She examines both normative and transgressive assumptions embedded within socially available narratives regarding women clients, and child sexual abuse, in order to expose therapeutic assumptions about pathology and normality. The implicit trajectories of accepted modes of recovery are then interrogated in order to evaluate their contributory effects in maintaining women's so-called pathological behaviours and emotions. This analysis is used to develop an alternative narrative strategy for understandings of, and practices around, women and childhood experiences of sexual abuse. This strategy directly addresses the socially situated production of symptomatic 'states' and behaviours and offers a means through which non-pathologising practices can be evaluated and developed. This new model termed 'Visible Therapy' provides a framework for the delivery of therapy, a framework for evaluating these practices and the specific contexts in which such practices operate.

References

Butler, J. (1990) *Gender trouble: feminism and the subversion of identity*, London: Routledge.

Foucault, M. (1978) *The history of sexuality, vol. one*, Harmondsworth: Penguin.

Hacking, I. (1995) *Rewriting the soul: multiple personality and the sciences of memory*, Princeton: Princeton University Press.

Reavey, P. and Warner, S. (2001) 'Giving up the cure: child sexual abuse and the construction of femininity', *International Journal of Critical Psychology* 3: 59–74.

Warner, S. (2000a) *Understanding child sexual abuse: making the tactics visible*, Gloucester: Handsell.

Warner, S. (2000b) 'Feminist theory, the Women's Liberation Movement and therapy for women: changing our concerns', *Changes: An International Journal of Psychology and Psychotherapy* 18, 4: 232–243.

Part I

Exploring the cultural and political landscape of child sexual abuse

Feminism's restless undead

The radical/lesbian/victim theorist and conflicts over sexual violence against children and women

Chris Atmore

In memory of Ruth Charters – proud radical feminist, lesbian, lawyer and activist against sexual violence

> It's enough to make a woman of the 1990s consider radical feminism all over again.
>
> (Sue O'Sullivan, *Where Does Political Correctness Come From?*)

I originally wrote most of this chapter for a conference in the early 1990s (Atmore, 1993b). It is difficult to say categorically, now in 2002, how much of a time capsule that paper has become. While I have made some transitions in my work against child sexual abuse and gendered violence more generally, these seem to further illustrate some of my earlier arguments. I use a series of italicised scenes from the 1990s to shape my reflections on that era, and end with an update of where they have led me now.

Introduction

1992. I am on a panel in an Australian cultural studies conference on 'pluralism and theory' (Atmore, 1993a). The speaker who has followed me is talking about the 'lesbian vampire murder' case in Brisbane. The media made much of the deviant figure of the chief protagonist, Tracey Wigginton, who murdered a man and drank his blood (Verhoeven, 1993a). Wigginton was described in the press as being dressed predominantly in black, during the court proceedings showing little emotion, and occasionally sipping water (ibid.: 276–277). On hearing this re-rendered, I'm discomforted by feeling momentarily in a too-public position as prize exhibit in a show-and-tell.

The descriptive resonances could be partly attributed to the demands of panel participation (and perhaps my dress sense). More pertinently, however, there seems to be a kind of tourist guide flow-on effect to a 'self-confessed lesbian' like myself that necessarily accompanies the re-articulation of the Wigginton discourses. Even the most well-meaning audience response to a minority group protesting against bad press includes the curiosity, even if politically embarrassing, to seek out hints that perhaps 'they' do indeed protest too much. But it doesn't seem adequate to account for my agitation by appealing to a simple sisterhood between Wigginton and me.

I want to use my discomfort in the above scene as an entry point into a debate whose terms seem at present largely set by popular figures like Camille Paglia, Katie Roiphe and Naomi Wolf (Atmore, 1999a). These critics argue that feminism falls into two camps: an older and now appropriately denigrated 'victim' feminism, and a more recent, valorised, 'power' feminism. My contrasting view is that this polarisation is inaccurate and inadequate, and I am particularly concerned with what interests may be served via such a characterisation.

For anyone entering the debate, local contexts, or more specifically, situated knowledges (e.g. Haraway, 1988), are important. With that in mind I will try to pick out my own interests and realignments as the result of geographical, intellectual and political migration: from a white, 'twenty-something', lesbian feminist active in 'grass roots' opposition to sexual violence in New Zealand's capital city, to more of a post-structuralist-influenced, 'thirty-something', feminist academic in Melbourne, Australia.

There seems more of a clue in that phrase, '"self-confessed lesbian" like myself'. I have spent some time since I arrived from New Zealand and the end of a PhD, in reassessing my intellectual–political interests as both lesbian and feminist – or rather being forced to recast them in the light of a culture which I (erroneously) anticipated to be essentially similar to the one I left, at least in terms of the circles in which I expected to be moving.

My work was concerned with finding a way to take lesbian/radical feminist theories and politics, and in particular their analyses of sexual violence, into some kind of productive relationship with my growing interest in post-structuralist ideas. With that kind of anti-dichotomising as background, I had presented as my panel contribution in the conference an analysis of how in New Zealand, a group of (unknown) women who accused a university lecturer of sexual harassment tied him to a tree, and were subsequently depicted as lesbian feminist man-haters in the media (Atmore, 1993a).

To the extent that the press representations in both cases focused on the 'monstrous' attributions of lesbianism, this might go some way to explain my uncomfortable identification. But both media cases centred not simply on female sexual deviancy, but on violent criminality. Despite my qualified support for the New Zealand attackers, I can make no serious claim to this form of outlaw status. So why might I feel cast in that fleeting moment as guilty by association?

I think that the more persuasive discursive link between the Wigginton fragments, the New Zealand controversy and my own position, is the threat of a kind of deadly seriousness. This threat links the 'vampire' figure of Wigginton to a more pervasive construction most strongly associated with 'victim' feminism, which Meaghan Morris (1987) has called the Humourless Feminist. Some of this figure's most prominent features include a censoring and authoritarian disposition, and a reputation for being 'constitutionally *heavy*' (ibid.: 176, Morris' emphasis).

I would like to retain an affinity with the vampire in thinking of the Humourless Feminist as herself a kind of restless undead. This archetype can be understood as not only the product of the success of public figures like Roiphe and Paglia, but as more broadly shaped by the interests of the mainstream media and a range of academic and 'grass roots' political contexts. It's helpful to trace some of the 'travels' of the Humourless Feminist depiction to show how present constructions are actually reactivations of supposedly 'dead' representations (Smith-Rosenberg 1989); and in the process to consider how the uses of this figure by different groups might overlap; and whether this could be significant. Or in other words, to speculate about what the 'stakes' might be, from my own partial viewpoint.

I will begin by tracing some of the incarnations of the Humourless Feminist in popular culture and outside explicitly feminist discourses.

The 'stakes': radical/lesbian feminism, sexual violence and the Humourless Feminist

While the Humourless Feminist has been associated with a range of feminist analyses and practices, she has been especially prominent in popular cultural responses to feminist work against sexual violence. It seems reasonable to make a few generalisations and say that the most systematic feminist theorising and activism against sexual violence is largely affiliated with radical feminisms. For example, while many Black feminists may not choose to identify with the tag of 'radical feminist' because of its public association with white-dominated feminism's tendency to emphasise gender at the expense of race, Black feminist traditions of organising against sexual violence have some important overlaps with what are more 'officially' known as radical feminist tenets (see e.g. hooks, 1990: 57–64, 112; Crenshaw, 1993).

I am not simply saying that anyone who does work which I might tag 'radical feminist' must be one. But any political manifesto which ranks taking sexual violence seriously as a key item has strong affinities with radical feminist thought and activities. Radical feminist theories take the view that sexual violence in any masculinist culture is both endemic and epidemic, and therefore will not be eliminated as long as the society concerned remains, in Catharine MacKinnon's (1983: 655) phrase, 'gendered to the ground'.

Of course it's only in our origin stories of 'how we got feminisms as we know them' that radical feminism can appear neatly as one arm which subsequently broke off into pieces. The image is even more inadequate when we try to talk about how feminisms are similar and different to each other now. One illustration is the way in which, via critiques from Black and working class feminists, feminists of colour, and other 'ex-centrics' (Anzaldúa, 1983; Hutcheon, 1988; Hartsock, 1989/1990), whatever we might call radical feminisms these days have to a great extent converged with similarly realigned socialist feminisms. So I am referring more to complex tangled strands, and fragments of these as radical feminist in their impetus.

A further complication in sexual violence work is the association of radical feminisms with lesbian feminisms. Partly this is due to the affinity between many of the leading figures active against sexual violence, and lesbian feminism as an identity politics. More significantly, lesbian feminism supplied the critique of heterosexuality as a compulsory institution which has both perpetuated and been sustained by sexual violence (e.g. Rich, 1987a).

Hence since the early 1970s there has been a sisterhood between radical feminist opposition to sexual violence, and lesbian feminism. It is also significant that in popular discourse, if one is perceived as too radical about sexual violence, the charge of lesbianism often follows. There are therefore some rather complex connections between radical feminist and lesbian feminist stances, making it difficult to separate them in analysing how feminist work on sexual violence is represented.

New Zealand, 1980s. The women who tie the university lecturer to a tree and those who support it are described by the mainstream media as lesbian fascists, totalitarian, thought police ... the long-running imported Australian television soap opera Prisoner *features a sadistic lesbian guard called The Freak; I add this to my childhood stock of James Bond (usually Russian) 'villainesses' ... As a feminist anti-pornography activist I am once referred to in the press as 'Atmore and her stormtroopers of the left' ... Popular magazines claim that professionals are being over-zealous in their efforts to protect children from abuse: this is blamed on biased lesbian and radical feminists who exaggerate the child sexual abuse statistics and put words in children's mouths (Atmore, 1996). One major newspaper runs a cartoon: two women in jackboots and military uniforms, women's symbols in place of a swastika, goosestep away from a prone man while in the background stand two other men, one holding the hand of a little girl. One man comments, 'They caught him giving his small daughter a bath ...' and the other replies, 'Really? ... Let go of Daddy's hand sweetheart ...'*

Australia, 1990s. The student newspaper at my university runs a major commentary describing as 'fascist' calls from feminists to remove sexist advertisements from the paper ... Major metropolitan newspapers and magazines run a spate of articles disputing radical feminist claims about date rape, sexual harassment and the truth of child sexual abuse allegations. These texts include prominent references to censoring from 'the lesbian left', and arguments that feminists who criticise sexist advertising are simply 'wowsers'.

While these popular constructions of radical and lesbian feminists are recognisable as part of broader anti-'political correctness' rhetoric, they do not seem to be challenged in left and queer networks to the same degree as other caricatures (cf. O'Sullivan, 1993; Wark, 1993). Rather, those who self-identify as 'progressive' often themselves subscribe to the Humourless Feminist depiction.

The sole female representative in a queer film forum disavows any connection to lesbians and thanks her 'gay brothers' for supporting her against 'the thought police' ... NZ friends of mine who complain about the sale of second-hand copies of *Penthouse* as part of a public gay fundraiser receive a Nazi salute. A refrain at several 1993 academic conferences and talks focusing on radical theories of sexuality is that political correctness is prescriptive, identity politics are repressive, separatism is defensive; and all of these are linked to the radical feminist bloc/lesbian feminist thought police.

The Humourless Feminist construction also circulates in a range of 'progressive' intellectual work. It often takes its crudest form in gay and queer texts: from Weeks to Watney (see especially Weeks, 1985: 19, 217–219, 235; Watney, 1987: 59, 61–63, 70–76), where lesbian theorists do rate at all it is as right-on rebel Rubin to denigrated Dworkin.[1] Lesbian and radical feminism are rarely discussed as coherent politics in such books.

The Humourless Feminist in/and feminism

In the last few years, resourcing of the Humourless Feminist figure seems to have taken a new turn – not just against and outside feminism, but from within it. Contemporary feminist theory in the university uses some of the same moves as media 'stars' like Roiphe and Paglia. Confining the Humourless Feminist to a populist rogues' gallery has its equivalent in taxonomies of social theory in which radical or lesbian feminist analyses are represented as diametrically opposed and inferior to approved ones. My experience of marking undergraduate essays is that they either routinely assume that radical feminism stopped with Shulamith Firestone, or effectively dismiss radical and lesbian feminism as offering only an intellectual living death. In most cases these views paraphrase recently published feminist sources, which offer at best secondary and somewhat one-sided critiques of radical and lesbian feminist work (cf. Bordo, 1990, 1992; Modleski, 1991, especially pp. 135–163; O'Sullivan, 1993).

This is especially obvious in feminist theories which engage with post-structuralist ideas. The unofficial narrative is often a search-and-destroy mission; or as Susan Bordo (1990: 154, n7) has called it, 'a demolition derby', the victors being 'the card-carrying deconstructivists' (Spivak, 1990: 166–168) who address to impress; the losers depicted as politically naïve overall-wearers, hopelessly theoretically inadequate, vulgar but not popular.

What finishes off our Humourless Feminist in this guise, as she is caught blinking earnestly in the dazzle of postmodern and queer hipness, clutching her faded banner, is terminal essentialism. For instance, I have read countless times recently, from feminists, the claim that radical feminists believe(d) that men and women are innately different. Especially common are jaw-droppingly wilful misreadings of the work of Adrienne Rich, Andrea Dworkin and Catharine MacKinnon (cf. Atmore, 1999a; Yorke, 1997).

Re-vamping the Humourless Feminist

The common rationale for a 'fascist' or 'thought police' characterisation of radical/lesbian feminisms is that these theories are totalising: pessimistically all-encompassing, inflexibly monolithic, impossibly universalist (the 'victim theory' charges) – and often prescriptive. Whether I like the style of such critiques, I am needled partly because, however inadequately, they do at least act as a focus for some crucial problems with many radical and lesbian feminist arguments, particularly around issues of sexuality, coercion and power (Atmore, 1999a, c).

It's perhaps easier with hindsight to appreciate how working against sexual violence can foster various solipsisms. The Humourless Feminist representation is also a family portrait, if badly done and with malice; we probably all know her, perhaps intimately. These themes have led me to try to incorporate some more post-structuralist forms of feminist theory into my own work on sexual violence.

It is difficult not to capitulate to the strong either/or pull that seems to characterise much feminist thinking around sexuality issues – a legacy from 'the feminist sex wars' (Rich, 1986).[2] The Humourless Feminist and the sex war polarities are affined with a larger set of dualisms that have stymied feminist theory – and which are particularly untenable from feminist positions claiming to appreciate this post-structuralist critique. Thus, Meaghan Morris supports feminist theory which might help also to make it harder for anyone of any sex 'in' feminism to think through difficult political problems (pornography and rape come to mind) by allocating rejected positions to the bad, the 'heavy' feminist.

(1987: 176)

Criticisms of radical and lesbian feminisms are often overstated. For instance, feminist work on 'the state' and its relationship to practices like 'family violence', has long acknowledged in activist and community service circles, if less forthcoming until recently in public and in written theory, how messy power relations can be.[3]

The dichotomising also glosses over the ways in which ostensibly opposed feminist theories actually share discursive strategies. For example, Carole Vance's (1993a, b) analysis of the proceedings of the US Meese Commission into Pornography raises some uncomfortable themes from my vantage point as a former anti-pornography activist. She develops the 'unholy alliance' and 'strange bedfellows' clichés of First Amendment absolutists into a more careful critique of the ways in which the strategies of moralists and anti-pornography feminists can converge, notably via a 'shock/horror' discourse. However, in the particular libertarian-oriented Australian context in which Vance presented her work, a dominant theme which emerged was of a litany of moralist and radical feminist transgressions to which many in the audience reacted as if they were indeed viewing an undesirably graphic slide show.

More generally, post-structuralist feminists tend to dismiss radical feminists, so that if a radical or lesbian feminist theory offers something seen as useful, it is claimed as a post-structuralist strategy and hence not really radical/lesbian feminist in origin. From the 'other side', radical feminists commonly oppose post-structuralist critiques of 'depth' by casting anyone engaging with this kind of thought as hopelessly shallow and irredeemably masculinist.

The Humourless Feminist as restless undead

If these dichotomies are unsustainable, why have they emerged? It is helpful to return to popular cultural representations. Recently 'lesbian chic' has made an appearance, particularly in glossy women's magazines. *Cleo*'s portrayal is fairly typical: the lesbianism endorsed is differentiated from 'the ultra-wowser radical lesbian separatists, who have done so much damage to the image of feminism' (Alderson, 1993). Radical and lesbian feminists play the 'cop' to their more palatable counterparts; or as the queer press would have it, to the much more desirable delinquent.

Australian national television, 1994. A 'forum' on the state of feminism, participants all women except for the 'host'. He continually brings the

discussion back to whether feminists are 'too hard on men', despite the
wide-ranging topics of the other contributors. The token lesbian feminist
offers a critique of compulsory heterosexuality, violence and reproductive
health; the camera lingers on the host's face contorted with incomprehen-
sion. He turns to another feminist who responds that the real problem is
women don't get enough sex. Laughter, applause.

It's tempting from my stance as 'activist turned academic', whatever that phrase might mean these days, to reinflect Barbara Smith's (Smith and Smith, 1983: 124) observation that 'there's nothing to compare with how you feel when you're cut cold by your own' – whatever *that* phrase might mean these days, to me.

'Restless undead' therefore has another connotation: the 'victim' or Humourless Feminist caricature tends to function as a legitimation of alternative ('power') accounts of women's sexuality; available for resurrection when necessary. This has a history, including Jacquelyn Zita's (1981: 186) description of a legacy from socialist feminism, in which the complexity of lesbian feminist politics tends to get reduced to 'a caricature of otherness, a lost coin for political exchange'.

But in a different reading, the Humourless Feminist *is* a currency, drawn on by some versions of feminism because it overlaps with other discourses which might then be enlisted as sympathetic. For instance, the distancing from the Humourless Feminist can be interpreted, in these times of the cult of the body, as yet again a defensive fear of women who are too much, of the emoting, corporeal, stolid earth-bound female.[4] Privileged in contrast is the lean intellectual rebel, traditionally (although not inevitably) coded as masculine (Bordo, 1989; Tetzlaff, 1992, especially p. 67).

In contrast, feminists wanting to theorise and oppose sexual coercion are in a particularly invidious position of trying to make 'stale old talk about male dominance and female subordination' (Bordo, 1990: 151; hooks, 1990: 52), in the face of demands for more open verdicts and playfulness. As Morris (1987: 175–176) points out:

> The very condition of the romantic game is that no one, whatever their position in political and social power, wants to be seen to be playing the cop ... If literary critics love to see themselves as criminals, what woman does not dread (whatever her occupation) being seen as some man's gaoler?

When the premium is entertainment value, the alternative for sexual violence theorists seems the not very successful stand-up routine of shock/horror (Merck, 1988; Smart, 1990).

1993. An Australian national television channel screens a documentary by a
male film-maker which argues that radical feminists have a stranglehold on

government policy on domestic violence. The documentary (somewhat iron-
ically) claims that any alternative perspective has been silenced and that men
are being blamed as innately evil beasts due to a tide of political correctness.
This point is made through an opening scene which juxtaposes women on a
Reclaim the Night protest with the marching of Mao's Red Guards.

Sue O'Sullivan's (1993) reflection on 'political correctness' is insightful
here. She argues that, at least in Britain and the United States, there are
two major realms of discourse around 'PC'. The first is associated largely
with the internal debates of various radical groupings; while the second is
more recent and mainstream, tending to use 'PC' as a term of abuse, and
generally hurling it at various minorities who threaten to rock the
conservative boat. O'Sullivan suggests that the two realms are therefore
extremely different in their political contexts, yet have become uncomfort-
ably linked.

How this might apply to the Australian context, and to what degree
'we' have 'imported' both realms of 'PC' discourse, is another essay. What
does it mean when *The Australian Magazine*, an insert that accompanies a
major Saturday newspaper, approvingly represents Jane Gallop's self-
description as a 'bad girl', pro-sex, pro-debate feminist? This is contrasted
to the 'good girl', anti-sex, pro-censorship feminist who is depicted as a
dinosaur outside the university, but wielding power in government bureau-
cracies (Lumby, 1993: 35–36).

Here there is a double resonance to Morris's (1987: 176) provocation
that the Humourless Feminist is 'really a helpful soul'. Again feminist politics and theories which 'make it' discursively rely on what they condemn to
do so. The dichotomisation is successful, at least in part due to the overlap
of anti-'PC' discourses in popular anti-feminisms, with those more recently
in feminist circulation.

However, the meanings of discourses are also dependent on specific
power-laden contexts, and so are neither absolute nor static. There are
constant shifts in what is 'fringe' or 'centre' in both feminist and mainstream cultural politics, and so in what we interpret as transgressive – a
'bad' or a 'good' girl? – and in whether this is marked as desirable.

At an early 1990s conference dedicated to the work of a key thinker for
post-structuralists, an entertaining and slick performance is given by the
kind of presenter most eligible for 'true' rebel status at such venues – as in
some variants of queer politics, straight but having a bit of the other. Then
in a throwaway remark calculated to offend and amuse depending on
one's positioning, he claims feminists just haven't understood the great
man. In question time a woman challenges this complete dismissal of a
sizeable chunk of feminist scholarship, and is given the brush-off; I try to
repeat the criticism and am told that my point has been taken. The
speaker now 'confesses' that he had been afraid of the politically correct

lobby and that this incident has caused his mouth to go dry (it is worth noting that he is a reasonably well-known and tenured academic and I am neither). Probably because the paper comes towards the end of a series of such conference incidents, I try again. This time the chairman interjects with 'steady on, steady on' and the presenter secures his victim status.

I am reminded of my work on the university lecturer, the angry women and the tree, which argued that the media gave him a largely sympathetic hearing because he claimed 'my present symptoms are those of one who has been raped' ... I am also transported to a forum involving a white male director who documented his relationship with a Thai sex worker, whom he set out from Australia to purchase and film. The forum began with the film-maker describing how he had suffered at the hands of 'fundamentalist feminists' and would-be censors. Needless to say, there he did not.

As my introductory identification with the vampire also suggests, it becomes very difficult to categorise outright just who is powerful and who is victimised, especially when it helps to dismiss 'victim' feminists by usurping the victim position for oneself.

There are other overlaps. Those of us working against sexual violence have been known to appropriate the lone rebel image, to provide partial consolation for activity which, if characterised by its critics as unremittingly negative, can be experienced by its advocates as unrelentingly grim. Hence in my own case, there has been a certain satisfaction along with the dismay in being described as 'a humourless history teacher with Stalinist leanings'. This appeal seems to go beyond the pleasures of Left retro memorabilia.

It does seem clearer that despite Australian comparative tolerance of homosexuality and the claims of gains from 'power feminism', 'man-hating' remains a great crime. But again, context is important. As far as I can judge, New Zealand seems to be more hospitable to strategic separatisms of various kinds (lesbian, feminist, indigenous) than does Australia, at least as I have experienced it; and the former is perhaps less sexually libertarian, so less hospitable to an opening up of at least some kinds of questions of sexual pleasure. If I had not left New Zealand, perhaps I would find myself more often arguing for the importance of both post-structuralist critiques and the impetus for some of the self-described media feminists' arguments; because in some quarters I would be assured of a taken-for-granted critique of sexual coercion. Here in Australia in my present locations, I'm not so sure.

Taking heart in a haven-less world

The legacy of the 1980s sex wars remains, in the sense that there is still an overwhelming temptation to reiterate important debates around sex and power in either/or terms. But at the same time, there have been major mitigating developments in feminist thought; via challenges to begin to seriously consider politics of difference, and the critical potential (without being too reverent about it) of post-structuralisms.

An epitome of these developments is the rethinking that has been going on about the concept of 'home'. Various forms of feminist thought have overlapped in their cautions against any appeal to a romanticised notion, because a safe haven in political and intellectual terms is always at someone else's expense (Pratt, 1984; Martin and Mohanty, 1986; Rich, 1987b; Haraway, 1988). For example, Teresa de Lauretis (1988) argues that feminist theory begins when it applies its critiques to its own assumptions and practices, which she associates with 'a qualitative shift in political and historical consciousness' (ibid.: 139). This must involve:

> leaving or giving up a place that is safe, that is 'home' (physically, emotionally, linguistically, and epistemologically) for another place that is unknown and risky, that is not only emotionally but conceptually other, a place of discourse from which speaking and thinking are at best tentative, uncertain, unguaranteed.
>
> (ibid.)

Monolithic accounts of all kinds therefore begin to break down. I am forced to begin to acknowledge more how my own partial perspective has shaped my view of sexual violence and its place in any larger social scheme, to the extent that at the height (or perhaps depth) of anti-pornography and anti-child-sexual-abuse activism, I operated from a kind of siege mentality (cf. Rich, 1987a: 74). Partly this has been due to my own knowledge of how the effects of sexual violence can flow into personal relationships, and shape in some important but not inevitable ways, the trajectory of lives. The research statistics condemned by Katie Roiphe feel like simple confirmation to me, not incitement to panic.

My attempt to secure this kind of theoretical and political home has also been produced via the broader dichotomised system of Western thought, in which the drive to unity insists on only one oppressed and one truth. Hence the kinds of feminist accounts of sexual violence which have been most visible, given the elevation of white women like myself within feminism, have mainly tended to privilege understandings of (white) gender over those of 'race' (hooks, 1990: 57–64; Crenshaw, 1993).

But this need not become a blanket categorisation of radical/lesbian feminism as inevitably solipsist. It tends to give too much to other white-dominated theories and politics like socialist feminisms, which tend to reproduce dualisms by legitimating themselves through singling out radical/lesbian feminisms as the only racists; and too little to those radical and lesbian feminist strands which have begun to address racism and their/our own privilege, starting from within their 'own assumptions and practices' (see e.g. Pratt, 1984; Rich, 1987b). Much of what I have learnt about racism has come from participation in a NZ discussion and activist group of women of colour (which in that context also means 'not indigenous') and white women. The basis for the group was to support Maori sovereignty and to try to begin to develop an understanding of racism in various forms, from our shared similarities and differences as tauiwi (nonindigenous) lesbians and feminists.

As I have suggested, a flat dismissal of radical/lesbian feminisms tends to marginalise sexual violence as a pressing feminist issue. Instead, critics like Kemberlé Crenshaw (1993) urge that sexual violence remain a crucial area of oppression for feminist attention, but not as simply a 'gender issue' – unless gender is redefined as always also racialised and enacted along other multiple dimensions of power.[5]

The ambivalent critique of 'home' also means that, at the same time, we cannot completely abandon systematic attempts to describe and change women's oppressions, both as sexual objects and (denied) subjects. For instance, it should be feasible to object to women's systematic victimisation without being dismissed as a 'victim' feminist. (I am reminded of MacKinnon's (1987: 220) remark on the double bind: 'If this [victim] stereotype is a stereotype, it has already been accomplished, and I come after'.)

If it is more difficult to try to think through questions of pleasure and coercion, victimisation and agency together; that they are entwined is often precisely the problem. Feminist post-structuralist theory can be helpful here (e.g. Gavey, 1989, 1992) but there remain many unsprung dualist traps. These are associated again with the urge for one clean truth, producing an 'innocence' requirement which rules out considering how the victimised might also be in a different way, or at a different moment, agents, oppressors or even perpetrators.

All of this postmodernist and feminist rethinking of 'home', and the consequent problematising of rigid boundaries with its simultaneous ambivalences, returns me to the Humourless Feminist in her 'restless undead', vampiric guise (see, e.g. Haraway, 1985; Verhoeven, 1993b, especially pp. 111–115). De Lauretis suggests that if the shift away from a secure home involves painful 'dis-placements', both personal and conceptual: 'the leaving is not a choice: one could not live there, in the first place' (de Lauretis, 1988: 139).

Afterword: loving another science

By the mid-1990s I began to see different aspects of my work as elements of a much larger project concerned with various forms of sexual violence and their different cultural representations (Atmore, 1997b, c, 1998, 1999a, c). The stories and images often jostle with each other for authoritative meaning, and that outcome is important partly because what is represented as 'sexual violence' also provides the ground through which other investments and interests are advanced (ibid.).

Such an approach led me into two areas. The first took the charting of some of the travels of 'the restless undead' of the Humourless or 'victim' Feminist, into a more detailed endeavour to understand the growing 1990s' typifications of many child sexual abuse conflicts as 'moral panics' (Atmore, 1996, 1997a, b, 1998, 1999b). The 'folk devils' in such panics were often represented as innocent families and parents being persecuted by a victimising and even abusive state. Liberal and left-wing academics added their own contributions, sometimes extending their folk devil defence to the bogey of the homosexual child molester, and to the satanist, who was usually regarded as akin to a heavy metal fan in having unpopular, but ultimately not harmful, interests (Atmore, 1999b). Most of the moral panic stories, liberal or otherwise, personified the state in the form of child protection workers, and/or feminists, and sometimes lesbians (ibid.; Atmore, 1996).

My discomfort as a feminist led me to trace this reappearance of the vampire to various iconographies and interests, to reformulate theories of moral panic, and so to the second area of work. I found a guiding framework in one of my favourite feminist texts, Donna Haraway's re-narrativising of primatology (Haraway, 1989), and her preference, aligned with her vision of feminism's love of another science, for heteroglossia and webbed accounts (Haraway, 1985, 1988). This science can be interpreted as referring to both the theoretical approach and where and how to go looking for relevant representations.

For my task, the 'material-semiotic' traffic (Haraway, 1989) among diverse fields includes: academic research and theory, particularly in sociology and cultural studies; the media; and feminisms, directly politically activist or otherwise. Some of these, and other relevant fields of power, are also explored elsewhere in this book. The 'traffic' approach is an illustration of the continuing need in work against sexual violence – child sexual abuse and other kinds – to problematise dualist thinking, emphatic categorisations and generalisations (see e.g. Gavey, 1999; Crossley, 2000).

For example, I cannot reject completely the moral panic theorists' criticisms of 'wrongful' state intervention. My own local context has a history of genocide against Indigenous people, which included systematic practices of the removal of a generation of children – ironically, sometimes on suspicion of monoculturally-defined child abuse – and often resulting in physical, sexual and emotional abuse of those children in white-run institutions (National Inquiry, 1997). Yet at the same time, family violence of all kinds is a serious and often unaddressed problem in many Indigenous communities (Bolger, 1991; Egger, 1997; Cultural Perspectives, 2000). As radical and lesbian feminists have long argued, home is often not a safe place for women and children, while Black feminists must remind some of us that it may be the only refuge.

Continuing with the 'home' trope, re-working at least some aspects of moral panic theories has led me to consider some child sexual abuse conflicts as panics about panics, deflecting concern towards other folk devils – social workers, psychologists, various feminists and lesbians. These figures are often versions of the Humourless Feminist, and along with the homosexual molesters and paedophile 'monsters' (Atmore, 1998), serve a 'good housekeeping' narrative in which the 'ordinary' and 'normal' are kept intact from contamination by sexual violence.

This is a theme all too well known by feminists, but it needs updating. As I have argued elsewhere (ibid.; Atmore 1999a), increased boundary crossing and unanticipated sharings of discursive space suggest that our conceptual tools need to catch up with profound cultural change (see also Crossley, 2000). The relevant contexts for anti-sexual-violence work in any general research or clinical practice, or theoretical approach, will often extend into the broader field of traffic, including cross-disciplinarily, -nationally and -culturally. At the same time, attention has to be paid to postmodernist and ex-centric stresses on positionality and situated knowledges in order to consider local settings, thereby pluralising our questions and strategies, including about sexual violences themselves (e.g. Gavey, 1999; Lamb, 1999; Warner, 2000).

For example, if we focus on the relationships between feminist and post-structuralist theories in the university, there seems still, in the twenty-first century, some tendency for radical feminisms and work on sexual violence to be mutually associated, while post-structuralist feminisms and queer theories get 'the rest' of sexuality. Of course this may be more true in some countries and tertiary institutions than others; and is also related to how, for instance, feminisms in different contexts have taken up post-structuralist theories; and how in turn this has re-positioned feminist work and the 'in' things to do in particular academic power nexuses.

Also relevant here are issues like the extent to which, and in what ways, feminists inside and outside universities are still working together; for instance, across academic publishing, government policy and community activist organisations. Work also remains to be done on how feminist activism against sexual violences, and mainstream responses to that, have been shaped by different national and local traditions like radical and socialist feminist, indigenous, anti-racist, lesbian, gay and queer politics. Is sexual violence any different from other areas here?

A recent further migration of my own – from the university environment to, in its own argot, the community sector; along with my typically late-twentieth-century shift to more coalition affiliations with various 'grass roots' activisms rather than identity politics – has given me more food for thought about sexual violence, and indeed, violences in general. Contracted to a domestic violence and incest centre which trains workers and provides resources, my impression has been that the community sector has changed since I last had contact as a much younger self (admittedly, not in the same country).

In my recent setting, 'academic' was not the 'outsider' word it once was. In the broader milieu of my work, I was slightly, if perhaps naïvely, surprised that some, especially younger, anti-violence workers are *au fait* with post-structuralist feminist theories and/or are keen consumers of postmodern-influenced popular culture. However, the domestic violence organisation I worked for may not be typical even of urban environments, and there often still seems in more direct services a 'them and us' divide between workers against violence and official, especially post-structuralist, 'theory'.

My work required me to address the (secondary research) issue of whether men can ever be regarded as victims of domestic violence by women. This is a question which I may not have been able to effectively explore without my previous migration experiences and reflections, and the inspiration of Mani (1990). It was a complex and challenging task, intellectually, politically and personally (Atmore, 2001a, b), and I was heartened in this area of traffic by Elizabeth Stanko (1997) and Claire Renzetti (1999).

That project has brought home to me the continuing relevance of the vampire figure to my ongoing involvement in the sexual violence field. While we might be more comfortable with the 'restless' aspect of this trope, the vampire also disturbingly connotes violence, blood and death. Keeping her status as a family portrait, albeit ambivalently, allows us to also acknowledge the still small but important contribution made by some feminists who theorise, research and work with and against violences *by women*, and which are potentially, in most if not all of their various forms, within us all.

Notes

1 Rubin's (1984) 'Thinking Sex', not Rubin's (1975) 'The Traffic in Women'.
2 We might have hoped that AIDS activism and cultural criticism, in engaging with threats to life and their entanglement with sexuality, would also contribute to sexual violence opposition; and vice versa. But the predominant presentation is one of 'competing' causes and mutually exclusive labels of sex 'positive' or 'negative'.
3 See e.g. Barrett and McIntosh (1982); Gordon (1986); McIntosh (1988). One could argue that this work is largely socialist feminist, but as suggested earlier, it also has radical feminist affiliations and influences.
4 See e.g. Bordo (1988, 1989); Morris (1987: 176). The fact that much of the vitriol is reserved for Andrea Dworkin, a big Jewish woman, is especially interesting.
5 There is also much work to be done on how depictions of the Humourless

Feminist are racialised (see e.g. hooks, 1981: 15–49, 1990: 89–102; Crenshaw, 1993, especially p. 432). This includes paying attention to the ways in which Black women and women of colour can function as the Humourless Other for white women.

References

Alderson, M. (1993) 'The new lesbians: sisters are doing it to themselves', *Cleo* October: 68–72.

Anzaldúa, G. (1983) 'La Prieta', in C. Moraga and G. Anzaldúa (eds) *This bridge called my back: writings by radical women of color*, 2nd edition, New York: Kitchen Table/Women of Color Press, pp. 198–209.

Atmore, C. (1993a) ' "Branded": lesbian representation and a New Zealand cultural controversy', in D. Bennett (ed.) *Cultural studies: pluralism and theory*, Melbourne: Department of English, University of Melbourne, Parkville, pp. 281–292.

Atmore, C. (1993b) 'Feminism's restless undead: the essential(ist) activist', unpublished paper presented at *'Bring a Plate': The Feminist Cultural Studies Conference*, University of Melbourne, December.

Atmore, C. (1996) 'Cross-cultural media-tions: media coverage of two child sexual abuse controversies in New Zealand/Aotearoa', *Child Abuse Review* 5: 334–345.

Atmore, C. (1997a) 'Rethinking moral panic and child abuse for 2000', in J. Bessant and R. Hil (eds) *Reporting law and order: youth, crime and the media*, Hobart: National Clearing House for Youth Studies, pp. 123–129.

Atmore, C. (1997b) 'Commentary: conflicts over recovered memories – every layer of the onion', *Feminism and Psychology* 7, 1: 57–62.

Atmore, C. (1997c) 'Loving another science: some musings on the complexities and productivities of cross-disciplinary feminist work against sexual violences', unpublished paper presented at *'Transformations: Thinking through feminism'* Conference, Centre for Women's Studies, Lancaster University, July 17–19.

Atmore, C. (1998) 'Towards 2000: Child sexual abuse and the media', in A. Howe (ed.) *Sexed crime in the news*, Melbourne: Federation Press, pp. 124–144.

Atmore, C. (1999a) 'Victims, backlash and radical feminist theory (or, The morning after they stole feminism's fire)', in S. Lamb (ed.) *New versions of victims: feminists struggle with the concept*, New York: New York University Press, pp. 183–211.

Atmore, C. (1999b) 'Towards rethinking moral panic: child sexual abuse conflicts and social constructionist responses', in C. Bagley and K. Mallick (eds) *Child sexual abuse and adult offenders: new theory and research*, Aldershot: Ashgate, pp. 11–26.

Atmore, C. (1999c) 'Sexual abuse and troubled feminism: a reply to Camille Guy', *Feminist Review* 61: 83–96.

Atmore, C. (2001a) 'Men as victims of domestic violence: some issues to consider', Discussion Paper No. 2, Melbourne: Domestic Violence and Incest Resource Centre.

Atmore, C. (2001b) 'Family violence perspectives and the conflict tactics scales', Reference Paper, Melbourne: Domestic Violence and Incest Resource Centre.

Barrett, M. and McIntosh, M. (1982) *The anti-social family*, London: Verso.

Bolger, A. (1991) *Aboriginal women and violence*, Darwin: Australian National University, North Australia Research Unit.

Bordo, S. (1988) 'Anorexia nervosa: psychopathology as the crystallization of culture', in I. Diamond and L. Quinby (eds) *Feminism and Foucault: reflections on resistance*, Boston: Northeastern University Press, pp. 87–117.

Bordo, S. (1989) 'Reading the slender body', in M. Jacobus, E. Fox Keller and S. Shuttleworth (eds) *Body/Politics: women and the discourses of science*, New York: Routledge, pp. 83–109.

Bordo, S. (1990) 'Feminism, postmodernism, and gender-scepticism', in L. Nicholson (ed.) *Feminism/Postmodernism*, New York: Routledge, pp. 133–156.

Bordo, S. (1992) 'Review essay: postmodern subjects, postmodern bodies', *Feminist Studies* 18, 1: 59–175.

Crenshaw, K. (1993) 'Whose story is it, anyway? Feminist and antiracist appropriations of Anita Hill', in T. Morrison (ed.) *Race-ing justice, en-gendering power*, London: Chatto & Windus, pp. 402–440.

Crossley, M. (2000) 'Deconstructing autobiographical accounts of childhood sexual abuse: some critical reflections', *Feminism and Psychology* 10, 1: 73–90.

Cultural Perspectives (2000) *Attitudes to domestic and family violence in the diverse Australian community*, Canberra: Commonwealth of Australia.

de Lauretis, T. (1988) 'Displacing hegemonic discourses: reflections on feminist theory in the 1980s', *Inscriptions* 3/4: 127–145.

Egger, S. (1997) 'Women and crime prevention', in P. O'Malley and A. Sutton (eds) *Crime prevention in Australia: issues in policy and research*, Sydney: Federation Press, pp. 84–104.

Gavey, N. (1989) 'Feminist post-structuralism and discourse analysis: contributions to feminist psychology', *Psychology of Women Quarterly* 13: 459–475.

Gavey, N. (1992) 'Technologies and effects of heterosexual coercion', *Feminism and Psychology* 2: 325–351.

Gavey, N. (1999) '"I wasn't raped, but …"': revisiting definitional problems in sexual victimisation', in S. Lamb (ed.) *New versions of victims: feminists struggle with the concept*, New York: New York University Press, pp. 57–81.

Gordon, L. (1986) 'Feminism and social control: the case of child abuse and neglect', in J. Mitchell and A. Oakley (eds) *What is feminism?*, Oxford: Basil Blackwell, pp. 63–84.

Haraway, D. (1985) 'A manifesto for cyborgs: science, technology, and socialist feminism in the 1980s', *Socialist Review* 15, March/April.

Haraway, D. (1988) 'Situated knowledges: the science question in feminism and the privilege of partial perspective', *Feminist Studies* 14, 3: 575–599.

Haraway, D. (1989) *Primate visions: gender, race, and nature in the world of modern science*, New York: Routledge.

Hartsock, N. (1989/90) 'Postmodernism and political change: issues for feminist theory', *Cultural Critique* Winter: 15–33.

hooks, b. (1981) *Ain't I a woman: Black women and feminism*, Boston: South End Press.

hooks, b. (1990) *Yearning: race, gender, and cultural politics*, Boston: South End Press.

Hutcheon, L. (1988) *A poetics of postmodernism*, London: Routledge.

Lamb, S. (ed.) (1999) *New versions of victims: feminists struggle with the concept*, New York: New York University Press.

Lumby, C. (1993) 'The new school/why the war isn't over yet', *The Australian Magazine* 4–5 December: 30–37.

McIntosh, M. (1988) 'Introduction to an issue: family secrets as public drama', *Feminist Review* 28, Spring: 6–15.

MacKinnon, C. (1983) 'Feminism, Marxism, method and the State: toward feminist jurisprudence', *Signs* 8, 4: 635–658.

MacKinnon, C. (1987) *Feminism unmodified: discourses on life and law*, Cambridge: Harvard University Press.

Mani, L. (1990) 'Multiple mediations: feminist scholarship in the age of multinational reception', *Feminist Review* 35, Summer: 24–41.

Martin, B. and Talpade Mohanty, C. (1986) 'Feminist politics: what's home got to do with it?', in T. de Lauretis (ed.) *Feminist studies/critical studies*, Bloomington: Indiana University Press, pp. 191–212.

Merck, M. (1988) 'Bedroom horror: the fatal attraction of *Intercourse*', *Feminist Review* 30, Autumn: 89–103.

Modleski, T. (1991) *Feminism without women: culture and criticism in a 'postfeminist' age*, New York and London: Routledge.

Morris, M. (1987) 'in any event . . .', in A. Jardine and P. Smith (eds) *Men in feminism*, New York: Methuen, pp. 173–181.

National Inquiry into the Separation of Aboriginal and Torres Strait Islander Children from Their Families (1997) *Bringing them home: report of the National Inquiry into the Separation of Aboriginal and Torres Strait Islander Children from Their Families*, Sydney: Human Rights and Equal Opportunity Commission.

O'Sullivan, S. (1993) 'Where does political correctness come from? Does it drop from the sky?', in D. Bennett (ed.) *Cultural studies: pluralism and theory*, Melbourne: Department of English, University of Melbourne, Parkville, pp. 189–196.

Pratt, M. (1984) 'Identity: skin, blood, heart', in E. Bulkin, M. Pratt and B. Smith (eds) *Yours in struggle: three feminist perspectives on anti-semitism and racism*, Brooklyn: Long Haul Press, pp. 11–63.

Renzetti, C. (1999) 'The challenge to feminism posed by women's use of violence in intimate relationships', in S. Lamb (ed.) *New versions of victims: feminists struggle with the concept*, New York: New York University Press, pp. 42–50.

Rich, A. (1987a) 'Compulsory heterosexuality and lesbian existence', in *Blood, bread and poetry*, London: Virago, pp. 23–75.

Rich, A. (1987b) 'Notes toward a politics of location', in *Blood, bread and poetry*, London: Virago, pp. 210–231.

Rich, B.R. (1986) 'Review essay: feminism and sexuality in the 1980s', *Feminist Studies* 12, 3: 525–561.

Rubin, G. (1975) 'The traffic in women: notes on the "political economy" of sex', in R. Reiter (ed.) *Toward an anthropology of women*, New York: Monthly Review Press, pp. 157–210.

Rubin, G. (1984) 'Thinking sex: notes for a radical theory of the politics of sexuality', in C. Vance (ed.) *Pleasure and danger: exploring female sexuality*, Boston: Routledge and Kegan Paul, pp. 267–319.

Smart, C. (1990) 'Law's power, the sexed body, and feminist discourse', *Journal of Law and Society* 17, 2: 194–210.

Smith, B. and Smith, B. (1983) 'Across the kitchen table: a sister-to-sister dialogue', in C. Moraga and G. Anzaldúa (eds) *This bridge called my back: writings by radical women of color*, 2nd edition, New York: Kitchen Table/Women of Color Press, pp. 113–127.

Smith-Rosenberg, C. (1989) 'The body politic', in E. Weed (ed.) *Coming to terms: feminism, theory, politics*, New York: Routledge, pp. 101–121.

Spivak, G. (1990) 'Criticism, feminism, and the institution', interview with Elizabeth Gross, in B. Robbins (ed.) *Intellectuals: aesthetics, politics, academics*, Minneapolis: University of Minnesota Press, pp. 153–171.

Stanko, E. (1997) ' "I second that emotion": reflections on feminism, emotionality, and research on sexual violence', in M. Schwartz (ed.) *Researching sexual violence against women: methodological and personal perspectives*, Thousand Oaks: Sage, pp. 74–84.

Tetzlaff, D. (1992) 'Popular culture and social control in late Capitalism', in P. Scannell, P. Schlesinger and C. Sparks (eds) *Culture and power: a Media, Culture & Society Reader*, London: Sage, pp. 48–72.

Vance, C. (1993a) 'The pleasures of looking', public lecture, Melbourne University, 26 August.

Vance, C. (1993b) 'Negotiating sexual images and sexual politics', *Island* 57, Summer: 20–25.

Verhoeven, D. (1993a) 'Great moments in mutual mastication: the trials of Tracey Wigginton', in D. Bennett (ed.) *Cultural studies: pluralism and theory*, Melbourne: Department of English, University of Melbourne, Parkville, pp. 272–280.

Verhoeven, D. (1993b) 'Biting the hand that breeds: the trials of Tracy Wigginton', in H. Birch (ed.) *Moving targets: women, murder and representation*, London: Virago, pp. 95–126.

Wark, M. (1993) 'Real victims of PC rhetoric', *The Australian Higher Education Supplement* 10 November: 20.

Warner, S. (2000) 'Feminist theory, the Women's Liberation Movement and therapy for women: changing our concerns', *Changes: An International Journal of Psychology and Psychotherapy* 18, 4: 232–243.

Watney, S. (1987) *Policing desire: pornography, aids and the media*, London: Methuen.

Weeks, J. (1985) *Sexuality and its discontents: meanings, myths and modern sexualities*, London: Routledge and Kegan Paul.

Yorke, L. (1997) *Adrienne Rich: passion, politics and the body*, London: Sage.

Zita, J. (1981) 'Historical amnesia and the lesbian continuum' *Signs* 7, 1: 172–187.

Chapter 3

Childhood, sexual abuse and contemporary political subjectivities

Erica Burman

This chapter addresses three main areas. First, it highlights the textualisation of childhood, within whose broader forms representations of child sexual abuse occur. Second, it explores some political consequences of some widely circulating texts of childhood to ward off the current political imperatives (towards action and intervention) attending these. Finally, the chapter ends by attempting to indicate strategies for the subversion of the models of development that discourses of child sexual abuse fracture, but equally by which they suffer.

Framing childhood texts

It is fitting that I start by clarifying the purpose of my own text here. Even though I am as subject as anyone else to the discourses of childhood I want to topicalise, I nevertheless want to offset the reproduction of their effects by commenting upon them. Of course I cannot prescribe how any reader of this text will interpret the arguments I present: whatever my intentions, my account will be understood differently according to readers' specific positions, histories and preoccupations. This reflects how, under late capitalism, authorial intention is rendered increasingly irrelevant in relation to audience receptivities (see discussion in Parker, 1998). But contrary to a relativist position, I want to assume some responsibility for interpretation that my speaking position here endows.

In relation both to child sexual abuse and the broader discourses or narratives of childhood to which this gives rise, my focus is on moral qualities that surround texts of childhood. So, since part of what I want to talk about is the emotionality surrounding children and childhood, let me make clear at the outset that my aim here is not to instil states of guilt, sentimentality, titillation, pity, horror or outrage. These are, however, well-rehearsed, culturally-sanctioned responses to children – whether the specific, individual children of our homes, schools, streets and shopping precincts, the children of our families, or more abstract, distant or even rhetorical categories of children. Notice how I am now speaking of the spaces of childhood, mapping the geography of childhood living, and the ways this intersects with other institutional arenas of production and consumption (Boyden with Holden, 1991). But outside the allocated spaces of childhood within Western industrialised life, children inhabit shadier places where they are regarded as not belonging. Here they appear as matters of management and policy – children in care, children in need, children subject to child protection legislation, children on behalf of whom we intervene to 'restore' the conditions of the kind of childhoods we approve. Moreover, beyond these, there are other children who are seemingly active agents in warranting these somehow 'abnormal' interventions; with such interventions formulated as 'in the best interests of' or 'on behalf of' children who work, children who have sex, children whose work is having sex; children who steal, bully, or even murder (see Burman, 1995a). Where, then, do children who have been sexually abused fit into this broader landscape? Are they damaged but innocent (but where does this leave those who might be 'culpable'?)? Are they tainted with the crime and offence that they themselves have been subject to? Let us pause for just a moment to take stock.

A first point to note is that I have hardly begun and yet we are already in the domain of normative prescription: the 'shoulds' and 'oughts' of what children are like, with correspondingly negative evaluation of children who don't 'fit' our notions.

Second, the much vaunted pleasure children bring seems to subsist within two sets of relations: for 'what children are' is constituted within sets of institutional relationships that are currently the site of much political focus – the family, schools, healthcare, etc. The uneasy relationship between children who have been sexually abused with the overall category of childhood is precisely what is at play here; for the above throw into question the viability of precisely those safe, comfortable spaces for children – family, schools, care – they are said to protect. Moreover I would also suggest that the 'right' kinds of childhood – innocent, playful, obedient, etc. – also exist because in some sense they repudiate, but at the same time require for their existence, the very stigmatised forms of childhood that they thereby display they are not (see Burman, 1995b).

So – to return to my initial comments about emotions and standpoint – even before we move to take account of the more metaphorical or rhetorical appeals to childhood, we are into affective domains that are highly politicised and highly emotionally charged (see also Burman, 1999). Even before we start to link children and development with broader social themes and trajectories it is clear that (what counts as) a desirable or undesirable childhood stands in a relation of mutual constitution: each in some sense relies upon the other.

I should perhaps make clear that I am not a child rights, child policy, or child services specialist. Nor am I even a specialist in development studies in the broader sense of international economic development – although I like to explore how the different notions of development are related to each other (see also Burman, 1995c). My interest lies in the claims made for and about children; and, beyond individually embodied children, in the notions of childhood these presuppose and their corresponding associations and reverberations. I want to discuss the political subjectivities mobilised by such notions, hopefully the better to determine which political subjectivities we should assume and which we should divest ourselves (and our children) of.

There are two additional points to note here. First, I am using the terms 'subject' and 'subjectivities' (as in my title 'political subjectivities') in the double senses highlighted by Foucauldian analyses, i.e. as subject *to* as well as subject *of* (Foucault, 1980). Hence I am speaking of forms of subjectivity or experience *as produced through* discourses or institutional frameworks of meaning, but also as functioning as – albeit circumscribed – agents within these (see also Fraser, 1989; Hekman, 1990; McNay, 1992; Bell, 1993). Such approaches have been taken up by feminists as helpful to analyse both processes of subjugation, but also how subjugated knowledges subsist whose expression and expertise can be mobilised. Hence although I will be concerned more in this chapter with the political subjectivities mobilised *around* children (including children who have been sexually abused), rather than by them, there are implications of this kind of analysis for highlighting and situating children's agency, of which I can only offer some indications here.

Second, it might be argued that such work is a luxury, the privilege of the academic who does not (have to) work with, or legislate about, the actions of, or care for, 'real children'. Even if this were true I would want to suggest that distance perhaps offers space for reflection that can be of value – for these analyses do offer a range of ways of thinking about the political and affective imperatives that surround children. In particular we can more easily ask questions about how things came to be this way, and thus come better equipped to policy and management development to ask whether these are the only, or best, ways of thinking *about* children, and our dealings *with* children.

Texts of childhood

Notions of childhood evoke concepts and practices such as nature, biology, stages, bodies, growth, (im)maturity, rights, vulnerability and innocence. These combine moral–political evaluation with apparently 'natural' terminology (of growth and maturity), but slip easily into consumer discourse (of value increase, as in the Laura Ashley children's clothes slogan of the mid-1990s: 'fashion for the upwardly mobile'). Additional associations might include childhood as a social category, or in relation to religious notions of original sin or anthropological notions of otherness – as well as other age-related categories such as baby, infant, newborn, neonate (the technical term) or toddler, of the kind that appear in developmental psychology textbooks.

All of this is even before we import the rhetorics of development associated with children and childhood. Here notions of progress, improvement, skill and adaptation emerge, words that migrate or even flow easily between the specific and the general, or from individual to social allocation. This happens whether we are talking about a single child or groups of children; or about descriptors of species as well as states or conditions. Or, further, from states of individual minds or bodies to evaluations of the relative status of nation states. Here we begin to see the political load carried by the discourse of development, and by children who are so often positioned as its bearers. Children thus provide the conceptual and emotional means by which contested social hierarchy can be perpetuated by being mapped onto an apparently natural asocial category (Burman, 1994a).

This is what I mean by the textualisation of childhood. For – irrespective of whatever children are 'really' like – we cannot know them or about them except through particular cultural and historical frames or discourses that structure that 'reality'. Moreover what really makes this matter is that these cultural and historical frames have varied and do vary quite considerably, with significantly different positions elaborated – not only for children and all those subject to the injunction to develop. Moreover there are others – girls and women, working children, black and working class people, people with physical or learning disabilities, gay men and lesbians – who are rendered invisible by their normalised (inferior) developmental status. Yet their positions and livelihoods are nevertheless constituted by (or perhaps it would be more accurate to say constellated around) our topic/subject. So there is a contest over *whose definitions* of development hold sway. It is part of the argument of this chapter that the dominant naturalised discourse of ('normal' or 'typical') development has obscured this contest, and so has helped to produce the position of the abused child as different, abnormal and outside prevailing discourses (including policy discourses) of childhood.

Hence, hierarchy is explicitly structured within the lexicon of age and life-stages (of baby-child-adolescent-adult, for example). But there are equivalent, if less naturalised, social and spatial distributions of 'differences' structured around gender, sexuality and 'race'. Such hierarchies clearly have important histories in colonialism and imperialism as well as current allocations (between the 'First' and 'Third' World, to take a very significant example of development discourse; see Sachs, 1999). But somehow the blending of history with hierarchy has been easier to recognise in talking about age. So we could conceivably consider the textualisation of the child as a paradigm case of other such ideological constructions.

At any rate let us consider five points: the special status of childhood, the gendering of the child; the child as true/lost self; contestations around the naturalness of childhood and the need to situate the contemporary 'crisis' of childhood.

I The special status of childhood

The UN Convention on the Rights of the Child as a piece of legislation was passed in record time (see my discussion of this in Burman, 1996). Yet this has been at a price. In some senses it can be argued that children – as the starting point or supposedly raw material for social development – are the victims of the asocial model of the bourgeois individual of modernity. For as the prototypical subjects of modernity – of the modern project of social improvement, it has been the fate of children to be talked of as though gender, culture and sexuality are additional qualities to be grafted onto some apparently prior or pre-given 'child'.

Thus the 'special'-ness of children seems to be at the expense of their being apart from the very social structures concerned with protecting or promoting them. The costs of this for the adequate analysis of, and engagement with, children who have been sexually abused are serious. For, once so identified, they seem neither to belong to the category of childhood (since this has been constituted as, by definition, safe and inno-cent), nor to the social structures that both constitute the domain of child-hood and accord them such anomalous status within it. Moreover the singular status of 'the child' confirms her or his position outside communit-ies. That is, outside not only cultural communities, but also communities of other children – including siblings who form significant, if not primary, caregivers for many of the world's children – and in particular *political* communities of other children. Here we might recall analyses of how 'the child' of developmental psychology and educational practices (including compulsory primary level schooling) emerged at a political moment within industrialising societies when children and young people were becoming economically active and increasingly organised (Hoyles, 1989; Hendrick, 1990). These indicate that the claims to the special protection with which contemporary childhood has been invested paradoxically correspond with the denial of children's agency.

So, to offer some crude but illustrative examples, currently in the UK our legal system does not regard young people as capable of democratic political participation (via casting votes) until the age of eighteen; of con-senting sexual activity until age sixteen, of earning a sustainable wage comparable to the minimum pay level, while the question of whether chil-dren and young people should be held legally responsible for their actions has been hugely exercised by the Bulger case (Burman, 1995a). Elsewhere in the world (and probably more within the UK than most people would like to realise) children bear arms, bear children and work long hours for little pay. Notwithstanding the reality of children's physical and emotional vulnerability, it seems there are broad cultural–political investments in maintaining children and young people as docile and dependent through educational, legal and welfare practices that portray them as deficient and therefore in need of training and/or protection. There may be practical political demands to be made, that correspond to the claims made for the movement for Democratic Psychiatry in Trieste, Italy (McLaughlin, 2000), of calling for legal responsibility as a means of warding off their status as asocial and disenfranchised.

2 Gendering the child

Children are generally treated as a unitary category unless marked explicitly by gender. Thus the new development category, 'the girlchild', produces girls and young women as both not quite child and not only woman, for as a new hybrid the 'girlchild' somehow represents a doubled position of vulnerability to abuse and oppression – whether in terms of labour or sexual services (see Burman, 1995b). Despite this, the qualities accorded children typically remain allocated according to conventional gender stereotypes. Thus the child of development, the developmental subject who is active, autonomous, playing, problem-solving and singular – is culturally masculine and often is portrayed as a little boy (as in Piaget's model of the child as mini-scientist, Piaget, 1957). Here it is also worth remembering that across the world it is boys who manage to access the efforts towards universal primary education better than girls; whereas the *state* from which development takes place is typically a feminised/infantilised arena. Thus girls represent childhood as a state of neediness or difference, including desirability, or sometimes supposedly inherent maternity; while boys represent a forward-looking potential (with the recent shift in aid imagery from girls to boys occupying an ambivalent place here).

However we should note that contexts of abuse fracture the dominant conception of childhood as devoid of gender, as much as of sexuality. For in understanding how sexual abuse comes about, we have to address the different (sexed and gendered) positions of boys and girls as subject to actual or potential abuse, and so begin to acknowledge the complex and constitutive intersections between these (Warner, 1996, 2000). Policy discourses of sexual abuse are themselves gender-stratified, with boys and girls being understood as being abused under different conditions (but with the abusers in both cases largely being men). But we should pause to note the potential conflation between vulnerability and feminisation that itself speaks of a culturally dominant discourse that transcends the gendered or sexed positions of actual children. Further, this not only implicitly pathologises their autonomy; it also discourages (attention to) their resilience and resistance.

3 The child as lost/true self

In the effort to repair the gap, to restore a subjectivity (and correspondingly a gender, culture and sexuality) denied to the child by virtue of the limitations of these prevailing models, many fictions and fantasies have been born. These fantasies indicate how children – especially little girls – signify not only the inner, fragile self, but also have come to express longing and loss within the modern Western imaginary. Carolyn Steedman suggests:

> The child within was always both immanent – ready to be drawn on in various ways – and, at the same time, always representative of a lost realm, lost in the individual past, and in the past of the culture ... The idea of the child was used both to recall and to express the past that each individual life contained: what was turned inside in the course of individual development was that which was also latent: the child *was* the story waiting to be told.
>
> (1995: 10–11, emphasis in original)

Hence the romance of the other is rendered docile and diminutive in the form of the little girl (who is positioned as in need of protection, or even covertly of seduction? See also Stainton Rogers and Stainton Rogers, 1994). This romance is written into models of psychological development as an origin story – a (cultural and individual) mythological narrative of (one's) beginnings, with development marking distance from a thereby inferior, devalued but also fascinating, place.

> The child was the figure that provided the largest number of people living in the recent past of Western societies with the means for thinking about and creating a self: something grasped and understood: a shape, moving in the body ... something *inside*, an interiority.
>
> (Steedman, 1995: 20)

It is a significant challenge to take seriously how deeply such gendered imagery informs not only concepts of childhood, but also Western subjectivity more generally. The figure of the little girl has come to function as both prototypical subject and object in ways that have not only normalised and naturalised exclusionary models of development, but have also obscured attention to the needs and capabilities of specifically gendered and embodied children and young people.

4 Contesting the naturalness of childhood

Thus the figure of the child – with its appeal to the natural, the divine and the taken for granted – has flourished precisely to the extent that it obscures its cultural and ideological origins. Herein lies the key to the current concern around children. The docile vulnerability accorded children, that prompts their protection and warrants their education, is thrown into confusion when some categories of children (notably working class and minoritised children, as well as those who have been abused) demonstrate themselves to be not so innocent; and the perplexity this generates is illuminating in two ways. First, not only is that protection conditional upon an injunction to be 'innocent' but, second, this clarifies how the very category of childhood presupposes the absence of all those ('knowing'/ 'knowledgeable') qualities of adulthood.

One political and psychological project of investigation that follows is this: if children are, after all, more like adults in matters of desires and complicities than had been supposed (or attributed), then what, if anything, develops? But while much developmental psychology preoccupies itself with this matter, I think the more important, because more easily avoided, topics to consider are just how and why we came to accord such different qualities and proclivities to adults and children (respectively). In particular we need to consider the investments underlying such distinctions, and how social–political questions are obscured by a contest for entitlements based on presumed constant and natural age or gender categories.

5 Situating the contemporary crisis of childhood

It seems that the contemporary policy (as well as representational[1]) crisis of childhood arises at a confluence of three key debates. First, there is unprecedented attention to the prevalence of the sexual abuse of children at local, national and international levels. While current reports of abuse both in private homes and residential care abound, there is a corresponding focus on those who abuse. But the emotional response unleashed towards those deemed at fault tends to resolve itself upon marginal individuals rather than institutional structures. This was graphically indicated by the disturbances in the British towns and cities in the summer of 2000, where Far Right groups mobilised, supposedly to support communities in the protection of their children, culminating in indiscriminate attacks on individuals rather than campaigning to improve services (see Bell, this volume).

A second context is the increasing publicity (and litigation) concerning people (mainly women) in therapy claiming to have recovered memories of abuse. This has thrown societal investments in constructing nostalgically happy childhoods and happy families into disarray (Burman, 1996/1997; Brown and Burman, 1997; Haaken, this volume).

Third, there are further ramifications surrounding the crisis of development and the project of modernity – both in terms of their manifest failure and in the sense of the rampant de-development (in the sense of active impoverishment of majority world nations, and imposition of dependency on the minority world/West) being perpetrated in the name of the benefits of globalisation and the free market. While most of the world still lives in acute poverty, notwithstanding the supposed cancellation of the world debt, the goals of sustainable, ecologically sound and equitable subsistence look more and more remote (see Sachs, 1999).

All of these factors give rise to an ever-increasing scrutiny of the supposed local index or representative of development: the child. For children form a key focus of intervention for all these disparate concerns. Moreover, these debates in turn relate to two other key contexts. First, there is an increasing professionalisation of talking and helping relationships within the condition of alienation in late modernity. Increasing social isolation and erosion of community/communal arenas for talk and support has fuelled the need to seek out professional spaces for intimate disclosure (Parker, 1997; Nicholson, 1999). Alongside this there is a correspondingly burgeoning bureaucracy around 'development' in the political sphere (think of how much supposed government international development 'aid' is spent on 'home' consultants and agencies). Second, in the contexts of increasing cuts in state welfare provision, there is a rampant proliferation of the privatised service sector (servicing both therapeutic and development studies needs) (Cooke and Kothari, 2001).

Traversing current texts

My arguments so far about the obscuring of culture within the discourse of nature may be familiar. They highlight how the naturalisation of childhood gives rise to corresponding pressures to homogenise all children and, by implication, developing subjects. But it is also worth noting their political significance in a number of ways. Hence, Valerie Walkerdine (1990) indicated how such naturalisation of gender also includes condoning gendered aggression. Moreover, as I will now discuss, the abstraction of the child affords a slippage from individual to society, from the child to the nation, from the lost to the true, authentic self; and – most significant in relation to child sexual abuse – from the feminised subject in need of protection, to the patriarchal superego urging action (or restraint from action). In short, ambivalent political agencies are constructed by, and in relation to, these texts of childhood. I turn now to discuss five illustrative examples.

I Originary state

There is emptiness about the originary state of childhood. Like many significant political spaces of occupation it is, conveniently, deemed to be without content or habitation. Similarly, the blank slate of childhood – within developmentalist accounts – is portrayed as empty, waiting to be inscribed by the social. The dependent, vulnerable condition of childhood calls forth all our practices of education, training and welfare intervention (including the policing of families, and stigmatisation of culturally minoritised practices, e.g. Phoenix, 1987). Here it is worth recalling that the political affiliations of environmentalists (as opposed to maturationists) in relation to child development have historically been directed towards public health rather than moral degeneracy positions. This social reforming, philanthropic position within the medical and mental hygiene movements of the early twentieth century marked out the medics from the budding psychologists. For it was the psychologists who were more inclined towards genetic determinist (and eugenic) positions – with all their attendant practices of classification, segregation and containment (see Rose, 1985).

Wiping that slate of development clean, producing that originary state, is not an obvious, innocent, or only rhetorical, activity. Similarly we might consider what racialised as well as gendered and sexualised positions are erased in keeping childhood safe, and what work of inscription belies its designated originary state of empty readiness. For it is this work that is highlighted by the position of children who have been sexually abused. Children who have been sexually abused perhaps 'hold' or represent the most stigmatised childhood knowledge that needs to be repudiated in order to safeguard prevailing power relations. As with black, working class and all other subaltern knowledges, this illustrates the discretionary character of our apparently boundless and unconditional indulgence to children.

2 Privileges/rights of childhood

Second, once childhood has been constituted as an original state, certain rights or privileges attend it. I have already mentioned the UN Convention on the Rights of the Child. This is as ambivalent a political document as any, in the sense that what counts as rights, and why, still has to be interpreted within each context and as such is amenable to considerable mediation and manipulation. But it is still a vital starting point for further mobilisation. Significantly, if predictably, though, protection rather than promotion figures most highly on the institutional agenda. This is seen worldwide in the difficulty of securing investment in promoting children's psychological and educational development, rather than only funding measures to reduce infant mortality (cf. Myers, 1992).

Once again, coming closer to my home, let me consider the little leaflet Manchester City Council delivered door to door in early 1999 entitled, *The Ten Things Children Need Most*. On the inside first page there is a list of children's needs:

- to feel safe and secure
- health and happiness
- cuddles and good touching
- lots of smiles
- praise and encouragement
- talking
- listening
- new experiences
- respect for their feelings
- rewards and treats.

(Manchester City Council/Area Child Protection Committee/
Manchester Social Services leaflet, 1999)

Who can fault these? It seems a comprehensive list – except that it fails to mention issues of power, consultation or authority. Moreover the rest of the leaflet is concerned with issues of safety and protection, and in particular is addressed to parents who might be experiencing difficulties, or want to intervene to help others in difficulty. Indeed the final page has a list of agencies for 'Getting Help'.

No wonder babies evoke such strong feelings, since they command such institutional support and intervention. But it is as if these babies exist either outside relationships, or within an adversarially constituted context of rights and responsibilities (which is of course the only way the individualist discourse of rights can conceive of relationships, Pateman, 1989).

3 'Giving children back their future' ...

Why do we rush to save children? Why should we pause to think about this, when the imperative to do so seems so strong, and indeed it has been called 'natural', or 'instinctive'? Yet the fact that this is not so, since the fact that certain cultural and especially economic conditions need to prevail before such 'natural' qualities are elicited or displayed is precisely what is at issue (cf. Scheper-Hughes, 1989). Let us pause a moment to consider Rahnema's advice:

Before intervening in people's lives, one should first intervene in one's own: 'polishing' oneself to ensure that all precautions have been taken to avoid harming the objects of intervention. Many questions should be explored first. What prompts me to intervene? Is it friendship, compassion, the 'mask of love', or an unconscious attempt to increase my powers of seduction? Have I done everything I could to assess the usefulness of my intervention? And if things do not proceed as I expect them, am I ready to face the full consequences of my intervention?

(1997: 497)

There is a lot of talk of lost childhoods and restoring childhoods. What is less often reflected upon is *whose* childhood we are referring to, or rather imposing, here. In the context of child (sexual) abuse, neglect or deprivation it is easy for these broader questions to feel like liberal agonisings, or inappropriate hesitations. Yet aid organisations have themselves become much more careful about, and critical of, the political positions mobilised for donor and recipient when images of children are used, especially in the context of international development causes (Black, 1992; Save the Children, 1992; see also Burman, 1994b).

Moreover, once we are outside the determinist discourse of original sin, what seems attractive about the modern developmental discourse of childhood is the indulgence or reforming 'understanding' it accords children. Recently in England the charity Barnardos was at the centre of controversy because of its new media campaign. This tried to ward off the discourse of blame attending various 'social misfits' through invoking the childhood history carried within, or alternatively conceived as producing, the adult. As a journalist commentator put it:

It's an advert based on the sort of solid truth that flashes through your mind every time you hand over 50p to a beggar – that everyone is born an innocent baby, and what is it that goes so wrong as to put that little ball of trust and love out on the Strand at midnight?
(Stephen Armstrong, in the *Guardian*, 24 January 2000: 4)

The images substituted a child for a young adult in a succession of contexts that included being in prison, homeless, on the streets, on drugs or alcohol, or about to jump off a skyscraper to a sure death. Thus they offered a dramatic invitation to see the inner needy or suffering child within the adult. These images of damaged children were invoked to account for socially useless, often morally degraded people. It is perhaps significant that the only girl/female image was also the only one specifically mentioning 'abuse'.

The small text beside the image in each case opened with a statement of original damage/trauma: 'neglected as a child ...', 'written off as a child ...', 'battered as a child ...', 'abused aged 5 ...', 'made to feel worthless as a child ...'. This was followed by an appeal for understanding and assertion of a 'possible' link between a childhood situation and the current situation of marginalisation/self-harm/destitution: 'it was always pos-sible ...', 'there was always a chance of ...', and, finally, 'it was hardly surprising ...' ('... that Carl would turn to alcohol', 'Martin could see no other way out', etc). The Barnardo's director of marketing and communi-cations behind the campaign, Andrew Neb, was reported as saying: 'Whenever you see a homeless person and sniff that it's all their own fault, it's worth remembering that it was probably something in their childhood that pushed them into it' (ibid.: 5).

So in terms of mitigating the discourse of blame or social responsibility, 'giving people back their future' is about attributing them with a trauma-tised past. This might in some circumstances be helpful, and perhaps *is* so if it prompts less stigmatising approaches to working with homeless people, people with mental health problems or drug users. However, there are two obvious problems. First, there is the familiar problem that once the past is seen as the traumatogenic place of origin it is all too easy to conveniently 'forget' present day sequelae/causative circumstances. In particular individualised, family-oriented explanations frequently function to exonerate state neglect or deprivations.

Second, the 'shock value' of this campaign relies upon a denial of what is actually the case: we are supposed to be shocked at these images pre-cisely because their estrangement relies upon seeing children (rather than adults) depicted as doing such things as taking drugs, and sleeping on the streets. That is, the assumption is that the people involved *were* the chil-dren these adults now *are*. What all the public debate and criticism gener-ated by this campaign failed to note was an obvious fact. This fact is that children, real chronological children, not metaphorically fixated or devel-opmentally arrested adults functioning *as* children, *are* in these states on streets the world over.

It seems, paradoxically, we are more willing to be sensitive to the damaged children *reconstructed* through contemporary adult damage/ failure than failing/deprived/abused children in the present. Irrespective of all the sentiment around babies and small children, they somehow fail to attract identification in the ways that adults, as more integrated, perhaps conventionally more morally accountable, social subjects do. Or perhaps if Winnicott (1958) is right about the hate that lies within sentimentality, it is precisely because of this lack of identification that such sentiment occurs. As I have already indicated, there may be political lessons here for ways of making children matter more – by being explicitly offered greater political involvement as actors rather than objects. In terms of child sexual abuse, we need to move beyond the portrayal of children and young people who have been sexually abused as 'victims', and instead acknowledge the more complicated but active strategies that enable them to survive, cope and even perhaps displace their abuse as a primary (historical or current) identity.

4 General culture of infantilisation

As I have already noted, children usually appear as talked about, rather than talked to, or indeed as the speakers. Within popular culture, where *we* are addressed as children it is often within the discourse of moral indulgence/desire for (escape from) responsibility. In the contemporary culture of infantilisation there is a representation of a pleasure-seeking child inside the reluctantly responsible (and productive) adult. Indeed many current advertising campaigns (especially for computers and cars) rely on just such an appeal to the inner child (in such contexts usually portrayed as a boy).

Entertainment itself can signify warding off an impending ageing/ maturing process. Indeed the 1999 Virgin advertisement displayed on hoardings all over Britain: 'delay becoming your parents', advertised website listings of shopping, cinema and shows to explicitly market consumption as the route to slow down the inevitable (now naturalised) process of becoming the responsible adults 'your parents' presumably are. It is naturalised by virtue of being a process that can only be 'delayed' rather than prevented or avoided, and also through both the use of the family kinship term 'your parents' and the generality of pronominal reference 'your' (since we all have, or have had, parents of some kind). The paradox here, as with all capitalist injunctions to 'enjoy' (cf. Zizek, 1991), is that 'you' need to do that supposedly very un-childlike (and therefore parent-like) activity, i.e. work/sell your labour, in order to generate the money to escape from the parental condition. We might further note here how an ideological rendering of history is presented, with 'our parents' portrayed as the boring, exploited classes, not the militant, class-conscious, struggling organisers they might well have been or, indeed, still be. But beyond this we could also acknowledge how children too are subject to such injunctions to demonstrate their (childhood or adult) social participation through consumption and leisure activities that require money. Hence as Mizen and Pole (2000) succinctly put it, working children in Britain 'work to play'.

5 Child as superegoic injunction

The final, fifth set of discourses I will discuss marks a shift from the cloyingly coy attribution of 'voice' to the child, although it is in fact only a particular variant of it. The moral injunction to action when spoken using the voice of the child, as in the widely available picture postcard: 'the planet is unique; it has to be protected', draws on a double notion of futurity. This is mobilised both by the explicit concern with planetary/ environmental future and by the commonly circulating discourse that '*children* are our future'. This device of being addressed *by* 'our future', and also advocating *for* our future, beats a powerful tune. The coy appeal here usually mingles with a faintly fascist air suggested by the image of a pale-eyed (boy) child's direct gaze. Could this hint at a discourse of the authoritarian personality being revisited upon the now terrorising child?

This seems to indicate a more general theme of the child as moral guarantor – the well worn 'out of the mouths of babes' narrative, 'the emperor's new clothes' (now turned into a typical Hollywood movie narrative), alongside the schlock film chestnut of the child's capacity to shame others into 'doing the right thing'. Yet there is a danger in over-playing this discourse of moral reproach or parental criticism, expressed in the words of the 'innocent' child. It could generate further resistance (rather than compliance) to its powerful combination of resources. For it invokes the forces of the past (as in the children we once were, or – especially in the context of the abused childhoods so many of us seem to have had – *wished* we were) with the moral responsibility for constructing the future we would like to secure/enjoy. This resistance is what (after Winnicott, 1958) fuels some of the sadism within the sentimentality surrounding children, which is perhaps what makes such campaigns that allow for multiple readings via humour more successful (as with the mid-1990s British Heart Foundation's campaign slogan: 'Send the money and the kid gets it').

Subverting developmental totalisations

I have been moving between texts of child development and economic and world development – arguably performing precisely the kind of reduction, or assertion of homology, that I seek to problematise within prevailing developmental discourse. However I want to finish by moving from these 'little' texts of child development to the broader discussions of economic development by way of indicating something of how such juxtapositions – although sadly too commonplace via their common political agendas – can be used subversively. It seems to me that those working with or around children have much to learn from the constructive and critical debates around the broader practices of world economic development. For these debates have come to produce the available discourses within which we think about *individual* developmental trajectories (whether normalised or – as in contexts of abuse – thereby problematised).

Connections include how the general models obscure the complexity of practices and contexts in which children survive, live and indeed develop, and the structurally diverse character of the economic, cultural and inter-personal relationships that produce these varied developments (see Crewe and Harrison, 1998). Our theories do not currently equip us well to do more than plot patterns that themselves reflect broader power relationships around what is deemed significant and what is not. Instead we need to attend to the question of compatibility versus divergence of interests between different parties (professional, stakeholder – including children), since (like international developers) within psychology and social welfare practice we are perhaps too quick either to assume the passivity of those rendered as objects of the psychological gaze, or else to identify their agency as pathology or deficit (cf. Phoenix, 1987). Perhaps this is because we overstate the extension and remit of the discourse of development we subscribe to.

Equally, like the children who form the topic of this chapter, and this book, there are no 'innocent' positions within these discussions. All of us are implicated in the discourses I have identified. There is no 'outside' to development discourse. Rather, in conclusion, I suggest, following critics of international development policy (e.g. Rahnema, 1997; Crewe and Harrison, 1998; Sachs, 1999), that – since we cannot entirely reject it – we practitioners of development should instead attend to the diversities of use, interpretation and incorporation of different discourses of development, as well as identify changing notions of intervention. We can do this whether we are practitioners of the individual, national or global varieties of development – and whether of its 'normal' or 'atypical' forms. Indeed this approach applies especially to those of us who concern ourselves with both, or all, of these.

Moreover, in terms of child sexual abuse, we need to analyse the interface between different groups of actors that surround caring as well as abusive relationships, and work to document the varying and contested accounts of what particular professional interventions mean, and what they achieve. Whether evaluating the success of an economic development intervention such as the introduction of a particular resource or technology or educational, care or health promoting practices, the same project of documenting diversities of perspective and interpretation of any intervention apply. This is one vital way, in my view, that we can begin to map what Katz (1996: 498) has termed 'renegade cartographies, rooted in experience and wrought of involvement [which] struggle to name a different spatiality and chart the politics to produce it'. By such means we may be better equipped to explore the range of political subjectivities mobilised and motivated by children and notions of childhood.

Note

1 The furore around the photographs by Sally Mann, for example, highlight the unease which apparently 'knowing', sexually aware children elicit – even, or perhaps especially, when we cannot resolve the ambiguities surrounding whether the sexualisation is generated by them or us.

References

Bell, V. (1993) *Interrogating incest*, London: Routledge.

Black, M. (1992) *A cause for our times: Oxfam – the first 50 years*, Oxford: Oxfam.

Boyden, J. with Holden, P. (1991) *Children of the cities*, London: Zed Press.

Brown, L. and Burman, E. (1997) 'Feminist responses to the delayed memory debate: an editorial introduction', *Feminism and Psychology* 7, 1: 7–16.

Burman, E. (1994a) *Deconstructing developmental psychology*, London: Routledge.

Burman, E. (1994b) 'Innocents abroad: projecting western fantasies of childhood onto the iconography of emergencies', *Disasters: Journal of Disaster Studies and Management* 18, 3: 238–253.

Burman, E. (1995a) 'What is it? Masculinity and femininity and the cultural representation of childhood', in S. Wilkinson and C. Kitzinger (eds) *Feminism and Discourse*, London: Sage, pp. 49–67.

Burman, E. (1995b) 'The abnormal distribution of development: child development and policies for Southern women', *Gender, Place and Culture* 2, 1: 21–36.

Burman, E. (1995c) 'Developing differences: childhood and economic development', *Children & Society* 9, 3: 121–141.

Burman, E. (1996) 'Local, global or globalized: child development and international child rights legislation', *Childhood: A Global Journal of Child Research* 3, 1: 45–66.

Burman, E. (1996/7) 'False memories, true hopes: revenge of the postmodern on therapy', *New Formations* 30: 122–134.

Burman, E. (1999) 'Appealing and appalling children', *Psychoanalytic Studies* 1, 3: 25–301.

Cooke, B. and Kothari, U. (eds) (2001) *Participation: the new tyranny?* London: Zed.

Crewe, E. and Harrison, E. (1998) *Whose development? An ethnography of aid*, London: Zed.

Foucault, M. (1980) *Power/knowledge: selected interviews and other writings*, Brighton: Harvester Wheatsheaf.

Fraser, N. (1989) *Unruly practices: power, discourse and gender in contemporary social theory*, London: Polity/Blackwell.

Hekman, S. (1990) *Gender and knowledge: elements of a postmodern feminism*, Oxford: Polity/Blackwell.

Hendrick, H. (1990) 'Constructions and reconstructions of British childhood: an interpretive survey 1800 to present day', in A. James and A. Prout (eds) *Constructing and reconstructing childhood*, Basingstoke: Falmer Press.

Hoyles, M. (1989) *The politics of childhood*, London: Journeyman.

Katz, C. (1996) 'Towards minor theory', *Society & Space* 15: 487–499.

McLaughlin, T. (2000) 'Psychology and mental health politics: a critical history of the Hearing Voices movement', unpublished doctoral dissertation, the Manchester Metropolitan University.

McNay, L. (1992) *Foucault and feminism*, Oxford: Blackwell.

Mizen. P. and Pole, C. (2000) 'Why work at the edge? Motivations for working among school age workers in Britain', paper presented at International Conference on Rethinking Childhood; Working Children's Challenge to the

Social Sciences, Institute de Recherche pour le Developpement (IRD), Paris, France, November.

Myers, R. (1992) *The twelve who survive: strengthening programmes of early childhood development in the Third World*, New York and London: Routledge.

Nicholson, L. (1999) *The play of reason: from the modern to the postmodern*, Buckingham: Open University Press.

Parker, I. (1997) *Psychoanalytic culture*, London: Sage.

Parker, I. (ed.) (1998) *Social constructionism, discourse and realism*, London: Sage.

Pateman, C. (1989) *The disorder of women*, Oxford: Polity Press.

Phoenix, A. (1987) 'Theories of gender and black families', in G. Weiner and M. Arnot (eds) *Gender under scrutiny*, London: Hutchinson, pp. 50–65.

Piaget, J. (1957) 'The child and modern physics', *Scientific American* 197: 46–51.

Rahnema, M. (1997) 'Towards post-development: searching for signposts, a new language and new paradigms', in M. Rahnema with V. Bawtree (eds) *The post-development reader*, London: Zed Books, pp. 377–404.

Rose, N. (1985) *The psychological complex: psychology, politics and society in England 1879–1939*, London: Routledge.

Sachs, W. (1999) *Planet dialectics: explorations in environment & development*, London: Zed Press.

Save The Children (1992) 'Focus on children', London: Save the Children.

Scheper-Hughes, N. (ed.) (1989) *Child survival: anthropological perspectives on the treatment and maltreatment of children*, Dordrecht: Reidel.

Stainton Rogers, R. and Stainton Rogers, W. (1994) *Stories of childhood: shifting agendas of child concern*, Lewes: Harvester Wheatsheaf.

Steedman, C. (1995) *Strange dislocations: childhood and the idea of human interiority 1780–1930*, London: Virago.

Walkerdine, V. (1990) 'Sex, power and pedagogy', *Schoolgirl Fictions*, London: Verso.

Warner, S. (1996) 'Constructing femininity: models of child sexual abuse and the production of "woman"', in E. Burman, G. Aitken, P. Alldred, *et al.*, *Challenging women: psychology's exclusions, feminist possibilities*, Buckingham: Open University Press, pp. 36–53.

Warner, S. (2000) *Understanding child sexual abuse: making the tactics visible*, Gloucester: Handsell.

Winnicott, D. (1958) 'Hate in the countertransference', in *Collected papers: from paediatrics to psychoanalysis*, London: Tavistock.

Zizek, S. (1991) *For they know not what they do: enjoyment as a political factor*, London: Verso.

Chapter 4

Problems of cultural imperialism in the study of child sexual abuse[1]

Ann Levett

Introduction

As a site in which to study the workings of power, child sexual abuse assumed a particular significance at the end of the twentieth century in the Western world and elsewhere. Despite the widespread publicity and due concern which childhood sexual abuse and its effects have evoked in recent years in Anglo-American communities, major conceptual and practical issues have not been seriously addressed. In this time, Western patriarchal social systems are easily able to take up and accommodate some liberal and feminist demands while giving minimal attention to the workings of power which led to the identification of social phenomena of concern in the first place. Appropriate remedies are difficult to devise and not seriously sought. There is selective neglect of important factors. I will briefly address these issues in order to prepare for an examination of the implications for current and imminent attempts to study child sexual abuse in southern Africa, in different speech communities. Patriarchy and other aspects of authority are played out in shared representations of everyday phenomena such as childhood, sexuality, human development and psychological disorder, although these may take distinctive forms in different social and historical contexts. Some dilemmas in current debates over protectionist policies and the abuse of power versus individual rights (and children's rights or needs) will also be briefly mentioned.

Hardly mentioned before 1970, child sexual abuse has been the focus of a huge outcry in English-speaking, especially Anglo-American, contexts in the past thirty years and is receiving increasing attention in South Africa in the 1990s and onwards, into the twenty-first century. Articles and reports are common in the news media, in weekly magazines and television programmes; parents and teachers are concerned and seek ways to prevent, recognise and deal with sexual abuse. In 2001/2002 the media has given particular prominence to situations where infants have been raped by adolescent and adult men, and in 2002 the South African Human Rights Commission has reported that the rights of children who have been sexually assaulted are not adequately addressed because of failures in the criminal justice system (E-TV news, 23 April, 2002).

Clinical and academic research has tended to take three forms. Prevalence studies have been conducted in different communities. However, it is interesting that another, larger body of literature concerns the 'damaging' psychological effects of such experience, and numerous reports on therapeutic interventions. In a third thrust, a handful of papers discuss attempts to prevent child sexual abuse – efforts described as largely ineffectual (Reppucci and Haugaard, 1989).

There are various reasons why childhood sexual abuse was singled out for attention at a particular socio-historical moment. Effects on children attracted attention first in the 1970s when American feminist and liberal human rights activitists took up the issue. Feminist writing around 1970 drew attention to male exploitation of structured power in relation to women and children, especially young girls, particularly in the context of sexuality (Millett, 1970; Russell, 1975). This led to research on child sexual abuse involving a growing range of professional mental health workers. Nelson (1984) and Hacking (1991) have documented the history of the category 'child abuse'. Nelson provides a fascinating analysis of the association between this preoccupation and the modern emergence of powerful lobbies of medical and legal institutions. The widespread belief that sexual abuse is psychologically damaging arose from these contexts and prompted demands for efforts to identify and redress such damage. All of this occurred in the wake of post-Second World War moves to increase professionalisation, along with the development of social policies highlighting the plight of various groups (the emergence of victimology), and the shaping of public policy and social interventions to improve the situation of such groups. It is conspicuous that there is almost no discussion of child abuse in the non-English literature and very little on this phenomenon in non-English-speaking communities, particularly in Africa.

In the twentieth century, children have assumed an increasingly important place in Western consciousness and in psychological theory and practice (Kessel and Siegel, 1983). Our models of psychology and of psychological development are inherently individualistic and assume that childhood experiences have a great deal of influence on adult behaviour. We have also tended to assume that Western studies are universally applicable. I use the term 'assume' advisedly because it has become apparent that much of what has been precious in psychological thinking, when subjected to closer scrutiny, is based on social constructions (Gergen, 1985; Arbib and Hesse, 1986) and rhetoric (Billig, 1987).

Child sexual abuse has assumed a particular significance as a consequence of many socio-political processes in a specific set of power structures, and of shifts in the position of women in Western societies. The term 'trauma', associated with child sexual abuse, is used metaphorically to convey various complex ideas and feelings about a set of Western, morally based ideologies (exploitation, abuse, the rights of individuals). Such metaphors arise in the context of particular discourses, in this instance those concerning the control of women and women's resistance to being controlled in certain ways. The development of gendered subject-ivity occurs in this context in a particular range of semiotic codes (Manning, 1987). Cross-cultural study of sexual abuse will have to deal with the problem of eliciting local sets of semiotic codes and counter-discourses in order to understand local circumstances, if we are to compare these with Anglo-American ones and work towards social change.

In the past decade, long-term effects on adults have also been studied (e.g. Wyatt and Powell, 1988; Beutler and Hill, 1992). Thousands of papers now discuss child sexual abuse and there are dozens of books on the subject, all published since the late 1970s. The majority of the authors are mental health clinicians and academic researchers. Although the issue is still associ-ated with feminist concerns about the abuse of girls and women, probably 95 per cent of this literature is only nominally feminist in the sense of offer-ing an articulated political analysis of sexual abuse. Liz Kelly notes:

> A new professional specialisation is emerging – people whose careers (and notice how many of the most 'successful' are men) have been built on the investigation, treatment and 'prevention' of child sexual assault. Within this group there are individuals who are passionately committed to supporting women and children, but very few have a coherent political analysis which would enable them to see just how challenging this issue is and, therefore, how difficult real change is going to be to achieve. The creation of this tier of 'experts' from within the profession means that many of the basic insights feminists developed concerning sexual violence and its impact have been lost, or deliberately ignored.
>
> (1989: 15)

The inescapables generally glossed over are that it is usually older or adult males who sexually abuse children, mainly girls and women, and that this proclivity is tied in with social constructions of male sexuality, gendered identity and patriarchal power. Furthermore, it is not generally noted that the research has focused on particular children – mainly those who live in the northern hemisphere in more or less Westernised, mainly urban con-texts (Burman, 1994).

How common is child sexual abuse?

The study of incidence (the number of new cases in a particular population in a stipulated period of time) has been reported for various populations sampled, almost exclusively in the USA. Studies of prevalence in a range of groups and communities, mainly in North America and in the UK, commonly suggest up to 54 per cent of women have been subjected to child sexual abuse, the most important difference being related to the definition of sexual abuse used by researchers and to the methods used to collect data. In a sample of women students at a South African university in 1986, the prevalence figure of 44 per cent was regarded as an under-report (Levett, 1989a). Although DeMause (1991) steps around difficulties in defining incestuous sexual abuse, he follows the current trend of a broad definition of sexual abuse, including not only cases of rape or attempted sexual intercourse but also genital fondling and other forms of unwanted and intrusive contact behaviours. In the USA at least 60 per cent of girls (and 45 per cent of boys) are likely to be sexually abused in childhood, 81 per cent before puberty and an equally large number within the family. He notes recent research with children from Berlin which found an 80 per cent child molestation prevalence, and comments that if children were surveyed in North America the figures are likely to be similar. He states that 'the incidence in countries outside the West is likely to be much higher', attributing this to an 'infanticidal mode of childrearing' and because, he claims, 'the use of children for the emotional needs of adults is far more accepted, an attitude that fosters widespread incestuous acts along with other child abuse' (1991: 142). De Mause is muddled in his use of terms such as incest (see La Fontaine, 1987) and in directly comparing human sexual behaviours of different socio-historical periods, with no discussion of the problems involved in over-simplified comparisons. However, in all probability the figures he cites for the Western world are possibly not far from the mark. There is little reason to argue that prevalence would be lower in Africa.

Given the high prevalence figures it is difficult to regard child sexual abuse experience as unusual. However, sexual abuse of children is generally studied as if these are uncommon events with specific outcomes even though a very large proportion of girls and women have been sexually abused under the age of eighteen years. One would call sexual abuse 'normative' with reluctance because there is a sense of moral indignation associated with such behaviour. It seems absurd then to talk about psychological damage when most women would be involved. Spaccarelli (1994) extensively reviewed the literature with a critical eye and highlighted the difficulties in researching a field where there is little consensus regarding definitions. Multiple factors affect situations of child sexual abuse.

The term 'psychological trauma' widely associated with child sexual abuse has been used metaphorically to convey the idea that, just as the body may be injured or bruised, so might the mind or mental sense of self (see O'Dell, this volume). Introduced initially in feminist counter-discourse as a critique of male and adult power over girls, the metaphor of damage has shifted. In the context of professional and protectionist discourses of regulation and social control, the damaging effects of child sexual abuse become as factual as a broken bone and the clinical elicitation of evidence lends itself to this usage. It has become a justification for interventions which are often counterproductive for the child and families involved.

The relationship to gendered subjectivity

For girls, experiences of child sexual abuse contribute to early notions of gendered identity based on semiotic systems of difference between the sexes. The particular overtones of difference involved in 'trauma' may serve to endorse stigmatised forms of gendered identity (Levett, 1992b).

In all socio-cultural contexts where men hold most public and economic power they also dominate the private sphere through their authority over women and children. This is linked with the finding that adolescent boys and men are almost invariably the perpetrators of sexual abuse and that most prevalence research concerns figures and consequences for girls and women. While a recent and growing literature suggests that boys are often sexually abused in contemporary Western society, it is not always clearly argued that the implications for boys and girls are different because of the association between gender and power. Boys grow into men and therefore into subjectivities in which coercive sexual relating and the active perpetration of sexual assault on children and women become a possibility (even if only in thought and fantasy). The claim that boys who have been sexually abused as children are the ones who become abusers as adults should be rejected as an oversimplification (see Widom, 1989). This idea of causation conceals the role of patriarchy – the social production and reproduction of male authority and normative conventions of male promiscuity. These, with the frequently hostile or ambivalent qualities sometimes involved in heterosexual relating, are all implicated in child sexual abuse, sexual assault and rape. Malamuth, Sockoskie, Koss and Tanaka (1991: 680) in a study of American college men, comment: 'Our findings on sexual aggression suggest that it results from the combination of relatively high levels of hostile masculinity and sexual promiscuity.' They mention elsewhere the significance of adversarial relating between men and a sense of shame and inadequacy involved in sexual coercion and aggression. The details of these aspects of male subjectivities require further, close psychosocial study in different contexts as it is likely that the dynamics which result in some men acting on ideas of sexually abusive behaviours may not be universal.

Although male–female dynamics are profoundly implicated, not all men are abusive; it is inescapable that child sexual abuse is an over-determined phenomenon with complex meanings. Generic factors include socially accepted idealisation of women as well as the degradation of them, both of which objectify women, and the unconscious confusion of women with children and vice versa, all of which are linked with certain forms of patriarchal power (the 'rule of the father').

Socarides discusses psychoanalytic understandings of child sexual abuse and adds that the current epidemic is not a clinical phenomenon but one which is related to 'times of social disequilibrium when there is no "authoritative prohibition by society" against such behaviour' (1991: 448). This assumes that such behaviour is 'naturally male' and that men have to learn to inhibit such behaviour through cultural constraints, an essentialist claim, although the widespread existence of patriarchal power makes it difficult to debunk. Fuss (1989) argues that the function which an essentialist claim serves should be questioned and, in this case, it seems that it serves to perpetuate the rule of the father.

Girls grow into women with gendered subjectivities in which sexual assault and harassment by males are part of everyday life. Although there has been a trend to research and discuss child sexual abuse as if it were a separate phenomenon (Russell, 1984, is a significant exception), experiences of sexual abuse in childhood must be seen as part of the broad processes in which male–female power and authority are epitomised. For both boys and girls who are sexually abused in childhood there is an exploitation of power differences between adults and children, but for girls the dynamics involved in male–female sexual relating also enter the picture, as Ennew (1986) has commented. I will be discussing child sexual abuse specifically in relation to girls because of the compounding of gender-linked power.

Child sexual abuse in African societies

There has been very little 'cross-cultural' study of child abuse and especially of child sexual abuse. The relative absence of research on child abuse in Africa is noteworthy but is also partly understandable in terms of the meagre resources available and because of the scarcity of feminist lobbies (Finkelhor, 1989). What exists are mostly attempts to reproduce Western assumptions and ideas, as though they are universal and unquestionable. Ennew (1986) provides a sophisticated commentary on the limitations of such work, and some more conventional difficulties of 'cross-cultural' studies are discussed by Korbin (1987), who also reviews international studies on child neglect and abuse (1991). She points to the importance of dealing with infectious diseases, diarrhoea, malnutrition and HIV and AIDS as primary problems in Third World countries, as distinct from child sexual abuse, and we need also to take account of the problems involved with poverty, malaria and basic struggles for survival (see also Burman, this volume).

Almost all research on sexual abuse initiated in South Africa, a country which is relatively wealthy in the African context, has simply emulated the conventions of North American research (Levett and Lachman, 1991), using a naïvely positivist empiricism. These studies import the assumptions and power structures of developed countries which still affect children in those societies (Sullivan, 1992). Today great concern is expressed about the sexual abuse of children in South Africa; there has been much media reportage and many people (at least of those who are literate) know that this occurs mainly within the familial environment, involving trusted males. However, 'stranger danger' is still also given emphasis in programmes for educating children and teachers. As in the USA and England, there has been some effort to facilitate assistance for those affected (e.g. in Cape Town there is RAPCAN, a feminist-informed NGO). As with South African social services in general, very little help is available; child welfare and social workers feel overwhelmed and helpless and the legislation and judicial processes are regarded as almost useless (Levett, 1991) – few allegations become charges, fewer reach the courts and there are very few convictions. The most effective legal procedures involve children who have been molested by strangers (Collings, 1989) although there is now a statutory obligation to report every instance of known or suspected child sexual abuse. Until recently, media attention was largely focused on boys sexually abused by paedophiles (misleadingly depicted as gay men) and on the brutal rape of infants and young children in poverty ridden black communities, sometimes by men who believe this is a cure for HIV/AIDS. Thus, links between male authority in the family and sexual abuse are obscured. The most common forms of child sexual abuse (within family relations) are curtained beneath myths of racism, heterosexism and stranger danger.

In South Africa, as in developed nations, the field has been largely co-opted by non-feminist professionals and the problems are generally depicted as individual or familial psychopathology, and class related (Kelly, 1989). Intervention is shaped by and thus limited by the dominant ideologies of the medical profession and the unwieldy efforts of the state and state-supported welfare services. The implications of patriarchal power in this sociohistorical process, the relationship of the 'incest industry' to professionalisation in the second half of the twentieth century, and the place of current ideas about the effects of child sexual abuse in the development of gendered subjectivity in contemporary societies demand serious and immediate attention at this significant period of transformation in South Africa.

Although one needs to be cautious in putting forward arguments about 'cultural differences' since this may be interpreted as racist in contemporary South Africa, it is necessary to make the socio-cultural and class contexts visible in terms of particular forms of patriarchal power and gendered subjectivities. Mejiuni (1991) addresses child abuse in Nigeria and the way it seems to have escalated there, arguing that although particular political and economic factors are implicated in the physical and sexual abuse of children in Africa, these find a fertile base in ideological facets of African patriarchal traditions of family life which facilitate the sexual objectification of women and girls. It might be added that there are prohibitions against acts and reactions which can be viewed as disrespectful of the age based authority system which forms a powerful part of the traditional African social framework in South Africa.

Bennett (1991) outlines specific forms of customary treatment of girls and women as male property in African communities. These local traditions were upheld by imported conventions and laws (introduced by the Dutch and British colonisers) and are perpetuated up to today. African women have been treated as minors in South African customary law and, generally, in common law as well, and there are major contradictions in the maintenance of customary law alongside the new South African Constitution. Bennett comments:

> On the one hand, the common-law categories of minor and major cannot reflect the nuances and flexibility inherent in customary law, and, on the other, these categories were imposed on women not with a view to protecting them but with a view to restraining them.
>
> (1991: 323)

He adds: 'No country in Africa has legislated with the sole purpose of ameliorating the civil-law status of women' (ibid.: 331). In fact this situation has been dramatically addressed in the new South African Constitution which was introduced in 1994 (adopted by parliament on October 11, 1996, taking effect from February 7, 1997) which specifically deals with human rights, and inequalities of power between social groups, including gender. The realities of daily life remain, in many ways, much the same as they were before and one can only hope that the rights entrenched in the Constitution are not eroded in future years.

It is particularly interesting to note that there are no stipulations in customary law to deal with the abuse or neglect of children, the sexual abuse of children or the sexual assault of women, except that there is a requirement of marriage or payment of lobola to the girl's father or male relatives if rape is involved, and any child which results from such an assault may then be taken into the paternal household. It is illustrative of the lack of awareness of issues raised by the women's movement that in an otherwise useful, critical set of interpretative comments, Bennett does not remark on these gaps in his chapters on children and on women. However, he notes:

> While [African] governments might have been sympathetic to the feminist cause, they could not afford to estrange the majority of their supporters, who in most cases were the conservative beneficiaries of the patriarchal tradition. Hence, even in countries espousing radical changes to the family structure, improvements to the status of women were incidental benefits, rather than a specific goal.
>
> (ibid.: 331–332)

Physical beatings are widespread and accepted forms of disciplining women and children although in urban areas this may be viewed as a rural and old-fashioned method (Bennett, 1991; Straker, Moosa, Becker and Nkwale, 1992). Furthermore the custom that prohibits any woman from disciplining boys and men once they have gone through male initiation rites associated with puberty has general effects which communicate a set of attitudes to male authority, even though fewer young men go through the initiation rites today.

Given the realities and ramifications of apartheid legislation and its aftermath, and current economic factors, over the last fifty years very large numbers of black men and women have attempted to move to cities to find work and opportunities to better their lives. For women there are extra benefits in escaping the older traditions of black patriarchy which were so constraining. In urban environments they escape more easily from both the customary authority of the father and husband and that of older, senior women, and often preserve their single status by resisting marriage arrangements. Increasing numbers of black women in South Africa remain single and live with children fathered by different men with whom they have chosen to associate, struggling materially but with relative independence. Through direct access to their own wages, minimal property rights, small savings co-operative schemes and personal initiative within the constraints of poverty and access to work, the number of women heading single-parent households has increased substantially (Bennett, 1991). In some ways this may safeguard some children from incestuous sexual abuse.

On the other hand there is an anecdotal tale of a black woman in a Cape Town squatter camp who discovered her prepubertal daughter being sexually abused by the woman's current lover and who reported this (and the child's account of previous such abuse) to the police, hoping for authoritative assistance. There was insufficient evidence to justify an arrest and the woman and her daughter were left to deal with the situation themselves (not in itself an uncommon situation in any part of the city). The accused man, ejected from the woman's home, rallied neighbourhood men to hound the woman and child out of the area.

It is difficult to interpret this anecdote without additional information. Is the man's behaviour acceptable to other men in this community? Was the reaction related to the police report? Was the perpetrator a member of a local criminal gang whose support he called on, or was he so respected by his peers that the woman's and child's story were disbelieved? How different is this story in its bare bones from accounts of child sexual abuse and male responses in other sections of the broader community? We need research to develop answers to these and other questions.

The difficulty of researching such material in contemporary South Africa is that it will conceivably be understood as a racist commentary, particularly if white researchers are involved, and could be seen as neglectful of the role which apartheid has played in the breakdown of family life, communities and social support, the emasculation of black men, the development of an exploited working class and the general escalation of crime and violence at the turn of the century. Such arguments do not give due consideration to the power of patriarchy and its local forms, essential for analysis concerning women in contemporary Africa. In workshops on child sexual abuse run in different parts of South Africa in recent years, various African men and women have often commented that men who sexually abuse children feel entitled to do so; this is true also of white men, although the excuses and justifications used may differ (Sterling, 1990). The analogy of a man who grows and cares for his maize patch and feels entitled to savour the crop first, when it is fresh and he chooses to do so, has been introduced by several unconnected African informants. In the early 1990s the concurrent notion was that his neighbours have no basis on which to regulate his behaviour and so, although perhaps they feel uneasy about what he does, they do nothing to admonish him. This absence of community sanctions is also found widely in white communities in South Africa: people do not feel they are entitled to interfere in a neighbour's family life. However, at the turn of this century there has been something of a shift in this attitude among black communities – in many instances reported in newspapers and TV since 2000, impoverished black communities have rallied to take issue with sexual assault and child sexual abuse, taking matters into their own hands, and there are reports of street justice with dire consequences for men so accused.

Through informal accounts and small local surveys discussed in conference contexts, the incidence of sexual abuse is described as widespread in the over-crowded and poverty-stricken urban communities which surround the cities of Southern Africa. Large numbers of children grow up in conditions which range from impoverished single-parent homes in shacks, or with mothers or fathers and occasionally with both parents, or a single grandparent, in urban or rural areas. Aunts and uncles often care for dislocated children who are frequently moved from one temporary context to another (Reynolds, 1991), a situation which increases the risk of physical and sexual abuse substantially. Violence is common and rape and sexual assault are endemic. However, although they are implicated in a range of ways which increase the complexity of the issues, it is a mistake to take the stand that racism, apartheid, capitalism, class and poverty are the main or sole reasons for sexually abusive phenomena. Sexual assault and abuse occur in all groups and through the entire class structure. The events which involve the wealthiest and the poorest families may be most invisible: the wealthy conceal these situations to protect the family, the perpetrator or the assaulted victim, being aware of stigmatic effects and wishing to avoid the public gaze. Poor people protect their tenuous material circumstances, especially if the perpetrator generates some income, and do not feel confident of assistance from the police and social agencies.

However, the power which males feel entitled to exert over females, the ways in which this is institutionalised (especially through access to economic resources), and the authority which older women accord men in African patriarchy, are fundamental and unavoidable aspects of the picture as they are in Western and developed countries, and must not be glossed. There may be a difference between black and white communities in prevalent rates of child sexual abuse (as some have argued for different social classes) but this is an empirical question which has not yet been addressed, is unlikely to be addressed and, in fact, is not really a useful question in the first place except as a statistic to be used in pressurising policy decisions.

Obviously the disruption and dislocation of everyday family life in consequence of apartheid labour and social practices has had something to do with violence and sexual abuse in contemporary South Africa. Any neighbourhood constraints and controls which may have operated within small, familiar community groups have largely been diluted or eliminated; and customary African conventions of respect for men and elders have declined (Viljoen, 1991) in some ways that are beneficial and in other ways not. South African women have not yet found ways to organise themselves into self-protective groups to deal effectively with sexual harassment and assault to which they are subjected by adolescent youths and men in their environments; there is very little feminist consciousness in southern Africa in terms of critiques of male–female sexual relating and this is almost as true of the progressive left as it is of nationalist liberation movements, educated middle-class women and working-class women. In general there is tremendous reluctance amongst South African women to 'organise against men' and the trend has been to organise with the support and involvement of men, an idealistic and only partially successful route, but one which better suits local political thought where 'There is no history or tradition within South Africa which recognises gender conflict as political conflict.' The construction of racism and class exploitation by the national liberation movements precludes a gender analysis of both class and race in South Africa (Charman, De Swardt and Simons, 1991: 12).

There has been a paradox between South African women's capacity to defiantly resist and bravely act against certain forms of patriarchal power while actively submitting to other forms (Posel, 1991; Walker, 1991). Posel comments:

> Arguably, the patriarchal 'contract' in African societies – pre-capitalist and beyond – has been successfully negotiated and redefined in response to a variety of pressures and opportunities – such as arrival of missionaries, insertion into capitalist relations of production, etc. In many cases, the scope of men's authority has been reduced, but in ways which redefine – rather than altogether overthrow – patriarchal norms.
>
> (1991: 26)

In a township in a small Karoo town where living conditions are cramped and privacy is rare, a social worker who had lived and worked in the area told of a widely accepted practice whereby daughters in the household are frequently involved by older brothers, cousins, uncles, cousins and neighbours in sexual activities from the age of five or six years. These activities are regarded as acceptable. The girls, as young adults, are often amazed and indignant to hear this practice described as 'child sexual abuse'. In an environment where this is widely accepted normative behaviour, girls learn at an early age that sexuality is perhaps one way to negotiate a special status or favours through an older or adult male figure in the household. The loss of the means to do so would be a loss of power to them, however problematic this power may seem to others. The high incidence of early teenage pregnancy and the fact that girls rarely manage to complete their education in these circumstances, are major costs: the notions of psychological trauma in the ways widely described in the psychological literature do not enter the picture.

At the same time, from preliminary data gathered among African and coloured women of little education in South Africa, it emerges that there is generally agreement that child sexual abuse is covered up and kept secret within the family. Stigma, shame and devaluation may be implicated for the girl involved, or for the perpetrator, and thus the perpetrator is protected. To break the traditions which prohibit talk about relatives who are perpetrators and about sex in general will require major shifts in consciousness among South Africans, although it may be that the current HIV/AIDS epidemic with the associated awareness and educational programmes will be instrumental in initiating such changes.

Although we need to study the detail of male authority in South Africa, the picture is not perhaps as different from the developed countries as the foregoing might suggest. Commenting on changes in Canadian legislation on child sexual abuse (then heralded as the most advanced in the world) Sullivan (1992) articulates some provocative questions. He draws attention

to the need to think carefully about the notion of children's rights in protectionist terms and cites pertinent criticisms by other Canadians regarding the neglect of contextual issues of structural power in the Badgley
Report (1984):

> Through the creation of 'sexual abuse' as a unified category to be
> treated as an empirical fact, the Committee precludes the investiga-
> tion of its social causes or attributes; for example, the patriarchal char-
> acter of family/domestic relations in this society, and the question of
> why in this context, sex-related violence is carried out primarily by
> heterosexual men.
>
> (Brock and Kinsman, cited by Sullivan, 1992: 99)

> New institutions must be developed, which embody a single standard
> of behaviour for all interpersonal and sexual relationships, based on
> the equality of men and women and their equal shared responsibility
> for ensuring that all children are given the opportunity to become fully
> actualised autonomous adults. These changes cannot be effected
> without facing the fact that patriarchy must be dismantled, and that
> paternalism must go with it. To fail to see that these problems are
> deeply rooted in patriarchal institutions related to the distribution and
> control of sexual property, and in the socialization of male sexuality
> appropriate to that system, is to mislocate the nature of the problem
> and the measures necessary to eliminate it.
>
> (Clarke cited in Sullivan, 1992: 100)

If we are to initiate the study of child sexual abuse in the wider communities of South Africa, the power of patriarchy and paternalism (protectionist policies) must be recognised and highlighted in the assumptions
embedded in current Western approaches to child sexual abuse, for they
have implications for those who have been sexually abused as children.

As argued elsewhere (Levett, 1992a), stigmatic effects associated with
difference and damage are produced and reproduced through the naïve
empirical study of 'facts' of prevalence and damage and in contexts of professional intervention. It is important to ensure that assumptions, which
are harboured in such research, are not transported, unquestioned, to
studies in different socio-cultural groups, contributing to the further cultural colonisation of girls and women.

Problems in the study of prevalence and consequences of child sexual abuse

Problems of methodology make it difficult to compare studies of prevalence and consequences of child sexual abuse (Spaccarelli, 1994). At the

most obvious level there are disagreements about definitions of sexual abuse, conceptions of childhood differ, and the significance of age differences between perpetrators and victims. The conventions guiding the gathering of data are a further source of difficulty related to sampling techniques, volunteer informants, unsophisticated questionnaires, etc. (Painter, 1986). A more serious problem is the absence of understanding and acceptance of the active sex life of children and their interest in adults and in taboo behaviours.

The research isolates particular events (child sexual abuse) and attempts to link these to specific patterns of effects or consequences. The only relatively consistent findings published are that experiences of violent sexual abuse, or repeated intercourse involving father and daughter, or situations which involved especially intrusive and insensitive interventions (by family or professionals), appear more likely to be associated with emotional disturbances in children (Browne and Finkelhor, 1986) at the time and in the following days or weeks. Since children who are not 'emotionally disturbed' have not been identified as sexually abused, and other variables usually confound the picture, the consistencies such as they are may well be spurious (Haugaard and Emery, 1989; Briere, 1992).

We need to be careful to avoid researching and dealing with child sexual abuse in ways which are not useful for changing the gendered systems of power and which fundamentally maintain patriarchal power. Russell (1991) has expressed criticism of my work, suggesting it is anti-feminist and anti-women. Whereas I am critical of non-reflective and naïvely liberal feminist approaches, as well as non-feminist research on child sexual abuse, Russell felt I had claimed that such abuse does not harm children. All forms of sexual abuse are expressions of power and the use of power to coerce, constrain and restrict is problematic and has ramifications; these must be examined in research and remedied through other means. However, the danger of adopting a simplistic empirical methodology is that this is another form of oppression unless very carefully conceptualised, and one which is detrimental to the interests of women and children (Levett, 1992a).

The most useful idea emerging is that a major effect in childhood sexual abuse is the stigma and disruption associated with the aftermath of such experience (Finkelhor and Browne, 1985) although process and outcome research in treatment of adult survivors (Beutler and Hill, 1992) and reviews (e.g. Briere, 1992) do not usually mention these problems. Interventions by welfare and other agencies, or the family discord following allegations of child sexual abuse, are complicated by a sense of betrayal (by parental or authority figures), and this is exacerbated when there is no retribution as a result of the intervention. Some therapeutic interventions may also involve a further experience of abuse (Reppucci and Haugaard, 1989).

Curiously, research rarely questions whether there are effects at all following child sexual abuse per se (without intervention and family disruptions) but rather what the range of effects may be. This style is characteristic of a great deal of applied psychology, a positivistic empiricism which reflects little awareness of its working assumptions. It is not surprising then that the range of 'consequences' which have been documented is vast. Assumptions of normal behaviour are heavily value-laden – implicit models of childhood, of development, of appropriate and inappropriate sexual behaviour in different age groups, are all invoked. The dominant discourses of childhood (James and Prout, 1990), of development (Shotter, 1984) and of sexuality, have not been understood to be discourses which can be examined and deconstructed, e.g. using the model of analysis introduced by Henriques, *et al.* (1984) as I have done previously (Levett, 1989b), and the seminal work of Parker (1992) and of Burman and Parker (1993). The term 'discourse' is used as a Foucaultian convention which draws attention to the significance of language practices in relation to other social practices, and of semiotic codes related to power, reflected in the ways we talk about and study social phenomena.

For example, if one assumes there to be abnormal behaviour and looks for it, it is likely to be found. Furthermore, dominant Western ideas about childhood are contradictory (Levett, 1989c). Psychological models of childhood, like lay models, hold for instance that there is a natural path for emotional and cognitive development; that children are naïve about sexual matters and can be precipitated into an abnormal route of sexual development; the 'proper' socialisation cloaks and harnesses the potential inherent sexuality of children which otherwise lies dormant; the gender development is based mainly on genetic or biological blueprints which can be upset, triggered or deformed by certain kinds of experience; that normal children are rarely anxious, depressed and that betrayals are not part of everyday life.

Ideas about psychiatric disorders (e.g. diagnostic categories derived from the American Psychiatric Association's Diagnostic and Statistical Manuals), about deviance (e.g. promiscuity or truanting), or psychological disorder (evaluations of self esteem, how sexual relationships should be) are based on implicit models of normal functioning relative to idealised behaviours. These can be termed 'discourses of psychological trauma' in relation to child sexual abuse (Levett, 1989b). Early in the twentieth century, many years before Foucault published his ideas, Ludwig Fleck discussed the influence of medical knowledge on popular ideas and vice versa, as social constructions reproduced by 'thought collectives' (Lowy, 1988). Because of the potency of everyday ideas in Western middle-class thought, perpetuated through the media and professional writings (the hegemony of tacit knowledge), it is extremely difficult to study child sexual abuse except in relation to prevalence and expected trauma.

Rules of behaviour render talk about child sexual abuse difficult, constrained or taboo – except in relation to those other than oneself, preferably strangers, reported in newspapers or professional journal articles. The belief that experience of sexual abuse causes psychological damage helps maintain the taboo (even among feminist researchers) and also makes it difficult to study. Ironically, feminist writing which drew attention to the extent of these phenomena has paradoxically added to the problem. Girls and women are likely to believe that they have been affected by such experiences and will attribute a range of current problems to them; they will not readily disclose or discuss the experience because of the expected stigma and shame. This makes the study of prevalence and of consequences extraordinarily difficult. Many parents and families also prefer to maintain a silence about sexual abuse and most commonly do not file reports or seek assistance. Partly this may be because they feel they have 'failed' as parents in not protecting the child from abuse, but it is also because they are aware of the likelihood of stigma for the family and child.

If a woman cannot connect specific current problems with childhood experiences she has come to identify as sexually abuse, in Western middle-class communities, she may re-label the experience ('perhaps it was not abuse because I allowed it to happen') or she may wait for the day when the 'delayed effects' widely believed to be inevitable may emerge; alternatively she may doubt her memories ('perhaps I imagined it'). It should be evident that what we are dealing with in this process of focusing on the damaging effects of child sexual abuse is a set of discourses which act as a self-fulfilling prophecy, common in stigma. If we label ourselves as damaged we will find evidence to support this view.

Stigma is difficult to study except through spoken discourse or the careful close study of social behaviours (unexplained avoidance, silence, protection of certain individuals). The way people talk about the significance of certain events or experiences in ordinary, everyday discourse requires a more ethno-methodological approach. We need to talk with girls and women about stigmatic effects and, even better, to find ways to document their talk among themselves about such experiences. The stigmatic associations of child sexual abuse are accessible through the conceptual schemas of adults, who communicate similar ideas to children through taboos and silences. Thus it is not essential to study the social representations of child sexual abuse and its effects among children per se, although this would also be useful. In fact, because of the widespread conviction that talk about sexual matters with children is potentially dangerous and thus taboo in itself (McKenna and Kessler, 1985) – perhaps as injurious as sexual abuse – it is not readily feasible to carry out such a study with children in general without some risk of accusations of unethical behaviour, and with considerable difficulty.

Gender differentiation

Contemporary models of damage in consequence of sexual abuse have assumed significance within the current climate of changing relationships between men and women in metropolitan society, as metaphorical representations of female distress or dysphoria, but it has not generally been recognised that these same models and representations of abuse/victims/exploitation also play a role in the development of gendered subjectivity for girls. The recognition of difference, and the playing out of male–female distinctions in terms of rules and restraints, are part of the social construction of identity and of sexuality during childhood.

From an early age girls in all societies are subjected to codes of behaviour and regulatory prohibitions which relate to the possibility of being sexually abused – boys are not. The exact codes and prohibitions may vary somewhat from one social context to another but for girls and women they have profound implications (1) for the effects of such experience when it does occur, (2) for the shaping of a sense of female subjectivity and relative powerlessness, whether or not there is an experience of sexual abuse, (3) for the maintenance of socially constructed differences between the sexes, and (4) for the maintenance of male power and authority.

Constructions of female gender development are related to child sexual abuse (among other processes) because instances of abuse are schematised by girls and women within semiotic systems of gender differentiation. The rules of behaviour for girls and women are elaborated around protection, prevention or avoidance of sexual abuse, partly because of the possibility of pregnancy after the onset of puberty.

The relevance of the study of all forms of child sexual abuse (including molestations, harassment and rape) lies in the close relationship which such experience, and how it is viewed by the community, is likely to have to the development of female gendered subjectivity. Even though these experiences may not be daily ones in actuality, in effect they are because girls have to shape their daily lives around choices which take account of the *possibility* of sexual abuse. Thus sexual abuse plays a role in maintaining existing power relations: female choices and positions from childhood are repeatedly subordinated to those available to men (see also Reavey, this volume). This contributes to the active participation of girls and women through self-subordination within gendered structures of power (Levett, 1989b).

Part of the process involved in the production and reproduction of gender differences is bound up with ideas about the damaging effects of experiences of childhood sexual abuse. This is not only in the Anglo-American psychological literature but also among people whose sense of identity is formed in a social context influenced by Anglo-American ideas. The folk models of Western societies, through professionalisation and the media, have absorbed ideas of damage which have become hegemonic and self-replicating. This cultural imperialism is perpetuated in unquestioned everyday talk about childhood and about sexual abuse.

A study of the constraints of discourses concerning childhood and child sexual abuse in different socio-cultural or linguistic groups may disclose a similar situation to the dominant Western discourses, but there might be distinctive differences which relate to local practices of childrearing, the development of gender, attitudes to children's sexuality and the acceptance or non-acceptance of adult–child sexual relationships. In Africa, where patriarchy is prevalent, significant aspects of gendered schema are likely to be reflected, and this will have implications for the participation of women in broader social change. It cannot be assumed however that stigmatic effects will necessarily be found following child sexual abuse experiences in all cases, nor in all speech communities. This needs to be studied. Further, it cannot be assumed that if there are consequences of such experience, these will be the same in all cultural groups. This also requires investigation. Third, more fundamental than ideas of damage or pollution may be the part which the sexual abuse of girls and women (if indeed there is sexual abuse) might play in the development of gendered identity and in the continuing domination of women by men in other societies. This issue needs to be addressed in its own right.

Discourse studies

What is required is an approach to the study of such phenomena and the ideas about them which is quite different from the simple empiricism which has characterised the study of child sexual abuse in English-speaking and metropolitan communities. One route might be by collecting common ideas as expressed in everyday language by ordinary people from different groups. As the chapters in this volume reiterate time and time again, dominant ideas and the way these are expressed in everyday spoken language shape emotional experience (Harre, 1986) such as involved in stigma. Interpretative analyses of discourse (Potter and Wetherell, 1987) or discourse analysis (Parker, 1992; Burman and Parker, 1993) may be useful in such research. My own work (Levett, 1989b) was based on the method of analysis used by Hollway (1984), where not only dominant discourses were examined but also coexisting muted contradictory themes, some of which might contain the seeds of alternative paths of resistance. Large numbers of adult women who were sexually abused as children are not psychologically disturbed, depressed more than most other women, nor are they delinquent, abusive, and so on – surely research which is not looking for such situations will not be likely to find them. It may be that it is an act of resistance to such categorisation that might lead many women to not disclose such experience although, paradoxically, such silence also protects patriarchy.

In the traditions of empirical psychology as outlined early in this chapter where a 'cross-cultural' study is proposed, the conventional psychological or psychiatric researcher takes little if any account of instructive recent writings in social science and anthropology which suggest that we present ourselves and our histories in terms of stories or narratives. Such narratives are available in each social community as what Jerome Bruner (1986) termed 'interpretative guides'. Geertz (1986) and Howard (1991) usefully discuss these ways of understanding human behaviours, but such authors appear to be unknown to those who are working and publishing in the 'incest industry'.

The importance of developing definitional clarity relates to a model of child sexual abuse which takes account of existing ideas – what Geertz (1983) terms 'local knowledge'. Local knowledge is to be found in the everyday talk and current social practices, e.g. childrearing, within a particular language or socio-cultural group, and needs to be identified in each speech community. Most significant are likely to be the dominant discourses concerning:

1   the nature of childhood and the kinds of relationship between adults and children which are seen as feasible and acceptable;
2   the development of female sexuality and expressions of sexuality which are viewed as 'natural' for girls;
3   the development of girls and women as gendered subjects in relation to experience of and ideas about sexual abuse
4   and, particularly, discourses concerning the consequences of such experience, if there are such discourses, and the role of stigma.

While acknowledging that cultural practices are never static and that each person's sense of self and choices of self-presentation shift from context to context (being related to time, place and person) we need to study these facets of human life within different language groups and social contexts, in order to establish the presence and form of stigma constituted – if indeed there is stigma – and to deconstruct how this relates to female subjectivity and deference to male authority in a range of instances, including child sexual abuse. At the same time we need to take seriously the consequences of such research, particularly if it is not interpreted in relation to patriarchal authority and power. For example, in Western societies the state has assumed power to regulate the daily life of families, to some degree, removing responsibility from adults, neighbours and communities, without dismantling patriarchy and without carefully considering the rights of children, including their right to sexual knowledge (Sullivan, 1992). There is a paradoxical conflict of interest between modern efforts to remedy injustice and eliminate the exploitation of children, including acting 'in their best interest' on the one hand, and the play of middle-class power in the medicalisation of social issues and extension of professional services, on the other. When the capacity of families and communities to find their own remedies for problems such as child sexual abuse is taken away, we find that the law and welfare procedures do not generally offer better remedies. An important reason is that structural power accommodates superficially; no fundamental changes are effected because the ones which are required concern deeply entrenched beliefs and normative systems.

We have little idea of how young people engage in sexual relationships, nor how adults and families in Western societies deal with children's sexuality (Sullivan, 1992). We have a long way to go in Western society towards understanding exactly how children and adolescents are recruited into discursive positions as sexual and gendered subjects, and how we insert ourselves within familial and local community patterns of gendered behaviours. Alternative solutions for the education of children in the area of sexual relating and in regard to child abuse, including sexual abuse, are long overdue but depend on research on these fundamental questions. Counter-discourses need perhaps to be developed in a collaborative process – investigations would be most usefully both research- and education-oriented. 'Solutions' found may turn out to be temporary and makeshift measures given the constraints of power of cultural colonialism, but our efforts need always to incorporate the re-visioning of alternatives in awareness of the subtleties of power. Recognition of strategies of resistance and survival, and building on these, will help. The breaking down of stigma through courageous self-examination and open accounts of our own experiences of childhood, including sexual explorations, sexual abuse and the development of gendered identities across a range of contexts should be envisaged. Theorising about these matters cannot be done without essential changes in consciousness of researchers. There will be no change in social practices, including child sexual abuse, without changes in the consciousness of large numbers of women and men.

However, the use of discourse analysis is not in itself the answer. Furthermore, there are major problems where cross-cultural research is envisaged. In communities with a colonial history, where there has been a struggle to resist the domination of colonialist groups, variously identified (and where a pride in local languages and categories of identity and experience is part of the resistance) complexities of human experience are not readily tapped through direct questioning, interviews or focused discussions with translation from English or some other northern language associated with dominant systems of knowledge (Levett *et al.*, 1997). There have been critiques of efforts to translate questionnaire research into black African languages (Kortmann, 1987, 1990), and Drennan *et al.* (1991) have discussed the subtle problems of interpretation in South African multilingual contexts, where apparently straightforward arrangements between researchers and interpreters are far from simple. Universalist assumptions have been exhaustively discussed by anthropologists (e.g. Sperber, 1985) – it could be a form of appropriation or neo-colonialism to 'name' a girl raised in this context as 'abused' or 'damaged' and to hold that a set of traumatic consequences is to be expected. Not all such experience is necessarily disruptive.

Furthermore, in my own research there were particular problems with the interpretation and translation of concepts which were assumed to be quite straightforward, such as 'pain', 'emotion', 'knowledge', 'talk', and 'shame', among many others. Cross-cultural research requires total submersion in the language community in which there is the goal to further a depth of understanding (the recent novel, *The Poisonwood Bible*, by Barbara Kingsolver (1999) gives one some inkling of the extent of the interpretive problems which are likely).

Are there ways in which discourse analysis can be useful in tagging and highlighting the invisible shackles of our assumptions around child sexual abuse without doing an injustice to the political goals of activists working on behalf of women and children? Although there are no clear answers to such questions, the beginnings of some answers may be attempted. The numerous complications of this methodology, problems of translation and interpretation, the need to use same-language speakers but to disrupt the effects of 'formal education', and so on, are discussed elsewhere (Levett *et al.*, 1997) and the possibilities of disrupting or elasticising our conceptual grids seem limited. Perhaps the idea of discourse analysis is one which has been valuable mainly in helping us to examine our own assumptions somewhat more critically and honestly, and this might enhance further attempts to make comparisons between the social practices and ideas of different language communities, providing us with a still tattered but richer patchwork of mutual understanding involving less exploitative processes.

Note

1 This is a revised version of a chapter of the same title (Levett, 1994). Acknowledgements and thanks are due to David Philip Publishers, Cape Town, for permission to use this material here.

References

Arbib, M.A. and Hesse, M. (1986) *The construction of reality*, Cambridge: Cambridge University Press.

Badgley, R. (1984) 'Report of the Committee on Sexual Offenses against Children and Youth', Ministries of Justice and Attorney General and Supply and Services, Government of Canada.

Bennett, T.W. (1991) *A sourcebook of African customary law for Southern Africa*, Cape Town: Juta.

Beutler, L.E. and Hill. C.E. (1992) 'Process and outcome research in the treatment of adult victims of childhood sexual abuse: methodological issues', *Journal of Consulting and Clinical Psychology* 60, 2: 203–212.

Billig, M. (1987) *Arguing and thinking: a rhetorical approach to social psychology*, Cambridge: Cambridge University Press.

Briere, J. (1992) 'Methodological issues in the study of sexual abuse effects', *Journal of Consulting and Clinical Psychology* 60, 2: 196–203.

Browne, A. and Finkelhor, D. (1986) 'Impact of childhood sexual abuse: a review of the research', *Psychological Bulletin* 99: 66–77.

Bruner, E.M. (1986) 'Ethnography as narrative', in V.W. Turner and E.M. Bruner (eds) *The anthropology of experience*, Urbana: University of Illinois Press.

Burman, E. (1994) *Deconstructing developmental psychology*, London: Routledge.

Burman, E. and Parker, I. (eds) (1993) *Discourse analytic research: repertoires and readings of texts in action*, London: Routledge.

Charman, A., De Swardt, C. and Simons, M. (1991) 'The politics of gender: a discussion of the Malibongwe Conference Papers and other current papers within the ANC', Paper presented at the Conference on Women and Gender in Southern Africa, University of Natal, Durban.

Collings, S. (1989) 'Social stereotypes and the likelihood of criminal conviction in cases of child sexual abuse: a research note', *Agenda* 5: 21–23.

DeMause, L. (1991) 'The universality of incest', *Journal of Psychohistory* 19, 2: 123–164.

Drennan, G., Levett, A. and Swartz, L. (1991) 'Hidden dimensions of power and resistance in the translation process: a South African study', *Culture, Medicine and Psychiatry* 15: 361–381.

Ennew, J. (1986) *The sexual exploitation of children*, Cambridge: Polity Press.

Finkelhor, D. (1989) 'Social and cultural factors in child sexual abuse', Paper presented at the 8th International Congress on Child Abuse and Neglect, Hamburg.

Finkelhor, D. and Browne, A. (1985) 'The traumatic impact of child sexual abuse: a conceptualisation', *American Journal of Orthopsychiatry* 55: 530–541.

Fuss, D. (1989) *Essentially speaking: feminism, nature and difference*, New York: Routledge.

Geertz, C. (1983) *Local knowledge: further essays in interpretive anthropology*, New York: Basic Books.

Geertz, C. (1986) 'Making experiences, authoring selves', in V.W. Turner and E.M. Bruner (eds) *The anthropology of experience*, Urbana: University of Illinois Press.

Gergen, K.J. (1985) 'The social constructionist movement in modern psychology', *American Psychologist* 40: 266–275.

Hacking, I. (1991) 'The making and molding of child abuse', in M. Douglas and D. Hull (eds) *Coherent worlds* (cited by Sullivan, 1992).

Haugaard, J.J. and Emery, T.E. (1989) 'Methodological issues in child sexual abuse research', *Child Abuse and Neglect* 13: 89–100.

Henriques, J., Hollway, W., Urwin, C., Venn, C. and Walkerdine, V. (1984) *Changing the subject*, London: Methuen.

Hollway, W. (1984) 'The power of women in heterosexual sex', *Women's Studies International Forum* 7: 63–68.

Howard, G.S. (1991) 'Culture tales: a narrative approach to thinking, cross-cultural psychology and psychotherapy', *American Psychologist* 46, 3: 187–197.

James, A. and Prout, A. (eds) (1990) *Constructing and reconstructing childhood: contemporary issues in the sociological study of childhood*, London: The Falmer Press.

Kelly, L. (1989) 'Bitter ironies', *Trouble and Strife* 16 (Summer): 14–21.

Kessell, F.S. and Siegel, A.W. (eds) (1983) *The child and other cultural inventions*, New York: Praeger Press.

Korbin, J.E. (1987) 'Child sexual abuse: implications from the cross-cultural record', in N. Scheper-Hughes (ed.) *Child Survival*, Dordrecht: D. Reidel.

Korbin, J.E. (1991) 'Cross-cultural perspectives and research directions for the twenty-first century', *Child Abuse and Neglect* 15, 1: 67–77.

Kortmann, F. (1987) 'Problems in communication in transcultural psychiatry', *Acta Psychiatrica Scandinavica* 75: 563–570.

Kortmann, F. (1990) 'Psychiatric case finding in Ethiopia: shortcomings of the self-reporting questionnaire', *Culture, Medicine and Psychiatry* 14: 381–392.

La Fontaine, J.S. (1987) 'Child sexual abuse and the incest taboo: practical problems and theoretical issues', *Man (N.S.)* 23: 1–18.

Levett, A. (1989a) 'A study of childhood sexual abuse among South African university women students', *South African Journal of Psychology* 19, 3: 122–129.

Levett, A. (1989b) 'Psychological trauma: discourses on childhood sexual abuse', unpublished doctoral dissertation, University of Cape Town.

Levett, A. (1989c) 'Children and psychological trauma', *Psychology in Society* 12: 19–32.

Levett, A. (1991) 'Contradictions and confusions in child sexual abuse', *South African Journal of Criminal Justice* 4, 1: 9–20.

Levett, A. (1992a) 'Regimes of truth: a response to Russell', *Agenda* 12: 67–74.

Levett, A. (1992b) 'Stigmatic factors in sexual abuse and the violence of representation', Paper presented at the Domestic Violence Conference, University of South Africa, Pretoria.

Levett, A. (1994) 'Problems of cultural imperialism in the study of childhood sexual abuse', in A. Dawes and D. Donald (eds), *Childhood and adversity: psychological perspectives from South African research*, Cape Town: David Philip.

Levett, A., Kottler, A., Walaza, N., Mabena, P., Leon, N. and Ngqakayi-Motaung, N. (1997) 'Pieces of mind: traumatic effects of child sexual abuse among black South African women', in A. Levett, A., Kottler, E., Burman and I. Parker (eds) *Culture, power and difference: discourse analysis in South Africa*, London: Zed Books Ltd/Cape Town: University of Cape Town Press.

Levett, A. and Lachman, P. (1991) *Child abuse research register. RAPCAN, Child Health Unit*, Cape Town: University of Cape Town and Red Cross Children's Hospital.

Lowy, I. (1988) 'Ludwig Fleck on the social construction of medical knowledge', *Sociology of Health and Illness* 10, 2: 133–155.

McKenna, W. and Kessler, S. (1985) 'Asking taboo questions and doing taboo deeds', in K.J. Gergen and K.E. Davis (eds) *The social construction of the person*, New York: Springer Verlag.

Malamuth, N.M., Sockoskie, R.J., Koss, M.J. and Tanaka, J.S. (1991) 'Characteristics of aggressors against women: testing a model using a national sample of college students', *Journal of Consulting and Clinical Psychology* 59, 7: 670–681.

Manning, P.K. (1987) *Semiotics and fieldwork. Sage University Paper series: Qualitative Research Methods, Volume 7*, Beverly Hills: Sage Publications.

Mejiuni, C.O. (1991) 'Educating adults against socio-culturally induced abuse and neglect of children in Nigeria', *Child Abuse and Neglect* 15: 139–145.

Millett, K. (1970) *Sexual politics*, New York: Doubleday.

Nelson, B. (1984) *Making an issue of child abuse: political agenda setting for social problems*, Chicago: University of Chicago Press.

Painter, S.L. (1986) Research on the prevalence of child sexual abuse: new directions, *Canadian Journal of Behavioral Science*, 18: 323–339.

Parker, I. (1992) *Discourse dynamics: critical analysis for social and individual psychology*, London: Routledge.

Parker, I. and Burman, E. (1993) 'Against discursive imperialism, empiricism and constructionism: thirty-two problems with discourse analysis', in E. Burman and Parker, I. (eds) *Discourse analytic research: repertoires and readings of texts in action*, London: Routledge.

Posel, D. (1991) 'Women's powers, men's authority: rethinking patriarchy', Paper presented at the Women and Gender Conference, University of Natal, Durban.

Potter, J. and Wetherell, M. (1987) *Discourse and social psychology*, London: Sage Publications.

Reppucci, N.C. and Haugaard, J.J.H. (1989) 'Prevention of child sexual abuse: myth or reality?' *American Psychologist* 44: 1266–1275.

Reynolds, P. (1991) 'Paring down the family: the child's point of view', Paper delivered at the Research Seminar on Children and Families, HSRC, Pretoria.

Russell, D.E.H. (1975) *The politics of rape*, New York: Stein and Day.

Russell, D.E.H. (1984) *Sexual exploitation*, Beverly Hills: Sage Publications.

Russell, D.E.H. (1991) 'The damaging effects of discounting damaging effects of child sexual abuse', *Agenda* 11: 47–56.

Shotter, J. (1984) *Social accountability and selfhood*, Oxford: Basil Blackwell.

Socarides, C. (1991) 'Adult–child sexual pairs: psychoanalytic findings', *Journal of Psychohistory*, 19, 2: 185–189.

Spaccarelli, S. (1994) 'Stress, appraisal and coping in child sexual abuse: a theoretical and empirical review', *Psychological Bulletin* 116, 2: 340–362.

Sperber, D. (1985) 'Apparently irrational beliefs', in *On anthropological knowledge. Three essays*, Cambridge: Cambridge University Press, pp. 35–63.

Sterling, C. (1990) 'Male accounts of child sexual abuse: excuses and justifications', unpublished Master's dissertation, University of Cape Town.

Straker, G., Moosa, F., Becker, R. and Nkwale, M. (1992). *Faces in the revolution: the psychological effects of violence on township youth in South Africa*, Cape Town: David Philip.

Sullivan, T. (1992) *Sexual abuse and the rights of children: reforming Canadian law*, Toronto: University of Toronto Press.

Viljoen, S. (1991) 'The nature of parental authority in family lives of black South Africans', Paper delivered at the Conference on the Child and the Family, HSRC, Pretoria.

Walker, C. (1991) *Women and resistance in South Africa*, Cape Town: David Philip.

Widom, C. (1989) 'Does violence beget violence? A critical examination of the literature', *Psychological Bulletin* 106: 3–28.

Wyatt, G.E. and Powell, G.J. (eds) (1988) *The lasting effects of child sexual abuse*, Newbury Park: Sage.

Chapter 5

Traumatic revisions

Remembering abuse and the politics of forgiveness

Janice Haaken

As a psychotherapist, I am interested in stories – or versions of the same story – repeatedly told. Included in my own stock of personal stories about sex is an entire sub-genre of memories about dancing prohibitions. I remember one episode during early adolescence where my friend Karla and I smuggled an Elvis record into my bedroom. Worldly music was strictly forbidden by my Christian fundamentalist parents, and Elvis was the embodiment of what 'worldly' meant. As Karla and I gyrated to 'Heartbreak Hotel', the towering figure of my father entered the room. He registered his disapproval with a stern glance, then turned and closed the door. Like two Eves caught in the Garden, my friend and I stiffened with shame. She left and I wallowed in my misery for the remainder of the day, even though my father had said nothing of our transgression. Sometime in my late twenties, I came across a diary from my early teens where this infamous day was minutely described. Contrary to my vivid memory, it was my mother who had entered my room that day to interrupt my furtive pleasures.

How do we understand such failures in memory, and what do they suggest about the narrative strategies available in constructing the past? One line of interpretation draws on findings suggesting that contemporary conflicts and social contexts retroactively shape the memory retrieved (Bower, 1981; Burman, 1996; Loftus and Ketchum, 1994). As a young woman, my father figured more prominently in my autobiography of barricades to freedom than did my mother. The parental substitution in the drama may have sacrificed a factual truth in an effort to represent this social truth. Yet the casting of my father in the role of prohibitive superego also may be interpreted as what Freud termed a *screen memory*, in this case a defensive construction of an event in the service of repression. For developmental and political reasons, the struggle with my father may have been more accessible to consciousness than was the struggle with my mother. On yet another level, this memory report may be interpreted as signifying a conflict between religious sanctions – the Law of the Father – and homoerotic desire. Women's consciousness-raising groups in the early

1970s opened up the cultural field for such valiant recollections – for stories of insurgent female desire defying the repressive codes of the patri-archs.

Many feminists position women – and the oppressed generally – as guardians of repressed truths, possessors of a language silenced but not destroyed. Adrienne Rich, for example, insists that 'whatever is ... is buried in the memory by the collapse of meaning under an inadequate or lying lan-guage – that will become, not merely unspoken, but unspeakable' (1977: 3). The politics of memory suffered a retreat in the 1990s, however, as public scrutiny of women's childhood recollections narrowly centred on the ques-tion of their literal accuracy. As therapists came to interpret a broad range of clinical indicators as signs of repressed memory of sexual abuse, incest emerged as the prototype of the unspeakable story. Allegations based on psychotherapeutically recovered memories of childhood sexual abuse were increasingly contested, with many feminists taking the position that any questioning of women's recollections was an act of betrayal.

For many years, I have been interested in narratives, particularly women's abuse and trauma narratives, and how to interpret them in ways that preserve the integrity of the story while going beyond simply 'validat-ing' them (Haaken, 1996, 1998). Particularly problematic has been the position that women's stories are transparent in meaning or that they are mere imprints of external events. This stance strips women's accounts of complexity, denying the role of imagination, symbolisation, displacements, narrative elaboration and social construction in speaking about disturbing experiences. Further, it downplays how official 'translators' on the scene (including women therapists) shape the transformation of inchoate, un-storied experience into narrative accounts.

My own interventions in feminist theory, including the emotionally charged atmosphere of the 'memory wars', draws on psychoanalytic social theory. While building on clinical traditions, psychoanalytic social theory situates unconscious processes, e.g., fantasies and defences, in historical and societal contexts.[1] This mode of inquiry takes into account objective constraints and structuring influences on group life, for example, differ-ences in power or access to the means of production. At the same time, psychoanalytic social theory attends to the non-rational or unconscious aspects of group life. To introduce this notion of the non-rational need not imply a pathologising of groups, nor does it suggest that the aims of groups or movements are irrational. Not unlike the oppressor, however, the oppressed may make defensive use of an enemy, either imagined or real, to create a sense of group unity, projecting onto an Other destructive cur-rents within the group. In the women's movement, for example, idealised representations of female culture may make it difficult to confront sources of conflict among women, including those based on class and other hierar-chical differences.

The concept of the unconscious, particularly, has been a fertile meeting ground for feminism and psychoanalysis in that it subverts patriarchal conceptions of the mind as coherent, rationally ordered and autonomous (see Rose 1986). While there are a range of psychoanalytic discourses concerning the dynamic unconscious, they share an emphasis on experiences at the margins of what is most readily noticed. This emphasis on group and individual defences requires us to attend to what is overlooked, omitted or marginalised in a given representation of human experiences.

This chapter makes use of psychoanalytic theory to explore some of the dilemmas that emerge for women – collectively and individually – in representing the past, and how these dilemmas emerge politically as a struggle over 'storytelling rights'. The psychoanalytic framework extends as well into a discussion of gender and the politics of forgiveness, focused on the limits of individualised denouements to collectively realised forms of suffering. In working through the problematics of reparation, I explore feminist ambivalences concerning clinical discourse on forgiveness. This section enlists the insights of women of colour in developing a critical social theory of reparation.

Feminism, psychoanalysis and collective remembering

Most stories have a beginning, a middle and an end. Storied events are organised according to a sequence of actions, with the first 'action' setting in motion and determining later actions. Experimental psychology is a pure form of storytelling in that it has a beginning, a middle and an end, with observed effects organised through this temporal framework. The beginning is defined as the independent variable, manipulated by the experimenter, and the ending defined as the dependent variable, thought to be an effect of this same manipulation. Mediating variables constitute the middle in that they modify the relationship between independent and dependent variables. In studying male violence, for example, an experimenter might tell the story as a sequence of actions originating in 'frustration' – or 'blocked goal attainment' and ending in variable levels of aggressive behaviour.

Many people think like experimentalists, even though they live in a densely correlational world. We rarely are able to hold single factors constant in order to assess their effects, separate from the complex web of influences that co-determine the impact of events. Nonetheless, searching for causality is a fundamental feature of human intelligence and this search often leads to the isolation of a primary cause, particularly in searching for the source of suffering. Sometimes we are correct in locating the source. But we may as easily be in error, misattributing the source of our misery.

While research inquiry on memory accuracy tends to hinge on the degree of correspondence between objective events and mental representations of them, feminist researchers insist that power relations must be taken into account. For oppressed groups, remembering involves a struggle to access more authentic versions of the past, against interpretations imposed by the more powerful. Peggy Miller (1995) makes use of this idea in her research on conflicts over 'storytelling rights' in families, attending as well to cultural contexts shaping what may be permissibly spoken about. In her research on class differences in storytelling rights, Miller challenges assumptions in the literature that middle-class families are more open and democratic than are lower-class families. She concludes that working-class families often allow more open expression of anger and aggression, and parents are less apt to censor what may be permissibly reported. In contrast to middle-class families, working-class families also express more pleasure in stories of open defiance: 'Many of the stories that the children heard their mothers tell were stories in which the mother described herself as speaking up, talking back, or otherwise defending herself in response to being wronged' (Miller, 1995: 178).

From a psychoanalytic perspective, stories about others are, in part, stories about the self – with other protagonists in the drama sometimes registering unconscious or split-off aspects of the patient's inner world. The victim's story about a perpetrator may be both an account of an objective event and a means of representing disturbing currents within the self. Dissociated images of beastly villains or scenes of violence may register split-off aspects of the self, just as well as they might indicate the emergence of traumatic memory. Ideally, therapists create a holding space for the emergence and integration of a wide range of mental imagery and self/object representations. If therapeutic attentiveness and empathy centre exclusively on the 'good' victim, however, the less culturally supported aspects of the female self may be smuggled into the clinical narrative through a perpetrator story.

Cultural narratives mediate the defensive elaboration of unconscious material, shaping what is more readily registered in consciousness and what is more apt to be dissociated, split-off or repressed. Multiple personality disorder, for example, emerged as a condition primarily of women in the late twentieth century as clinicians grappled with their own anxieties about the fragmented, unintegrated aspects of female identity (see Haaken, 1998). During periods of social change, we might expect greater discontinuities in the autobiographical record as groups struggle to create more authentic versions of the past, over and against authoritatively received accounts.

In the context of psychotherapy, the structuring effects of culture and history often operate unconsciously. Moving from individual to collective forms of remembering, we may recognise multiple functions of incest accounts within feminist-informed practices. On the one hand, movements provide a holding ground for recollections – one that goes beyond the capacities of individuals and families to contain disturbing experiences. Within feminism, the incest survivor's story was a project of stripping patriarchy of its figleaf of benevolence to expose the violations of individual and collective father figures. But the father's dirty secret – asserted as a memory born of struggle – acquires new meanings as it circulates as a marker of an emergent female authority. Further, this emergent female authority carries myriad defensive possibilities, including reliance on the villainy of patriarchs – or the enemy camp – for the maintenance of vital psychic and social borders.

Similarly, clinical reliance on stock scripts – the standard melodrama of a virtuous female protagonist and a one-dimensional male villain – strips women of complex subjectivity. In enlisting schema for recollecting the past, many feminists have cautioned against this romanticising of women, including over-emphasis on an inherent female 'goodness' (Minsky, 1998; Westcott, 1998; Lamb, 2002). Breaking out of domesticated scripts means claiming a broader range of idealised female images than those culturally authorised for women. Much like other social movements, feminism requires access to aggression and stories that explore moral dilemmas associated with fighting back. If women are cast as good by nature, if all acts of female resistance are portrayed as just and noble, the drama collapses into a morality play.

Trauma and reparation: the gender politics of forgiveness

On a social psychological level, the disputes over factual claims and counter-claims in the recovered memory debate might be viewed as an obsessive defence against deeper anxieties over the shifting boundaries of gender relations and intergenerational ties. While public outrage focused on false allegations and legal actions against fathers, there was a palpable intergenerational crisis animating the memory controversy – a crisis that lapsed into hysterical fear of an epidemic of prodigal daughters, abandoning their ageing parents. Indeed, one of the more vitriolic charges in the recovered memory debate centred on the power of therapists to break up families, seducing grown daughters from the loving folds of their families. Cheery scenes of Norman Rockwell childhoods emerged in the FMS literature, in stark contrast to the Gothic scenes excavated from the memories of many of these same daughters (see Haaken, 1998).

In interpreting the recovered memory debate, it is important to keep in view the disturbing incidence of child sexual abuse and to preserve the ground that has been won in addressing this pervasive social problem. So, too, the quasi-religious claims of family and kinship must be resisted, along with the disproportionate burdens women face in rehabilitating fractured relationships. Women do have the right to sever family ties, as do men, even though there is a place in any society for moral and emotional injunctions against doing so. Rather than casting it in either/or terms, we need to confront the issue more dialectically. Specifically, we must address the dilemmas that emerge as women negotiate the tension between freedoms and obligations.

While second-wave feminism produced a critique of the patriarchal family, the 'third wave' includes palpable resistances to any form of universalising about women's experiences, including those within the family. Some of these differences centre on degrees of ambivalence over the patriarchal family, and the extent to which traditional kinship structures oppress women. For many women of colour, escaping the binding ties of family confronts more complex countervailing pressures and ideals than it does for many white women. While women share a common cultural position in preserving kinship ties, the project of emancipation from the patriarchal family is a more ambivalent one for women of colour than it is for white women (Collins, 1998; Crenshaw, 1994). The source of hardships is less readily located within the family structure, and broader contingencies controlling the fates of family members impose themselves more forcefully on daily life. The cultural ideal of the autonomous nuclear family, like that of the autonomous individual, is more apt to be recognised as an illusion.

I was particularly aware of these complex currents in the stories of women confronting a legacy of racism and colonialism when I was carrying out my research in West Africa in the summer of 1999. As part of a larger project on cultural contexts shaping women's understandings of family violence, I visited refugee camps in Guinea to interview women who had fled the civil war in Sierra Leone. As I talked with women about their experiences of the war – a brutal conflict that included reports of women raped by their own sons – discussion turned to the meaning of forgiveness. Some women stressed the importance of forgetting the past and looking to the future. 'We have to put it at our backs,' one woman insisted. 'If you dwell on the past, the trauma will never leave you. The way we do this is by engaging in activity together, by working together.' Other women stressed remembering as vital to the project of recovery. As one of the Sisters at a centre for child soldiers explained, 'we have to understand why this happened to us. If you do not deal with the past, it will never leave you.' While these prescriptive statements seem contradictory, I came to see them as a necessary contradiction. In the refugee camps, children and adults came together to create theatre re-enacting and reworking memory of the war. But they also taught each other skills and found creative ways of remembering the positive side of the cultural past. Remembering meant recovering the good as well as the bad within the past, and finding collective means of 'holding' the trauma.[2]

Talk of forgiveness also led to the issue of how responsibility for suffering should be socially distributed. For Sierra Leonean women, identifying the enemy – the perpetrators of the war – defied the individualist categories that prevail in Western discourse on victimisation and forgiveness. Women struggled with the question of who to hold responsible as the primary perpetrators of this war. Is it the young men and boys who joined a violent rebel movement and turned brutally on their own communities? Is it corrupt government officials who made deals with foreign governments and investors while turning their backs on their own people? Is it the International Monetary Fund, the institution that forced the government to lay off a third of its public sector workforce just prior to the outbreak of the war? Is it the continuing impact of colonialism? Is it the international diamond trade and the global economy – systems that extract raw materials from Africa without building the productive capacities of its peoples? While women differed in where they placed most blame, there was considerable agreement that the villainy behind the war was not readily located. Some of the perpetrators of the war were more easily identified than were others. But social understandings predominated over individualistic ones, as women struggled to find some transcendent means of bridging the war that was still all too present, and prospects for peace that seemed all to remote.

For many women in oppressed communities, the family is not as apt to be viewed as the primary site of oppression, nor are men – as fathers or husbands – as apt to be cast as the singular source of villainy. Just as feminism offered a redemptive framework for re-interpreting child abuse committed by women, women in communities of colour introduce a wider set of contingencies in explaining the failures of men. In both contexts, groups are able to work through some of the effects of abuse by placing some of the 'bad' outside the boundaries of kinship ties and onto an external oppressor. At the same time, this group defence may be a means of avoiding intra-group conflict, particularly if the grievances of subordinate groups, such as women, are routinely attributed to external agitators, e.g. 'Western feminists'.

It is not surprising that the clinical discourse on forgiveness is regarded with wariness by many feminists, however, who are more concerned with giving voice to what has happened than with making reparation (see Lamb, 1996, 2002). The suspicion is that the valorising of forgiveness is a seductive demand on victims to redeem their oppressors, relieving them of the burden of guilt. As oppressed groups gain the strength to speak up and claim new rights, including the right to disengage from abusive relationships, the powerful rediscover the salutary virtue of forgiveness (Keene, 1995).

I share much of this wariness, even as I believe that the capacity to forgive is integral to many other capacities, including the self-reflective capacities of social movements. So what might be learned from psychoanalytic theory in uncovering the conflicting motivations and defences of projects of reparation? Is there a productive middle ground between an over-idealisation and a devaluing of forgiveness?

One way of entering into the conundrum is to begin with the experience of victims – with those who have been injured, and particularly with those whose complaints are more likely to be silenced by the more powerful. In arguing for the benefits of forgiveness for victims, Sue Walrond-Skinner states that:

> forgiveness acts as a temporary agent of empowerment because it dramatically changes the balance of power within the relationship in some mysterious way, shifting it initially in a straight exchange from the previously empowered offender to the previously disempowered victim ... This dramatic exchange of power is however often such a shock that its effect is to liberate both parties from their entrenched positions.
>
> (1998: 16)

But what is this 'mysterious' effect of forgiveness that liberates both parties? And under what conditions does forgiveness shift the balance of power in oppressive relationships? Like many other Christian counsellors in the forgiveness literature, Walrond-Skinner embraces the idea of mystical transformation, invoking it as a means of fortifying the resolve of ambivalent participants. Reconciliation in the Christian literature tends to be understood as a form of emotional surrender – a dramatic change of heart in both the transgressor and the transgressed. From a psychoanalytic perspective, however, the concept of mystical transformation may be understood as a form of magical undoing, the hypnotic effect of a ritual or authoritative influence. From a more political perspective, reconciliation means addressing the conditions under which families are able to resolve difficulties, move beyond stalemates, and work together more co-operatively. These conditions would include confronting the double standard that permits men greater sexual freedoms and places women in the position of bearing primary responsibility for children, often with minimal social supports.

Walrond-Skinner (ibid.) goes beyond Christian pieties, however, in grounding the process of forgiveness in a developmental framework. The process of trying to reach forgiveness arouses our earliest experiences of loss, she suggests, particularly the loss of an infantile sense of grandiose control over the mother. The capacity to weather early losses and to make reparation depends on how the infant navigates through early experiences of separation.

Though she cites the work of feminist relational theorists, Walrond-Skinner does not discuss the gender dynamics of forgiveness. Mothers are often at the centre of our first images of betrayal, as Walrond-Skinner suggests, but they also are at the centre of our deepest representations of reparation. While God the Father grants forgiveness in Christian theology, it is the mother – both the material mother of childhood and the fantasy representation of her – who represents possibilities for restored connection.

Carol Gilligan (1982), a leading relational theorist, concludes from her own research that women approach moral conflict differently than men and are more apt to engage in the work of reparation. Whereas men focus on an ethic of individual rights, women are more apt to invoke an ethic of care in negotiating moral conflict. Building on Nancy Chodorow's (1978) work, Gilligan argues that female development is directed towards preserving relational ties whereas male development is oriented towards separation from others. In societies where women are responsible for the care of children and men dominate public life, male gender identity comes to be constructed around defensive dis-identification with the mother and a corresponding repression of dependency needs. Female gender identity, on the other hand, allows for a greater integration of dependence and independence needs. This gender distinction implies that women tend to develop more flexible ego boundaries, a deeper capacity for relatedness, and less fear of yielding to others than do men.

One of the main criticisms of feminist relational theory, however, is that it downplays the costs of feminine 'peace-making' and the costs to women in striving for the restoration of 'connection' (Westcott, 1998). Further, relational theory does not place much emphasis on female aggressive impulses and thus colludes with domesticated cultural representations of femininity. From a psychoanalytic feminist perspective, we would want to attend to collective defences against female outrage and how these same collective defences operate in censoring women's stories.

Oppressed groups – that is, those who have had less power in defending against victimisation – have expressed the greatest wariness concerning the valorising of forgiveness. The literature on abuse victims – particularly the vast literature on sexual abuse survivors – routinely cautions against forgiveness (see Bass and Davis, 1988; Burstow, 2002; Lamb, 2002; Walker, 1984, 1989). Forgiveness is viewed as either condoning abuse or repeating an oppressive pattern of enlisting the victim, often a woman, in taking care of the perpetrator, who is often a man.

Those who promote forgiveness as a mental health practice typically respond by pointing out that these dynamics need not be part of the process of forgiveness. Indeed, terms such as 'pseudo-forgiveness' and 'conciliatory forgiveness' pervade the literature as caveats against the potential replay of these oppressive interactions. The literature abounds with recommendations and criteria for distinguishing between 'authentic' forgiveness and various counterfeit versions (see DiBlasio, 1998; Ferch, 1998; Freedman and Enright, 1996).

This focus on authenticity is continuous with a longstanding Western emphasis, particularly within the middle classes, on expressive states as markers of individual identity. With the decline of traditional practices which located personal identity in a matrix of kinship obligations and ritualised practices, the achievement of social identity in the bourgeois era came to rest more heavily on the capacity to transform oneself and to master emotional states (Hochschild, 1994).

One could say that forgiveness is a 'feminised' subject position in that it is associated with traditional female gendered attributes, e.g., yielding, empathy and responsiveness to others. The feminising of the capacity to forgive in Western discourse is also related to the heightening of the division, particularly in the nineteenth century, between private and public life (Epstein, 1981; Hoeveler, 1998). The emergence of a market economy organised around the negotiation of impersonal contracts left domestic life as the site of personal fulfilment and the nuclear family as an idealised sanctuary from public life. Barbara Epstein (1981) describes the nineteenth-century 'cult of domesticity' which placed women in the position of guardians of virtue, family togetherness, and emotional harmony. In presiding over this place of respite from a competitive world, middle-class women became the embodiment of unconditional love, turning the other way when confronted with the infidelity of husbands. Women's economic dependency granted men automatic rights to forgiveness, even though women resisted more openly as the century wore on. There are also longstanding cultural scripts inscribing forgiveness, as an emotional state, with femininity. The God of the Hebrew Bible is less forgiving than is the Christian Son of God, with the latter expressing a more accepting, yielding image of a deity. Even the Christian portrait of a forgiving Christ impaled on a cross, surrendering to his fate, assumes what is culturally coded as a feminine posture. For every unforgiving Medea, there is a chorus of forgiving Corinthian wives, ready to make adjustments for the failings of men. To forgive may be divine, but it is also often thought to be a feminine spiritual craft.

The emergence of a contemporary discourse on forgiveness may register cultural anxieties over the adequacy of traditional means of containing conflict, particularly within the family. The social movements that achieved momentum in the 1970s destabilised traditional hierarchies, particularly patriarchal control of the family. At the same time, women continue to carry disproportionate responsibility for the emotional labour of relationships, including the work required in yielding to the interests of others (Hochschild, 1994). One of the social consequences of feminism, then, is that women are no longer assumed to be the loyal guardians of family togetherness. Emotional labour may still be women's work but female resistances are changing the terms of the contract.

From a feminist perspective, the question is not whether forgiveness is good or bad, nor is it a matter of simply calibrating the dispensary of forgiveness in some rational proportions to the scales of justice. The more important issues concern the interplay of gendered positions, and the range of freedom for women in negotiating the terms of their fate. Given the standard patriarchal plotline, with a long-suffering wife bestowing mercy on her prodigal husband, it is not surprising that feminists have been among the more vocal critics of forgiveness rhetoric. Indeed, the emergence of interest in this topic during the 1980s and 1990s may be read as a collective appeal for the 'forgiveness' of women. At the same time, incest emerged as the one sin from which fathers could not expect to be pardoned. For women struggling to break free of familial entanglements, the incest narrative carried a particular social symbolic loading, making some women responsive to therapeutic probing in this area. There are few culturally redemptive stories of women who walk away from their families without looking back, and incest most certainly is among them.

While daughters and wives continue to navigate a world of constraints, contemporary discourse on forgiveness also registers the distance women have travelled in resisting patriarchy. Capitulation and accommodation are no longer assumed to be women's lot, nor is it assumed that only the powerful are in the position of granting forgiveness. Yet in coming down on the side of forgiveness and reconciliation, we are emphasising the value of reintegrating transgressors into the community. As an ethical ideal, it represents a flexible morality, grounded in acknowledgement of weaknesses and failings as fundamental to the human condition (see Douglas, 1966). If we are all 'sinners saved by grace', we share a common heritage of guilt and a shared mandate to make reparations with others. There is implicit knowledge of these processes in many cultural practices, including the emotional malignancies associated with revenge and enemy-making. Culture equips individuals with practices for resolving disputes, including treatment of various bilious emotional afflictions associated with the failure of such cultural mechanisms.

Women – as wives, mothers and daughters – carry much of the responsibility for maintaining emotional attachments and thus are under considerable pressure often to forgive their abusers. Yet, capitalistic societies exacerbate this tendency towards social fragmentation and isolation of families, even as they allow more space for women's mobility. But for many women, this mobility circles back to the same place of bondage. The abusive actions of fathers, husbands or boyfriends are also understood within a wider world of contingencies that allows some 'redistrubution' of blame. A recurring theme in the literature of women of colour concerns this difficulty in drawing the boundary between daily hardships and domestic abuse, on the one hand, and in locating a single source of villainy on the other (Crenshaw, 1994; Lockhart and White, 1989; Richie, 2000).

In addressing cultural dimensions of family violence, Evelyn White emphasises the difficulties black women face in acknowledging their own vulnerabilities and in extricating themselves from the pain of men. While this is a consistent refrain in popular literature on the psychology of women, White does not lose sight of the social forces impinging on women's ambivalence about leaving abusive situations. She makes a distinction between empathising with the oppression black men face and taking responsibility for it:

> You don't have to become your partner's target because the bank didn't give him a loan. You do not have to become the scapegoat when the landlord raises the rent. And you do not have to become the punching bag because he can't afford to take the children to Disneyland. Physical and emotional abuse are not acceptable demonstrations of Black manhood ... Black men will not heal their wounded pride or regain a sense of dignity by abusing Black women.
>
> (1994: 26)

In the abuse recovery movement, it has been difficult to acknowledge the damaged humanity of men without yielding to the seductive pull of another stereotypical drama, where woman is cast as perpetual nursemaid to an injured manhood. The ideology of romantic love, realised in the context of the nuclear family, intensifies these emotional demands placed on women. But finding a new denouement need not require us to demonise abusers. By focusing on group interventions with abusive men, women – as individual partners of abusive men – bear less of the load.

In laying out a framework for 'justice-making', Traci West goes beyond the idea of individual accountability for abusers to include the community's responsibility for family violence and for supporting women's resistance to it:

> Because of the potent relationship between social and intimate violence, this formula must not rely upon an individualistic understanding that isolates 'incidents' of sexual and physical assault for redress. Justice-making action calls for a continuous struggle with the manifold cultural assaults that reproduce the conditions of male violence ... Those who benefit from and perpetuate the ongoing social subjugation of African–American women must be held accountable in the justice-making process for women.
>
> (1999: 197)

West calls for local tribunals, similar to international tribunals for war crimes, which would place on trial those who benefit from violence against women. This strategy is meant to raise consciousness about how dominant institutions, for example, the banks, the local Housing Authority, companies that close operations in poor communities, are deeply implicated in violence against women in poor communities. Family violence programmes must include anti-poverty measures that would give women meaningful alternatives to abusive situations and resources to rebuild communities devastated by capital flight and underemployment.

In contrast, based on their extensive experience with tribal councils, Native American women assume a more ambivalent stance towards community-based interventions in situations of abuse. In Canada, women in First Nations organisations emphasise that 'there is "good medicine" and "bad medicine" in Aboriginal communities' (McGillivray and Comaskey, 1999: 51). While tribal councils sometimes intervene on women's behalf, they as readily rule in favour of abusive men. Even though Aboriginal women tend to favour mediation and alternative remedies to the criminal justice system, researchers Anne McGillivray and Brenda Comaskey found that others preferred outside police intervention to the local councils. This conflict is not surprising, however, particularly in that many of these councils continue to be patriarchal. In spite of revitalised traditional practices, Native American/Aboriginal peoples continue to have the highest poverty and unemployment rates in North America.

Cultural practices offer means of ritually working through tensions in group life and sustaining human connection. But they also may operate repressively, or permit the deliverance of one group at the expense of another. Those who refuse to forgive may serve a vital social role in keeping tensions alive, preserving social space for the emergence of alternative, better forms of resolutions. Without Malcolm X refusing to forgive the 'white devils', Martin Luther King's message of non-violence and reconciliation may not have been so persuasive. King could pray for the salvation of racist oppressors and have mercy on their souls because the black power movement threatened to bring the white devils to their knees.

Conclusions

The pronouncement of forgiveness is like being told the ending of a story. It may serve as a foreclosure, a denouement, a resolution, but nonetheless suggests that something disturbing has happened. The recovered memory debate that raged in the US and parts of Europe during the 1990s opened up questions over 'storytelling rights' and the uncertainties of memory, questions that burst the bounds of readily available scientific or clinical explanations. What was required, I argue, is a theory of storytelling – one that bridges clinical and scientific discourse, on the one hand, and cultural theory on the other.

The incest story emerged as a unifying narrative within feminism in the

1980s and 1990s, not simply because the daughter revels in her victimhood, as critics suggest, but quite the opposite. The narrative is one of latent rebellion, of righteous rage in exposing the father. As it traversed across the cultural landscape, the incest story acquired social symbolic loadings. It moved from the particular to the universal, from the concrete to the mythic. By mythic, I do not mean *untrue*, but rather that the truth encompasses more than its factual correspondence to an event or its persuasiveness as an individual account of experience. Its meaning resides in what it reveals about a larger world of forces, a universe of contingencies operating beyond the protagonist's immediate control.

To what extent does the child sexual abuse story – as Every Woman's story – serve to disguise or displace the outrage of women, however, even as it illuminates a primary source of women's oppression? The most common, everyday effect of women's oppression is in the *absence* of vital supports for wellbeing. It is the *insufficiency* of male responses to women's needs, rather than violence or abuse per se that is the most ordinary and pervasive effect of women's oppression. But it is much harder to fight an absence than a presence, and the incest story does palpably register the malevolent, destructive side of men.

There are other cultural factors that contribute to the leading role of childhood sexual abuse in feminist storytelling as well. In the United States, particularly, anxieties about sex and violence are palpable, particularly within the middle class. Such anxieties do have a reality basis, in that sexual exploitation of women and male aggression are glorified in advertising, the media and popular culture. The revulsion expressed towards sex and violence – often paired as instinctually-driven vices with equal moral loading – often contains more than a modicum of voyeuristic pleasure.

Just as the fixation among many Christian fundamentalists on homosexuality permits forms of pleasure in the pursuit of banishing them, there was a pornographic substrate to clinical preoccupation with gothic scenes of sexual torture in the recovered memory literature. Women, including many feminists, learned that women's stories must, above all else, arouse interest in their listeners. Stories of sheer need – poverty, homelessness, neglect – became even less enchanting in the 1980s as the United States moved politically further to the right. Fewer victims were judged worthy of public concern, in an era of heightened 'personal responsibility'. Feminists, too, were able to employ this discourse in confronting male irresponsibility. There was a unifying picture that emerged of the perpetrator in the feminist literature, stripped of his arsenal of 'excuses'.

Social movements give rise to forms of collective remembering that do establish unity around common struggles. They create valorised accounts of what the oppressed has endured, and the rich knowledge that has survived such hardship. But idealised representations of group experience become repressive if they disallow the full range of humanity – destructive and noble – that is part of the history of struggle. For if only noble representations of the past are integrated into group consciousness, the less noble elements of human experience may find their way into group life disguised as the oppressor.

Feminism introduced the idea that the personal is the political, but this need not mean that the two dimensions of experience are one and the same. The personal is more of a given than is the political, the latter of which must be acquired as a form of consciousness. But the two interact in complex ways. From a psychoanalytic perspective, we may recognise how the torment and tormentors of childhood are displaced onto more impersonal enemies such as a dominant or ruling class. But this same displacement – the transfer of intimate struggles into group life – may also permit means of 'holding' disturbing affects and memories associated with early experience. The holding framework of a social movement may permit a working through of the good and bad elements of the personal past. Rather than God the father serving as the projective container of infantile longings, the concept of kinship, the working class, or Earth goddesses may be created as the idealised, mythologised protector. The movement – the history of struggle and the ideals it embodies – may also contain empirical and fantasy elements as the 'container' of myriad threats, both intrapsychic and social. Unlike religion or mythology, however, movements for social justice do not satisfy the regressive wish for an Ultimate Protector so fully. We can never escape knowledge of the movement's vulnerabilities, defeats, nor the necessity of action in the world. Appeals to an Almighty to intervene in our suffering are met with the cold silence of the universe. We can only achieve what we are able to collectively bring about.

Notes

1 For examples of psychoanalytic social theory, see Michael Rustin, *The Good Society and the Inner World*, and Rosalind Minsky, *Psychoanalysis and Culture*, and Radhika Mohanram, *Black Body: Women, Colonialism, and Space*. For an overview of concepts and issues in feminism and psychoanalytic cultural studies, see Kathryn Woodward, *Identity and Difference*.
2 Interviews of women are included in the documentary film, *Diamonds, Guns, and Rice: Sierra Leone and the Women's Peace Movement*.

References

Bass, E. and Davis, L. (1988) *The courage to heal*, New York: Harper-Perennial.
Bower, G. (1981) 'Mood and memory', *American Psychologist* 36: 129–148.
Burman, E. (1996/1997) 'False memories, true hopes and the angelic: revenge of the postmodern in therapy', *New Formations* 30: 122–134.
Burstow, B. (1992) *Radical feminist therapy: working in the context of violence*, Newbury Park: Sage.

Chodorow, N. (1978) *The reproduction of mothering: psychoanalysis and the sociology of gender*, Berkeley: University of California Press.

Collins, P.H. (1998) *Fighting words: black women and the search for justice*, Minneapolis: University of Minnesota Press.

Crenshaw, K.W. (1994) 'Mapping the margins: intersectionality, identity politics, and violence against women of color', in M.A. Fineman and R. Mykitiuk (eds) *The public nature of private violence: the discovery of domestic abuse*, New York: Routledge, pp. 93–118.

DiBlasio, F.A. (1998) 'The use of a decision-based forgiveness intervention within intergenerational family therapy', *Journal of Family Therapy* 20: 77–94.

Douglas, M. (1966) *Purity and danger*, New York: Praeger.

Epstein, B.L. (1981) *The politics of domesticity: women, evangelism, and temperance in nineteenth-century America*, Middletown: Wesleyan University Press.

Ferch, S.R. (1998) 'Intentional forgiveness as a counseling intervention', *Journal of Counseling and Development* 76: 261–270.

Freedman, S.R. and Enright, R.D. (1996) 'Forgiveness as an intervention strategy with incest survivors', *Journal of Consulting and Clinical Psychology* 64: 983–992.

Gilligan, C. (1982) *In a different voice: psychological theory and women's development*, Cambridge: Harvard University Press.

Haaken, J. (1996) 'The recovery of fantasy, memory, and desire: feminist approaches to sexual abuse and psychic trauma', *Signs: Journal of Women in Culture and Society* 21: 1069–1094.

Haaken, J. (1998) *Pillar of salt: gender, memory, and the perils of looking back*, New Brunswick: Rutgers University Press.

Hochschild, A. (1994) *The managed heart: commercialization of human feeling*, Berkeley: University of California Press.

Hoeveler, D.L. (1998) *Gothic feminism: the professionalization of gender from Charlotte Smith to the Brontes*, University Park: Pennsylvania State University Press.

Keene, F.W. (1995) 'The politics of forgiveness', *On the Issues*, Fall: 32–35.

Lamb, S. (1996) *The trouble with blame: victims, perpetrators, and responsibility*, Cambridge: Harvard University Press.

Lamb, S. (1999) *New versions of victims: feminists struggle with the concept*, New York: New York University Press.

Lamb, S. (2002) 'Women, abuse and forgiveness: a special case', in S. Lamb and J.G. Murphy (eds) *Before forgiving: cautionary views of forgiveness in psychotherapy*, New York: Oxford University Press, pp. 155–171.

Lockhart, L. and White, B.W. (1989) 'Understanding marital violence in the black community', *Journal of Interpersonal Violence* 4: 421–436.

Loftus, E. and Ketchum, K. (1994) *The myth of repressed memory*, New York: St. Martin's Press.

McGillivray, A. and Comaskey, B. (1999) *Black eyes all of the time: intimate violence, Aboriginal women, and the justice system*, Toronto: University of Toronto Press.

Miller, P. (1995) 'Personal storytelling in everyday life: social and cultural perspectives', in R.S. Wyer Jr (ed.) *Knowledge and memory: the real story*, Hillsdale: Earlbaum.

Minsky, R. (1998) *Psychoanalysis and culture*, Cambridge, UK: Polity Press.

Mohanram, Radhika (1999) *Black body: women, colonialism, and space*, Minneapolis: University of Minneapolis Press.

Rich, A. (1977) 'It is the lesbian in us', *Sinister Wisdom 3*.

Richie, B.E. (2000) 'A black feminist reflection on the antiviolence movement', *Signs: Journal of Women in Culture and Society* 25, 4: 1133–1137.

Rose, J. (1986) *Sexuality in the field of vision*, London: Verso.

Rustin, Michael (1991) *The good society and the Inner world: psychoanalysis, politics and culture*, London: Verso.

Walker, L. (1984) *The battered woman syndrome*, New York: Springer.

Walker, L. (1989) *Terrifying love: why battered women kill and how society responds*, New York: Harper & Row.

Walrond-Skinner, S. (1998) 'The function and role of forgiveness in working with couples and families: clearing the ground', *Journal of Family Therapy* 20: 3–19.

West, T.C. (1999) *Wounds of the spirit: black women, violence, and resistance ethics*, New York: New York University Press.

Westcott, M. (1998) 'Female relationality and the idealized self', in B.M. Clinchy and J.K. Norm (eds) *The gender and psychology reader*, New York: New York University Press, pp. 396–406.

White, E.C. (1994) *Chain, chain, change: for black women in abusive relationships*, Seattle: Seal Press.

Chapter 6

Creating discourses of 'false memory'

Media coverage and production dynamics[1]

Jenny Kitzinger

The role of 'naming' and what we commonly call 'memory' has become a highly contested space in debates around sexual violence across many parts of the world. Feminist activism and cultural changes during the last thirty years have allowed women to address or reconstruct events in their lives in unprecedented ways. Experiences of sexual violence have been re-defined, re-called, re-membered and re-constituted as ideas about what is possible, acceptable or normal have been transformed. Alongside this, the line between knowing and not knowing, forgetting and remembering, avoiding and confronting, has become a dynamic and often explicitly negotiated one. Nowhere has this been more marked than in the field of childhood sexual abuse. As the philosopher, Ian Hacking, comments:

> You might think that the experiences speak for themselves, at least for the victims. Yes – and yet events, no matter how painful or terrifying, have been experienced or recalled *as child abuse* only after consciousness-raising. That requires inventing new descriptions, providing new ways to see old acts – and a great deal of social agitation.
>
> (Hacking, 1995: 55, emphasis in original)

New description can thus beget new events:

> Old actions under new description may be re-experienced in memory. And if these are genuinely new descriptions, descriptions not available or perhaps non-existent at the time of the episodes remembered, then something is experienced now, in memory, that in a certain sense did not exist before. The action took place, but not the action under the new description.
>
> (Hacking, 1995: 249)

Outright opponents of feminist cultural transformations argue that such re-definition is a distortion of the truth based on mislabelling, fantasy or ideological bias (as if the 'correct' way to experience an action lay beyond cultural repertoires). More sophisticated concerns are raised by those sympathetic with feminism. Hacking's comments, quoted above, are presented in the context of his attack on the fashion for diagnosing multiple personality disorder – a dangerous tendency that has flourished alongside the discovery of sexual abuse. His concerns echo those of many feminists, including many of those who fought to create awareness about sexual abuse in the first place, but who now feel that the issue has been co-opted. Louise Armstrong, author of the groundbreaking exposé of incest, *Kiss Daddy Goodnight* (1978), challenges the subsequent growth of an abuse 'industry' which feeds into, and off, the proliferation of victims (Armstrong, 1994). Others question the popularising of sexual abuse as a trivialised catch-all cultural explanation and 'master narrative' (Haaken, 1999). Many feminists have also critically analysed the implicit ideologies in the psychiatric, therapy and self-help literature through which women are encouraged to process their experiences (Kelly, 1988; Kitzinger, 1992: Reavey and Warner, 2001).

The naming, definition and recall of sexual abuse needs to be understood in this context: a context of multi-layered disputes about the meaning of abusive experiences and their relationship to language, interpretation, reality, identity and politics (see, for example, Brown and Burman, 1997; Huntingdon, 1999; Lamb, 1999; Scott, 1997, 1998, 1999). Yet these sophisticated debates from *within* feminism rarely surface in the mass media and wider popular discourse. Instead, false memory syndrome has become the main way of understanding, typecasting and dismissing memories of abuse recovered in adulthood. The mass media have played a vital role in this, providing a mechanism through which false memory syndrome was created as a social issue and pushed into the public domain. This chapter examines how this happened.

The chapter draws on an empirical study of the 'false memory' story as it evolved in Britain. In addition to examining media coverage I also interviewed fifty-eight key actors from within the media (e.g. journalists and editors) and source organisations (e.g. the press officers of psychological societies and those involved with relevant pressure groups such as the British False Memory Society). My argument highlights the ways in which coverage of false memory syndrome was influenced by gendered power relations. I point to the selective privileging of 'masculine' over 'feminine' discourses, asymmetrical judgements about men's and women's emotions and credibility, the gendered operation of media formats and the impact of gender hierarchies within media organisations. The chapter concludes by arguing for feminist media analysis that includes attending to the context and practices that inform the production of media discourses.

The 'discovery' of false memory syndrome

The concept of false memory syndrome originated in the USA. In 1990, Jennifer Freyd, a cognitive psychology professor at the University of Oregon, began to recall incest. Her parents denied her memories and, by 1992, they had set up the False Memory Syndrome Foundation which attracted international attention. The 'false memory' argument is that, particularly as a result of therapy, people (usually women) can recover memories of abusive childhoods which are inaccurate and untrue. The proponents of false memory syndrome (FMS) argue that it is impossible to repress memories of repeated abuse in childhood, and then to recall them correctly as an adult. The issue is deeply embedded in debates about how the human brain evolves, and about the practice and regulation of therapy. However, the argument involves much more than this – the conflict reaches beyond the science of memory or disputes about professional training and qualifications to address far more fundamental struggles. Above all, the false memory debate is intimately intertwined with gender politics.

False memory syndrome rapidly shot to public prominence during the early to mid-1990s. The very first mention of this issue in the British media appeared in January 1993 (*Daily Telegraph*, 17 January 1993). This article referenced the debate already raging in America and continuing media interest was quickly fuelled by accounts from an accused father in England (e.g. 'When a Father Wakes up to his Worst Nightmare', *Sunday Telegraph*, 7 March 1993). This media attention facilitated accused parents contacting each other and mobilising into the British False Memory Society which, in turn, generated further reporting. In 1994 and 1995 there were over 125 items about FMS in just three daily and three Sunday broadsheets (*The Times, Independent, Guardian, Sunday Times, Observer* and *Independent on Sunday*). This coverage included front-page stories, editorials and lengthy features in the weekend supplements. For example, the *Sunday Times* invited reader empathy with their report entitled: ' "Memories" that surface to destroy us' (15 May 1994) and the subject was the cover story of the *Guardian Weekend* on three separate occasions: 'Total recall? How false memory syndrome reveals a past that never was' (6 January 1994); 'What memories are made of' (23 July 1994); 'Remember Daddy' (28 December 1995). The tabloids also eagerly pursued the story with headlines such as 'Therapy of danger: how this sick girl came to believe that her loving parents abused her.' (*Mail on Sunday*, 5 December 1995), 'Father's nightmare: daughter made up rape story after therapist's counselling' (*Mail*, 29 March 1995) and 'Mind-bending treatments need testing' (*Mail on Sunday*, 5 December 1995). False memory syndrome was also discussed in chat shows and documentaries and was aired on national TV news, including two lengthy discussions on the flagship BBC news programme *Newsnight* (17 February 1994; 12 January 1995).

There are four key features worth noting in addition to the breadth and extent of media reporting. The first feature is the *speed* with which the issue attracted attention. The rapid media response is particularly noticeable if one compares it to other social problems, such as attempts to highlight male violence in the first place. During the 1970s many women's organisations had been working around such issues long before journalists became interested (Tierney, 1982). By contrast, press and TV attention to FMS was simultaneous and symbiotic with pressure group activity. The second key feature is that the majority of coverage promoted the idea that false memory syndrome was a real and common problem, in spite of the, at that time, lack of official endorsement. The third noteworthy feature was the priority given to lay opinion. In a break with usual journalistic practice, lay people (accused parents) were actually more likely to be quoted in the press than professional experts (Kitzinger and Reilly, 1997). The fourth and final point to note is the privileging of the voices of those denying abuse over the voices of those recalling abuse. For example, accused parents were seven times more likely to be quoted in the newspapers than the person recalling the abuse. In addition, when the experiences of those recalling abuse *were* reported, this was often based on descriptions by sceptical members of their family who presented them only in order to discredit them.

The extent, timing, form and trajectory of media coverage of FMS raise some obvious questions. How was a small and unofficial organisation (the BFMS) able to achieve such remarkable success in defining a new social problem? Why did journalists disregard their traditional respect for the authority of experts over lay people? How did accused parents manage to dominate the media coverage – ensuring their own voices were heard, and controlling the voices of their accusers? I will explore these questions through looking first at the strategies adopted by the BFMS and then at the internal dynamics and response of media organisations. In each case I will focus on how gender operated as one crucial element.

Pressure group strategies and resources

There were three gender-related factors crucial to the operation of the British False Memory Society as a media source. The first important factor is the rhetoric and history surrounding the relationship between science, emotion and women. The terminology of 'false memory syndrome' is itself a good marketing tool. It is a catchy and 'media-friendly' phrase which spotlights and problematises the Daughter's accusation rather than the Father's denials and draws on a long tradition of dismissing women as suggestible, unstable and prone to hysteria (Chesler, 1989). The importance of using (pseudo)psychiatric terminology was recognised early on by parents confronting accusations from their grown-up children. The BFMS was originally called Adult Children Accusing Parents, until quickly renaming itself in a way which made it sound more like a learned society than a pressure group. In addition, proponents of FMS constantly allied their perspective with a traditional image of masculine science (hard, objective, providing direct access to truth) and accused their opponents of being biased and led by emotion rather than 'facts'. This division inhibited some female psychologists from adopting a high public profile in opposition to the FMS hypothesis. In interview with me, several commented that it was particularly dangerous for women academics to associate themselves with any position seen as scientifically marginal. Any woman who did this risked being typecast as a feminist instead of an intellectual (as if the two categories are mutually exclusive).

The second key factor in the success of the BFMS was its practical and social resources. At first glance this pressure group had none of the 'source capital' traditionally associated with professional or government bodies who are able to influence the media agenda (Miller *et al.*, 1998). This was a small group with no established contacts with the media and lacking any official status. It was not part of journalists' routine beat and had few actual events to offer as news hooks. However, unlike the professional therapy or psychological organisations, the BFMS was able to respond quickly to the media and to initiate its own publicity in a very focused and effective way. In fact, although resource poor in traditional terms, the BFMS drew on highly motivated activists and had the support of eminent upper class and professional allies. As a representative explained:

> The nucleus [of the BFMS] was accused parents so there was a mother who was accused by her son who herself worked for a charity. There was a solicitor, ... there was a minister [of religion], ... There was a peer who'd been accused ... You name it, we've got it – judges, barristers, solicitors, doctors ...

In addition, the BFMS set up a scientific advisory board involving senior academics in psychology, psychiatry and psychoanalysis. When I interviewed some of these individuals they emphasised that their motivation for involvement with the BFMS was based on their assessment of the science. They talked about their reservations about the evidential status of repressed memories, concern about the damage done to families and worries about the professional status of psychiatry and psychotherapy. However, one member of the BFMS advisory board also commented on his reactions to the first meeting of the board in the following terms:

> I sat and looked around this table ... I couldn't help but be struck with what seemed to be the relative ease with which [the BFMS] ... had gathered this incredibly impressive bunch of academics. ... I think we

are very sensitive, males, ... about the feminist agenda. I can't believe that this assembly of figures of approximately 20 men and one woman isn't something to do with men, if you like, rushing in to protect their image.... I think it's a defensive operation. That is to say recovered memories has as part of its hidden agenda the demonisation of men.

The third and perhaps most important resource that the BFMS were able to tap into was the power of their own stories: stories of irrational accusations and innocent families torn apart. The BFMS were acutely aware of the impact of such personal accounts on several levels. As a representative of the Society explained: 'with every journalist that comes here we offer to put them in touch with other families and ... they realise that these are perfectly decent, normal people, and they see that something strange is going on.' It was not only that meeting parents helped convince journalists of the justice of the BFMS cause, such interviews also provided valuable bases for feature articles and human-interest profiles. It is noticeable that the early reporting about FMS was not predominantly in 'hard news' form (event-oriented, front-page coverage). Instead, FMS entered the mass media through feature articles, television chat shows, discussion and magazine programmes and coverage on women's pages: often relying heavily on personal accounts from accused parents. One of the very early articles appeared on the women's page of the right-wing tabloid paper, the *Daily Mail*. The headline asked, 'Did this man abuse his child?' and declared 'New theories suggest that some women who claim they've been sexually molested by their fathers are, in fact, making it up' (3 March 1993). The picture showed a disguised image of an accused father with the caption, 'I'm the only one who really knows the truth'. The article was entirely devoted to his challenge to his daughter's perceptions of reality – without any response from her being included. This account ironically appeared under the page heading, 'Femail Testimony'. Clearly *'femail* testimony' can be the antithesis of *'female* testimony'.

The style of such reporting, combined with comments from journalists I interviewed, highlights an interesting double standard around men's and women's emotional reactions. Journalists routinely referred to men's feelings to signal these men's sincerity. They made comments such as: 'he was so obviously totally bemused and confused' or 'their distress is quite terrible to see'. In one television programme the father himself highlighted the unusual status of men admitting emotion. He detailed the accusation against him, and expressing his despair, provided his own commentary: 'I've cried and cried and cried, and that, for me, that's an admission I would never have ... I ... I can hardly believe I'm saying it' (*Strange Days*, BBC2, 2 June 1996). By contrast, women's emotionality was often used to discredit them. Journalists in interviews with me, and in their writing, dismissed women's accounts of remembered abuse through descriptions of their 'obvious vulnerability', 'fragility' and 'near hysteria'. This double standard was pointed out very concisely by one woman I interviewed whose father had publicly accused her of suffering from FMS. She was extremely angry about the media representation of her case: 'He can use his suicidal thoughts as proof of his innocence,' she commented, 'my suicidal thoughts are proof of my guilt.'

Media production processes

The supportive media reporting was partly related to the BFMS's resources and strategies but it was also related to complementary dynamics within the media at the time. Without a receptive media the BFMS would have been powerless to make the impact that it did. I will therefore now go on to discuss factors within the media that complemented the strategies of the British False Memory Society, making media outlets particularly receptive to the FMS story and inform the positive nature of the coverage.

Story fatigue and the potential of FMS to provide a 'new angle'

False memory syndrome was introduced to the media at a time when media attention to the standard sexual abuse story was waning. By the beginning of the 1990s there was a general feeling among both journalists and press officers that sexual abuse was no longer considered news. There was a declining interest in sexual abuse, pointing to what one reporter called 'child abuse fatigue' (Kitzinger and Skidmore, 1995).

The media's fatigue with sexual abuse was accompanied, according to some journalists, by a desire to challenge old established truths and a feeling that the problem may have been exaggerated. As one journalist pointed out: 'the whole boredom factor on child sexual abuse means that ... there's a general climate of let's find out this isn't true.' A point reinforced by a second journalist who commented that: 'everyone was getting sick with the child abuse story. They were sick to death of it, every day another celebrity popped up saying they had been abused as a child and people wanted something new.'

When, in the early 1990s, fathers (and mothers) began to protest about being falsely accused by their grown-up offspring this then was seen to provide a 'new angle' and be a 'hot topic'. Not only this, but FMS could also be seen to illustrate a growing 'problem of our time'. This gave it extra value to journalists for whom capturing the Zeitgeist is an important professional aim.

Capturing the Zeitgeist and challenging the 'matriarchal terror squads'

False memory syndrome was often used to illustrate newspaper or television reporters' general theories about the state of contemporary society. FMS was, for example, addressed in *Strange Days*, a TV series of polemical explorations of 'superstitions in the 1990s' (*Strange Days*, BBC2, 2 June 1996). It was also often used by right-wing newspapers to illustrate a growing social problem: the threat of political correctness, inappropriate intervention into family life and the power of feminist ideology. The *Daily Telegraph*, for example, informed readers that false memory was a product of a society 'run by vengeful maniacs, who more than condone the explosion of parent abuse in this country' (5 February 1993). In *The Times* the cultivation of false memories was associated with 'the still blossoming cult of "sexual harassment"' (2 December 1993). Its sister paper, The *Sunday Times* cited the spread of false memories as evidence of a 'shift in the collective psyche'. 'Stand up the usual suspects,' declared the journalist, 'an unstoppable child abuse industry; a feminist agenda that regards all men as bogeymen; a climate in which people are encouraged to see themselves as victims' (17 April 1994). One commentator even presented FMS as evidence that 'We live in an age of matriarchal terror squads' and concluded: 'How was it possible, we all asked, for people to watch what was happening in Germany during the 1930s? Open your eyes and look around' (*Sunday Times*, 15 May 1994).[2]

Gendered identification and judgements of source credibility

The third factor influencing the profile of FMS and, in particular, the dominance of the voices of accused fathers (and some mothers), is the issue of 'journalistic intuition' and identification. Journalists emphasised that they relied on a 'sixth sense' in assessing the validity of their sources' accounts. This journalistic 'nose' for a source's credibility is a valued professional skill. As one journalist commented:

> You actually have got to make an assessment quite quickly, do I find this person credible or not? ... What I'm doing is watching the way they talk, I'm watching their mannerisms, I'm watching the way they construct sentences, what they say and what they leave out. How are they trying to relate to me? ... Because when you get back to the office what your editor says is, 'Well, did you find them credible or not?' and you have to say 'yes' or 'no'.

In documenting the personal account of an accused father (or the person who is accusing him) journalists make judgements based on their reaction to the protagonist(s). This is crucial in the false memory debate, given that the credibility of the parents proved to be much greater than that attributed to their offspring. The FMS debate is characterised by parents (usually fathers) who are white, heterosexual, successful, middle class, professionals. They are often rather like the journalists who are interviewing them and they certainly do not conform to the stereotypes associated with child abusers (Kitzinger, 1996, 1999). Several journalists emphasised in interview the nice and plausible nature of the BFMS parents. They made comments such as: 'They were a lovely couple … my gut reaction was positive' and 'these particular parents, I just believed instantly'. Often there was an explicit empathy with the parents, a feeling that 'there but for the grace of God go I'. Thus, for example, one *Sunday Times* journalist recorded his sudden concern about being naked with his young daughter. He speculated whether this moment might be 'unwittingly filed away, just one fragment for a mosaic of repressed memories to be unveiled in all their awful wonder by a psychotherapist 20 years hence' (17 April 1994).

Such empathy and identification was often in sharp contrast to journalists' reactions to the adult offspring who were accusing their parents of abuse. Often their access to these sons and daughters was, in any case, very limited or indirect. For example, several journalists were influenced by one father playing them the message left on his answer phone by his daughter – her tone of voice and nature of her accusations made them feel she was 'clearly disturbed' and 'hysterical'. Those asserting that they have been victims of abuse may also have low credibility, because as one television reporter commented: 'They may have taken drugs, they may have gone into alcohol, they may be slightly unbalanced. So we never quite trust them.'

The importance of such judgements is quite explicit in an article about FMS by Simon Hoggart. 'There is a new witch hunt in Britain: to root out child abusers,' he wrote, 'But are some "victims" just having ideas put into their heads?' He went on to describe his visit to one accused father: 'We are in a pleasant middle-class sitting room in Southern England, and Ronald is playing back his daughter's voice from the answer phone. Hoggart acknowledges that 'of course' the accusations 'may be true' but:

> As one talks to him, a mild-mannered former naval officer, it doesn't seem awfully likely, however, and the less so because the daughter's voice has that quality one associates with the care-in-the-community lunatics sometimes heard in the street or on station platforms: a flat, unchanging aggression which claims to be directed at the outside world, but which is clearly fomented by an inner turmoil.
>
> (*Observer*, 27 March 1994)

Male-dominated media organisation

Credibility judgements are not just made by the individual journalist doing the interview; senior editorial staff may intervene at a later stage in proceedings. While both male and female journalists used their 'gut feelings' in judging source credibility, some female journalists who were critical of the BFMS claimed that their gut feelings were dismissed by male editors as 'subjective' or 'biased'. By contrast, they thought that their male colleagues' gut feelings were seen to constitute 'common sense' or 'professional instinct'. Women journalists who felt uneasy about the accused fathers or attempted to analyse the BFMS's 'power base' and 'dubious connections' sometimes felt that they were dismissed as promoting 'simplistic conspiracy theory'. One female journalist also commented that her very expertise in the area of sexual abuse was seen to disqualify her as biased (Kitzinger, 1998). By contrast, some journalists who were more sympathetic to the BFMS were aware that this met with approval from senior male colleagues. One female journalist described the 'total glee' with which editorial staff responded to her own article attacking psychotherapy. In their view, she commented, 'therapists are kind of weak-minded and they're in the business of feelings, which in journalism is the bloody last thing that you would ever express in the office.'

The importance of a male-dominated hierarchy within media organisations was vividly illustrated by one case in which there was explicit conflict between the male and female staff. It is this example which I will use to conclude this chapter.

In a key potential development in the FMS story, a woman journalist, with the support of the women's page editor, gained interviews with two daughters of one of the leading members of the BFMS. This man's story had appeared repeatedly in magazines, newspaper articles and television reports. Two of his daughters decided they were prepared to tell their side of the story. The two women disputed their father's description both of their childhood and adult relationship with him and challenged his account of the way in which their memories were recovered. In straight news value terms interviews with these particular sisters clearly had the potential for a good story. It was a scoop and was new in that it overtly contradicted a series of accounts which had appeared in other newspapers. Their accounts not only provided a different perspective on an individual case but also implicitly challenged the validity of the FMS movement. As the journalist concerned commented: 'At its absolute basis people just said "it's a good story and nobody else has got it".'

However, in the event this story never reached the public. Although the father's story had repeatedly appeared in the media without any rebuttal from his daughters, the newspaper's lawyers advised against publishing the daughters' accounts, without allowing the father a parallel right of reply in an article of equal length. An interviewer was duly dispatched to provide this 'balance' and that second article was drafted. However, the two sisters refused to have their accounts appear in this way. The journalist who had originally interviewed them was unable to persuade her paper to compromise in spite of the full support of the editor of the woman's page. 'Legally we could not persuade the lawyers,' she commented:

> And it was really interesting that the whole massed male ranks of the paper were just saying 'Well, this guy seems alright ... what's the matter with him? Yeah, well, this girl has been to see a therapist you know, are you sure she's alright?' [...] I remember just sitting there in the office with this gaggle of suits around me, and they're going: 'You can't run this, you know, seems like a decent chap.'

Conclusion

The media have a key role in how we understand the world around us and even the landscape inside our own heads. Media coverage can influence our identity, how we talk with each other, how we interpret other people's stories and the very ways in which we experience our lives (Kitzinger, 2001). Yet what is represented in the media, whose voices are heard, and how they are portrayed, is a highly selective process. This is why feminists have for so long been interested in analysing media representations. I hope that this chapter has shown the value of such analysis and, in addition, highlighted the value of going beyond the analysis of media texts and towards exploring how journalists and their sources operate and interact. Media reporting is influenced by news values, hierarchies of credibility, journalistic routines and dominant cultural assumptions (Hall *et al.*, 1978; Schudson, 1989; Tuchman, 1978). Coverage is shaped by struggles within media organisations as well as competition between diverse pressure groups seeking to influence public perceptions (Ericson *et al.*, 1989; Schlesinger, 1990; Miller *et al.*, 1998). The arguments presented here highlight the gender politics running through these processes. I have shown how media attention to FMS was influenced by factors varying from the masculine values of the newsroom and the gut reactions of journalists to the differential assessment of men and women's anger and distress. Gender politics ran through all elements of the story's production, from the resources and strategies used by the proponents of FMS through to journalists' gendered judgements about source credibility. Indeed, it would be impossible to tell the false memory syndrome story without attention to the gender politics within which it is embedded.

The analysis presented here also raises crucial questions about the role of diverse TV and press formats. In the 1970s, Tuchman asked whether women's pages could be a resource for the women's movement (1978). In the new millennium, other questions may now be equally pertinent. What are the limits of the woman's page as a non-autonomous space within a male-dominated newspaper and can the woman's page sometimes be used against women (especially in right-wing newspapers where the interests of women, men, children and the family are seen as coterminous)? My research also raises more general questions about the role of 'soft' outlets in the media. Mainstream media analysts have often disregarded soft and low-status media formats but it is becoming increasingly evident that this is an important site of cultural influence (Henderson and Kitzinger, 1999). Certainly, as the FMS story highlights, 'soft' formats may act as a crucial point of entry for the emergence of new public issues. The way in which the proponents of FMS used human interest stories and exploited the asymmetrical status of men's and women's emotions highlights potential problems in such forms. At the very least the FMS story highlights the dangers of formats which offer raw experience without social analysis or simply encourage a theatre of feeling (whether that is endless accounts of the trauma of sexual victimisation, or of false accusations).

This chapter began by commenting on the need for increased feminist analysis of news production processes, and I hope that it has illustrated the continuing importance of this area of enquiry. I have sought to explore the *processes* and the *extent* to which 'the group which dominates newsrooms ... also dominates news judgements' (Gist, 1993: 109). Organisational hierarchies are clearly important; however gender politics do not simply operate though structures, but through a whole series of discourses, norms, unspoken assumptions and empathetic identifications. Critical analysis of news production should include unpacking the relationship between 'femininity', 'femaleness' and 'feminism' and, indeed, analysing the operation of men and masculinities as they act upon, and are constructed across, the pages of newspapers and on television. This is an urgent task for all those interested in the operation of media power and anyone concerned with the construction and location of women and men in contemporary society.

Notes

1 This chapter is adapted from a chapter that originally appeared in Carter, C., Branston, G. and Allan, S. (eds) *News, gender and power*, London: Routledge. Thanks are due to Routledge for permission to reproduce these sections. Thanks are also due to the ESRC for research grant no. L211252010.
2 The emergence of 'false memory syndrome' as a public issue built on the source networks and news agenda established after Cleveland, Rochdale and Orkney (scandals involving disputed allegations of abuse and professional malpractice). In fact, the very first report about false memories in the British press drew on a statement from Parents Against Injustice, a group which came to prominence after the Cleveland case (*Sunday Telegraph*, 17 January 1993). 'False memory' thus did not emerge out of nowhere. It neatly fitted in with a media 'template'

emphasising a series of previous 'scandals' and drew on previously established source organisations as well as the 'collective memory' of both audiences and journalists (Kitzinger, 2000).

References

Armstrong, L. (1978) *Kiss daddy goodnight*, New York: Profile Books.

Armstrong, L. (1994) *Rocking the cradle of sexual politics: what happened when women said incest*, New York: Addison Wesley.

Brown, L. and Burman, E. (1997) 'The delayed memory debate: why feminist voices matter', *Feminism and Psychology* 7, 1: 7–16.

Chesler, P. (1989) *Women and madness*, London: Harcourt Brace Jovanovich.

Ericson, R., Baranek, P. and Chan, J. (1989) *Negotiating control,* Milton Keynes: Open University Press.

Gist, M. (1993) 'Through the looking glass: diversity and reflected appraisals of self in mass media', in P. Creedon (ed.) *Women in mass communication*, London: Sage, pp. 104–126.

Haaken, J. (1999) 'Heretical texts: the Courage to Heal and the incest survivor movement', in S. Lamb (ed.) *New versions of victims: feminists struggle with the concept*, New York: New York University Press, pp. 13–41.

Hacking, I. (1995) *Rewriting the soul: multiple personality and the sciences of memory*, Princeton: Princeton University Press.

Hall, S., Critcher, C., Jefferson, T., Clarke, J. and Roberts, B. (1978) *Policing the crisis: mugging, the state and law and order*, London: Macmillan.

Henderson, L. and Kitzinger, J. (1999) 'The human drama of genetics: "hard" and "soft" media representations of inherited breast cancer', *Sociology of Health and Illness* 21, 5: 560–578.

Huntingdon, A. (1999) 'A critical response to Sara Scott's "Here be dragons; researching the unbelievable, hearing the unthinkable. A feminist sociologist in unchartered territory"', *Sociological Research Online* 4, 1: [www.socres-online.org/uk/socreonline/4/1/huntingdon.html].

Kelly, L. (1988) 'From politics to pathology: the medicalisation of the impact of rape and child sexual abuse', *Radical Community Medicine* 36: 14–18.

Kitzinger, J. (1992) 'Sexual violence and compulsory heterosexuality', *Feminism and Psychology* 2, 3: 399–418.

Kitzinger, J. (1996) 'Media representations of sexual abuse risks', *Child Abuse Review* 5, 5: 319–333.

Kitzinger, J. (1998) 'The gender-politics of news production: silenced voices and false memories', in C. Carter., G. Branston and S. Allan (eds) *News, gender and power*, London: Routledge, pp. 186–203.

Kitzinger, J. (1999) 'The ultimate neighbour from hell? Stranger danger and the media representation of paedophilia', in B. Franklin (ed.) *Social policy, the media and misrepresentation*, London: Routledge, pp. 207–221.

Kitzinger, J. (2000) 'Media templates: patterns of association and the (re)construc-tion of meaning over time', *Media, culture and society* 22, 1: 64–84.

Kitzinger, J. (2001) 'Transformations of public and private knowledge: audience reception, feminism and the experience of childhood sexual abuse', *Feminist Media Studies* 1, 1: 91–104.

Kitzinger, J. and Reilly, J. (1997) 'The rise and fall of risk reporting', *The European Journal of Communication* 12, 3: 319–350.

Kitzinger, J. and Skidmore, P. (1995) 'Playing safe: media coverage of the prevention of child sexual abuse', *Child Abuse Review* 4, 1: 47–56.

Lamb, S. (ed.) (1999) *New versions of victims: feminists struggle with the concept*, New York: New York University Press.

Miller, D., Kitzinger, J., Williams, K. and Beharrell, P. (1998) *The circuit of mass communication*, London: Sage.

Reavey, P. and Warner, S. (2001) 'Curing women: child sexual abuse, therapy and the construction of femininity', *The International Journal of Critical Psychology* Special Issue on Sex and Sexualities 3: 49–71.

Schlesinger, P. (1990) 'Rethinking the sociology of journalism: source strategies and the limits of media centrism', in M. Fergurson (ed.) *Public communication: the new imperatives*, London: Sage, pp. 61–84.

Schudson, M. (1989) 'The sociology of news production', *Media, culture and society* 11, 3: 263–282.

Scott, S. (1997) 'Feminists and false memories: a case of postmodern amnesia' *Feminism and Psychology* 7, 1: 33–38.

Scott, S. (1998) 'Here be Dragons: researching the unbelievable, hearing the unthinkable. A feminist sociologist in unchartered territory', *Sociological Research Online* 3, 3: [www.socresonline.org/uk/socreonline/3/3/1.html].

Scott, S. (1999) 'Dancing to different tunes: a reply to response to Here be Dragons', *Sociological Research Online* 4, 2: [www.socresonline.org/uk/socreonline/4/2/scott_sara.html].

Tierney, K. (1982) 'The battered women movement and the creation of the wife-beating problem', *Social Problems* 29, 3: 207–220.

Tuchman, G. (1978) *Making news: a study of the construction of reality*, New York: Free Press.

Chapter 7

The vigilant(e) parent and the paedophile

The *News of the World* campaign 2000 and the contemporary governmentality of child sexual abuse

Vikki Bell

Introduction

This chapter is informed by the work of Michel Foucault in so far as it is a contemporary study of bio-politics.[1] Foucault's term 'bio-politics' (1981; see also Bell, 1995) refers to an analytical perspective that comprehends the politics of governing as reliant upon the disciplined modes of embodiment and styles of judgement that the populus are invited to 'freely' adopt. Attention is therefore given both to forms of conduct at the local embodied level and to broader strategies of 'power/knowledge' whose development describe more general patterns of socio-political change. In particular, bio-politics focuses attention on the regulatory strategies by which processes of normalisation are maintained and which extend one's analysis beyond state power. This is the lead that is taken up by Miller and Rose (1992; see also, e.g. Rose, 1999) under the term Foucault proposed: 'governmentality'. Within neo-liberal societies, this argument runs, people are governed at a distance and through their freedom, positioned within regulatory strategies that operate within the many intersecting domains we pass through in our lives. Within this chapter, I am interested to take a look at the furore that took place in Britain in the summer of 2000 around child sexual abuse by locating it within contemporary modes by which people have been invited to think about the risk of child sexual abuse. Importantly, if one is thinking through the lens of a 'governmentality analysis' it would not be sufficient to consider in isolation the figure of the 'paedophile' who emerged within these public debates. The problematisation (Foucault, 1988) of 'the paedophile' has to be understood within the normalising strategies of power/knowledge that produce him, and would therefore include a relation to other figures who will surround and 'support' this production,[2] as well as the contemporary modes of bio-political government that form the wider setting within which these figures emerge. All of these lines of analysis are parts of the analytic puzzle.

Looking remarkably like Lombroso's table of criminals,[3] a table of photographs appeared in a British national Sunday newspaper in the summer of 2000. The table was presented with the ostensible aim of informing the public of the appearance, age, crime, punishment and whereabouts of those who had been convicted of a variety of sexual offences grouped (by the newspaper and the ensuing furore) under the term 'paedophilia'. The *News of the World*'s campaign, which came to be known as the 'name and shame' campaign, presented these tables as neither scientific evidence nor within a theory of insanity, but as a form of public information, information that had been deemed by official bodies involved in governing child sexual abuse(rs) too dangerous to be made publicly available. The newspaper's intervention caused a storm of controversy in Britain, which focused principally on the contested rationalities of present modes of government of child sexual abuse and abusers. Politicians, journalists, police chiefs, lawyers, pressure groups and parents engaged in protracted and vociferous debates.[4]

The campaign was launched in the aftermath of the abduction and murder of Sarah Payne, an eight-year-old girl in West Sussex, England, who went missing on the short walk across a field to her grandparents' home after playing with her siblings. Every day the national media reported on developments in the search to try to find her, and her parents and siblings made appeals to her and to the public to help in her safe return. The discovery of Sarah's body on 18 July was met with widespread sorrow, and an estimated 30,000 people visited the site where she was found, many to lay flowers in her memory. In this period of heightened emotion, the *News of the World* published the photographs to which I refer to above with the front page headline reading: 'If you're a parent you must read this: Named, Shamed' and the text continuing 'There are 110,000 child sex offenders in Britain, one for every square mile. The murder of Sarah Payne has proved police monitoring of these perverts is not enough. So we are revealing WHO they are and WHERE they are ... starting today' (23 July 2000: 1).

This was the beginning of the campaign which saw the weekly newspaper publish the photographs, names and locations of convicted child sexual offenders and which it vowed to continue: 'week in week out we will add to our record so that every parent in the land can have the RIGHT to know where these people are living.' (23 July 2000: 2). As well as publishing these 'tables', as it turned out on only one further occasion (30 July 2000), the *News of the World* made certain demands for legal changes, specifically public access to the sexual offenders register, a form of the USA's 'Megan's law', which the paper called 'Sarah's law'. Furthermore, despite the newspaper's request for readers not to engage in vigilante actions, one group of mothers on the Paulsgrove housing estate in Hampshire received much media attention as they organised local parents in nightly marches, holding 'vigils' outside the homes of those known 'pae-dophiles' on their estate and protesting at the housing of those convicted of child sexual offences in their locale. One mother explained that, in the wake of Sarah Payne's murder, 'The mums decided we had to do some-thing. Someone said that one lived there and we started marching' (the *Mirror*, 11 August 2000: 9). Each night over the course of the next week, they marched through their housing estate. Over the next few weeks, stories of the actions of mothers 'turned vigilantes' were widely reported, mostly focusing on the Paulsgrove estate but also elsewhere, as well as stories of convicted sexual offenders fleeing their homes, being confronted by angry mobs, having property or relatives attacked and, a fortnight or so after the *News of the World* campaign began, taking their own lives. Offi-cial response, and that of the 'quality' newspapers, was to express sym-pathy with the mothers' sentiments but to decline to support the campaign's demands or the actions of the mothers and their prompting of 'vigilante' attacks.

Pressure mounted on the *News of the World* to halt the campaign, which they did, claiming victories at least in terms of the level of public support received and the discussions they had instigated between 'power-ful agencies' such as the Association of Chief Police Officers, the NSPCC, NACRO and the Association of Chief Officers of Probation (*News of the World*, 6 August 2000: 6). The parents at Paulsgrove also suspended their protests, but gathered at least once more, holding a candlelit vigil, as well as discussing strategy and taking part in meetings with their local council.

It is important how we remember these events, and to recognise that there is never just one account. Thus although it would not be untrue to argue, as does Haug (2001), that this was an occasion on which the public were whipped up by the newspaper in question into a storm of anger in the midst of which the figure of 'the paedophile' became a monster for our times, such an account does not give attention to various other aspects of the wider bio-political context. Nevertheless it is, of course, important to look at the way the figure of 'the paedophile' emerged in these debates. In particular I would argue that it is important to note that no one ventured an interpretation of the images in terms of *types* and indeed, the images themselves received no comment, suggesting that, in the public imagina-tion at least, the 'paedophile' has lost any ability to be rendered into cred-ible knowledge; no one seemed to be interested within this debate in pursuing a theoretical explanation of child sexual abuse, psychological, feminist, cultural or otherwise, that might be able to make pronounce-ments on the characteristics of the child sexual abuser as a type beyond the fact that he was understood throughout as likely to commit repeated offences.[5] He has become, once again, an individual instance rather than an example of a type or an illustration of a theory. This was true both within a 'populist' discourse and an opposing 'liberal' one. In the first, 'the paedophile' was referred to by many as unintelligible, monstrous, evil, diseased, and perverted – e.g. amidst the many examples, in the *Mirror*: 'these people ... are inflicted with an incurable disease, the most terrifying disease there is' (18 July 2000: 4); in the *News of the World*: 'for these evil perverts there must be no hiding place' (16 July 2000: 6) and 'Does a monster live near you?' (23 July 2000: 2) – in ways that drew a line between him and normal individuals casting him as a constant and irredeemable danger, existing within the realm of the inhuman and the unknowable. In the opposing 'liberal' discourse, he was understood as an offender who like any other, the sexual nature of the crime notwithstanding, has human rights such that he should be given the benefit of attempts at rehabilitation and resettlement with anonymity.[6] Furthermore, it is important to note how notions of home and the family, cornerstones of ideologies that feminists have repeatedly critiqued, emerged intact, with 'the paedophile' understood as a figure existing outside the home, where the main danger to children was understood to lie by the dominating discourses.[7]

However, as I've indicated, it is also important to consider the context in which this figure appears, and to connect his appearance with other figures who appear simultaneously within the problematisation of child sexual abuse. In this chapter, I want to suggest that a focus on the figure of the mother/parent, and these parents' actions, is as significant in the analysis of these events as a focus on the constitution of 'the paedophile'. Moreover, it is incumbent upon a feminist analysis to consider the actions of the women protesters beyond an understanding of them as the reactionary dupes of a profit-seeking media. And this especially so given the fact that feminism has wanted to get child sexual abuse understood as widespread and as a serious matter, and the fact that feminist politics often implicitly endorses forms of direct action by women 'doing something' by taking up public space and the attention of the public sphere. In this chapter, therefore, I will follow a few of the many avenues of exploration that one might pursue in relation to the contemporary problematisation of child sexual abuse through these events, with a focus on the parents/mothers. First, I argue that one can understand the episode in terms of a legitimation crisis in the contemporary governmentality of child sexual abuse which resulted from the questioning of the specific role that parents are required to adopt within its rationalities. The depiction of the parents' protests as vigilante action is overdetermined by the contemporary position in which parents are required to act as risk-assessing – and therefore as ever-vigilant – parents. I argue that how the line between the vigilant and the vigilante is constituted and governed in 'normal' circumstances depends upon the level of trust that is generated in parents, understood in turn as their faith in both a basic general level of security of the society in which they parent and the information that is available to them by which to make risk-assessments with regard to their children's safety. Second, I argue that this 'crisis' was averted by the re-establishment of lines of government between parents, the public sphere, public agencies/institutions and government so that the danger posed to contemporary rationalities passed over. As well as drawing upon the depictions of the parents as irrational, this re-establishment involved interesting discursive manoeuvres with respect to notions of 'the public'. Third I pose the question suggested above: given the image of strong women challenging the state, what happens if we attempt to view the mothers' actions through a feminist lens?

Legitimation crisis in a 'risk' society

Within sociology, much has been written about 'risk society' and its operations. According to the thesis proposed by Ulrich Beck in *Risk Society* (1992), the language and procedures of our government and self-government in the developed world can be characterised as forms of risk assessment. Decisions made at the level of government, community or individual tend to be approached as, and couched within, the terms of risk, so that, *inter alia*, the effect is such that in order to make and to articulate a decision in life, individuals receive and respond to abstracted forms of knowledge, calculate risk and respond according to that calculation. Decisions ranging from whether to immunise our children to whether to take an umbrella on our walk involve balancing risks and making judgements based on probabilities. To put a Foucauldian gloss on this argument, one might say that individuals are encouraged to constitute themselves as risk-assessing subjects who receive knowledge, whether bidden or unbidden, and who proceed according to their response to that knowledge. Nikolas Rose has drawn attention to the 'relentless imperative of risk management' (1999: 160) as it has spread to encompass not only matters of personal insurance (pensions, health insurance and the like), where it has belonged historically, but also matters of lifestyle management.

Reading these trends towards 'risk assessment' culture through the prism of Jacques Donzelot's (1979) *The Policing of Families*, furthermore, one begins to develop a perspective on them as they relate to the government of families and the constitution of the modern parent. Donzelot argued that the position of the parent within governmental strategies has developed historically as the functions of parenting have transferred to the state, while the latter relies on the family as a principal site through which to deliver its good government of the citizenry and future citizens (children); the state therefore governs through the family and promises a certain autonomy to the family in return for its co-operation. Within the recent and contemporary government of the family, one could argue, the parental role has remained key for the implementation of policy decisions and political imaginations generally, while parents are invited to consider themselves independent of the state at least in familial matters.

Within contemporary Britain, one could argue, parents and especially mothers, are invited and expected to engage in an escalating number of risk assessments in relation to their children's health, education, psychological development and safety, and to practise rational parenting. Enabled in their task by information from a variety of official and unofficial experts and their range of knowledges (doctors and health visitors, OFSTED tables, developmental psychologists, pamphlets suggesting healthy eating and home safety tips, advice columns and websites for parents, self-help books and groups and so on), parents are entrusted with the care of the future generation while the government, relieved of the close management of this task, has only to provide a context of basic security, the institutional settings required (e.g. for health and education) along with general standardised forms of guidance from a distance. No one is unaware that the whole system operates with a certain level of threat. The consequences of approaching the parenting role inadequately would mean the balance of power becomes sharply asymmetrical. But for the most part this mode of government works not by surveillance and dictate but by encouraging adults to approach their parenting and their risk-assessing rationally.

The events of summer 2000 can be understood as what one might term a legitimation crisis, in the Habermassian sense, around this risk-assessment culture. This was a legitimation crisis in so far as there was a questioning of state legitimacy expressed by a public withdrawal of support from the official understanding of the parents' role by a small but voiciferous group; for a while, the mode in which the parents' rational risk-assessing role was being constituted was shaken. The *News of the World* campaign envisioned a mode of government whose rationality was dramatically at odds with the ways in which the British public have been officially invited to respond to child sexual abuse since it became an issue spoken about in the public sphere at all. As opposed to an official account that asks parents to engage in a rational assessment of risk (which they are advised is small) and to adopt a range of techniques for themselves and their children,[8] the newspaper campaign implied that the risk is in fact great and the perpetrators so numerous that parents need *specific* information about individuals in their local area so that they can teach their children to avoid *specific* individuals, not (just) specific types or categories (such as strange old men with sweets, or those who have unsupervised access to their children). According to this reading, the parents involved in the Paulsgrove protests and their supporters were staging a protest that contested the positioning of parents within the rationalities by which child sexual abuse and abusers are governed. The challenge was levied, first, on the basis that generalised information and statistics do not give *enough specific* information to assess the localised risks that faced their children. Second, it was levied on the basis that the parents no longer had faith in the government's own assessment of risk from those individuals already criminalised for sexual offences. Consequently they no longer had faith in the provision of a basic level of security within which parents are supposed to make their assessments.

As such, the campaign and the members of the public who protested, according to its logic, were not only attacking the sources of the danger, as they understood it, embodied in the 'paedophiles' but were also explicitly attacking the governmentality by which child sexual abuse and abusers are presently governed. In order to be good parents and to safeguard our children, they argued, we need the hard facts – the who and where – of individual threats, not the interpretation of aggregated national statistics and expert guidelines for creating good parenting techniques and safe neighbourhoods. The *Mirror*'s editorial, which wavered in its reaction to the *News of the World*'s campaign, nevertheless stated the point clearly: 'Ordinary families want one thing and one thing only – the right to know if their children are in danger from convicted perverts. The only way to deliver that assurance is to open the sex offenders register to public scrutiny' (4 August 2000: 6).

To fuel its demand for specific information through access to the public register, the *News of the World* reported stories from various states in the USA where access is more publicly available and in which children had been 'saved' from paedophiles in their area, including one of a woman who had recognised a neighbour on a police Internet site. He was subsequently arrested for violating his probation and admitted fantasising about children in the area (23 July 2000: 4). In contrast to these stories, reports reminded readers of cases in Britain where children have been killed by known abusers. For example, the *Mirror* carried the story of a ten-year-old girl who was killed in West Yorkshire by a known paedophile who had moved onto her estate, and contrasted 'Megan's law' with a Britain where 'we tip toe around criminals with grandiose plans of rehabilitation' (26 July 2000: 9).[9]

Despite the resemblance between the *News of the World*'s pages of photographs and the tables of Lombroso, therefore, the former appeared within a very different power–knowledge complex. These images appeared without any resultant argument about 'types' theories or causes. Indeed, theories such as Lombroso's are rejected in the presentation of the criminal as *unknowable* through general information such as that which founds 'expert' knowledge. Besides, the argument ran, in terms of giving the public information, generalised theories of atavistic leanings, or of abusers' childhoods or Oedipal difficulties for that matter, are unimportant; all the public needs, they declared, is the simple information as to which particular neighbours to avoid.[10]

Given that the contemporary rationalities by which child sexual abuse and abusers are governed are profoundly at odds with the way the *News of the World* campaign and its supporters were figuring the need for information and the possibilities of risk assessment, one would expect the official response to be dismissive. In the debates that followed, the task facing the 'official' line, and the one taken by the Home Secretary Jack Straw and Home Office Minister Paul Boateng, was to reaffirm the need to limit public knowledge to anonymised and generalised knowledge, with access to detailed knowledge reserved for governmental and legal bodies. In countering the fundamental challenge that the newspaper and the protesting parents represented, their response was to present the campaign and the protests as themselves representing the danger, both to individuals and to democratic justice. The parents, mostly mothers, who were arguing that their desire to be vigilant parents was being undermined by policies which refused them information, were quickly cast as vigilantes. Acting as they were from their personal situations of emotional connection with their own children, they were easily cast as having a volatile interest that was properly distinct from the overall and sober view that government must take.

Other newspapers tended to report the protests along these lines, depicting them as excessive eruptions of ungovernable irrational sentiment. The day after the *News of the World* began its campaign, for example, the *Guardian* reported several incidents, under the headline 'Innocents suffer when law of the lynch mob takes hold' (24 July 2000: 3), where child sexual offenders had been attacked or had killed themselves, where men had been wrongly identified as 'paedophiles', and where mobs had acted 'irrationally', in order to argue that the campaign would lead to 'vigilante actions'. A week later, the *Guardian* reported a group of sixty people waving banners, throwing paint and shouting abuse at a house in Plymouth that was wrongly identified as home to a paedophile (31 July 2000). The *Guardian* leader on 11 August 2000 made reference to the lessons to be found in Shakespeare's *Julius Caesar* – 'a mob, once roused, will not easily be stood down' – and reflected on the Paulsgrove 'anti-paedophilia protests' arguing that while there was justification for their anger and fear, their actions were both dangerous and *uncivilised*:

'Either way we just want them out of here,' said one of the protesters' leaders on Wednesday. What might be the evidence against someone convicted of no crime? 'Word of mouth,' she said. *What might count elsewhere as the basic principles of civilised society are a foreign language in Paulsgrove.*

This, then, is the real meaning of social exclusion. Thousands of estates have been allowed to become dustbins for the rest of society, out of sight and, until a moment like this one, out of mind. Now they are getting together, bonding as a community – if not quite the way the Prime Minister and all his communitarian rhetoric envisaged. *There are dangers here*, and not just from those who abuse children (emphasis added).

On 9 August 2000 a headline in the *Mirror* read: 'Vigilante Britain: paedophile kills himself after mob attacks his home,' reporting on the suicide of a fifty-year-old man the day before he was due to appear in court accused of assaulting a girl of four. Although he was not named in the *News of the World* campaign, he had been subject to threats and an angry crowd had gathered outside his home in North Manchester after he had appeared in court admitting three indecent assaults on young girls. His lawyer said he was 'terrified out of his wits by a newspaper name and shame campaign in the wake of Sarah Payne's murder' (p. 17). On the same page a photograph depicts three of the mothers and a man at the Paulsgrove estate, arms crossed in defiance, displaying a Union Jack flag on which is scrawled 'Paedophiles – a child never forgets why should you'. Two days later, the newspaper writes: 'Police have pleaded for an end to this vigilante action but the women here are a force to be reckoned with' (the *Mirror*, 11 August 2000: 9)

The parents' group protests were understood by no one as serious political engagements, but as either reactive protests or vigilante actions, depending on one's point of view, performed by those who felt threatened and decided instead to be threatening. One woman, 'Angela Pettinger, 46, a tough-talking mother of four' who became 'a figurehead in the nightly demonstrations' reportedly said that if the mothers laid their hands on a suspect, he 'would be lynched'; 'if they touched one of mine,' she continues, 'I'd do time for it' (the *Mirror*, 11 August 2000: 9). Another woman, speaking after a crowd had attacked the home and car of a man who had 'abused 140 youngsters', said 'we'd have ripped him to pieces' (the *Mirror*, 5 August 2000: 8). The language and provocative tactics of the mothers, that were potentially and actually violent in direct and indirect ways, meant their actions were presented as irrational, uncontrollable and indeed, as pre-modern, as outside the realm of 'the political' altogether. It was the mothers, in short, and no longer 'the child sexual abuser' who were depicted as atavistic.

Not only were they denied status as *political* comment, the *News of the World*'s campaign and the protesting parents were themselves depicted as abusive, especially in the sense of abusing childhood innocence, and the latter especially in relation to the involvement of children in the protests and in the chanting of violent slogans and taunts. For example, the *Guardian* reported a case in Greater Manchester where a '300 strong mob' surrounded the house of a man shouting 'paedophile, rapist, beast, pervert'. The man alleged that a group of kids had 'backed a six year old

child halfway down the path to my door shouting "do you want this one?" '
(25 July 2000: 7). Similarly, the *Mirror* journalist Barbara Davies reported
children joining in the Paulsgrove protests alongside their mothers who
'laugh at the youngsters who have just finished stuffing a life-size doll and
hung it from a noose on a lamppost' and who say 'we'll lynch the pervs'
(11 August 2000: 9). The tone of these reports is clearly condemnatory,
with an explicit point about the 'irony' of such actions in terms of caring
for children.

My contention here, therefore, is that these events can be seen to
demonstrate the position in which parents, especially mothers, and especially those who are less well off and therefore less mobile, are placed.
That is, they highlighted the way that parents are expected to trust that a
certain level of security is provided, to make risk assessments based
on generalised information and expertise, and to communicate to their
children safety techniques based on this general information. Neo-
liberal government runs smoothly only if parents can trust that the state
is indeed providing both a basic level of general security and trustworthy
information by which to make their risk-assessments. Both of these
fundamental beliefs were being questioned, and the protesters' disquiet
was focused on the resulting precariousness of their position. The
state's ability to guard against real dangers was under question, because
it seemed to them that convicted sexual offenders were not being re-
habilitated or adequately monitored when released. Further, although
relevant information was being collected, it was not being made available
to those who were most in need of it, that is, parents. Their ability to fulfil
their roles as rational risk-assessing parents was thereby rendered impossible.

The 'state', for its part, was left in the position of having to argue
against the transparency of information, despite the general governmental
trend to require parents to assess risks according to more and more
detailed information and to act rationally in relation to that information.
Aided by media representation of the protesters as themselves anti-
democratic, emotional, violent, pre-modern, as acting out of proportion
(to the real risk) and as out of place, the state reaffirmed its role as the
provider of a general context of public security and of sober, non-emotive,
rational, modern, democratic government.

Representing 'the public' and re-establishing the lines of government

[O]ur critics are a tiny minority. An unknown MP, a judge ... and two
newspaper editors, Simon Kelner of the *Independent* and Charles
Moore of the *Daily Telegraph*. This arrogant lot have ventured from
their cosseted, cloistered and comfortable worlds just long enough to

> show their contempt for your opinions. They know nothing of the real
> world and show no concern for real people.
>
> (Rebekah Wade, editor, *News of the World*, 13 August 2000: 2)

Running through the debate was, interestingly, a battle around the representation of 'the public' – who they were, who was 'in touch' with them, how their interests were best known and provided for – that was crucial to the momentum of the newspaper's campaign. As the *News of the World* moved away from its originally stated intention to present information direct to the reading public as parents, it began to figure its campaign less provocatively as an intermediary role between public opinion and official bodies. As such it became more and more concerned with public opinion and gathering evidence of their support for the demands of the campaign. This was crucial to its rhetoric. As well as asking readers to call a hotline to pledge support, and to sign a petition to the Home Secretary asking him to introduce 'Sarah's Law', they commissioned random telephone surveys by an independent polling group (MORI) reporting in one, for example, that 76 per cent of the 1004 people interviewed agreed that people should know if a convicted paedophile was living in their area (20 August 2000).

The *News of the World* maintained throughout that public opinion was on their side. Even a man who had been wrongly attacked as a direct result of being misidentified as the man in a photograph published in their table of faces was triumphantly reported as agreeing with the campaign's ends: 'Iain Armstrong was a victim of vigilante attack because he bears a striking resemblance to pervert Peter Smith, but he BACKS our campaign'. The newspaper quotes him as saying: 'I suffer from spondilitis and wear a neck brace like him. But I'm no pervert. As a father myself I would want to know if there are any perverts nearby so I can keep an eye on what they're up to' (30 July 2000: 3).

The official response was one which had to perform the potentially difficult (discursive) task of arguing that even if the concerns and demands made through the *News of the World* may have represented public *opinion* they were not in the democratic public *interest*. The means were denounced as provoking vigilante attacks, as we've seen, and the specific end (public access to the Sexual Offenders Register) was denounced for its potentially deleterious effect, most often understood as 'driving paedophiles underground where they cannot be monitored' (the *Guardian*, 31 July 2000, and 11 August 2000). When Paul Boateng refused to support 'Sarah's Law', arguing that it was not in the public interest for these reasons, Sarah Payne's parents were reported as reacting angrily, suggesting that he should 'take a look at public opinion' (the *Mirror*, 8 August 2000: 8). While the 'quality' newspapers were on the whole extremely critical of the *News of the World* campaign, seeing it as irresponsible, wrongheaded and as a cynical ploy to improve declining sales (the *Guardian*, 24 July 2000: 17), the newspaper retorted that their critics were cloistered and cosseted in comfortable worlds, out of touch with the 'real world' and therefore the public's concerns.

The eventual reframing of the campaign, however, and the Editor's turn to the relevant national organisations and agencies as the focus of seeking changes that would ameliorate public anger and anxiety about child sexual abuse, meant that the newspaper's radical challenge dispersed as it returned to the terms and the logic of the present modes of government of child sexual abuse. In the paper's editorial printed on 13 August 2000, the issue the 'naming and shaming' campaign was suspended, the public's protests became depicted as inchoate 'direct action' – this despite the fact that the same issue reports the Paulsgrove parents holding meetings, discussing strategy and entering negotiations with local authorities – with the *News of the World* then presented as stepping in to give voice to the public sentiment. This move from action to speech is figured as one from potentially violent emotion to calm rationality:

> pushed to the extreme otherwise reasonable citizens are forced into vigilante action. . . . Concerned parents who believe they have no voice see the only way forward as direct action . . . Now they have a voice. The *News of the World*. And already they can see the results [in the meeting between principal agencies].
>
> (13 August 2000: 2)

By the end of the campaign, therefore, with the move from action on the streets to the 'high level summit' between the experts and officials presented as a victory – and thereafter the petition to government (which Sara and Michael Payne later presented to Jack Straw) the main focus of the campaign – the lines of governmentality were re-established. Communication, expertise and information flows between parents and government were no longer to be circumvented by the newspaper's offer of full specific information direct to parents. Instead the newspaper positioned itself rather differently, arguing that the public had been *represented* by the *News of the World*, who had achieved the aim, in the final analysis, not of being the alternative and direct source of public information, as they had originally presented it, but by being the conduit of information and facilitator of proper democratic process between the public and government. According to the newspaper's own representation of events, levels of trust were re-established so that the public interest would now be attended by policy makers and their initiatives, and parents need no longer be in direct protest with government. Parents' demands on government could be mediated, first, by the agencies whose role it is to provide basic levels of security and of care, and second, via the newspaper's route of petitioning the Home Secretary whose role, in turn, would be to consider their concerns. What had begun as a challenge to these intermediary levels and routes of government, therefore, and an explicit challenge to contemporary governmentality of child sexual abuse, came to claim victory in the reinstating of those rationalities.

Reading for a feminist politics?

> When Sarah Payne was killed we all thought that could have been one of our kids. When we went to the council to get one paedophile removed they fitted his home with a fire door. It was as if their main concern was to protect the paedophile, not our kids. That's why we took to the streets.
>
> (*News of the World*, 13 August 2000: 4)

It was remarkable, given the image of strong women taking to the streets making demands around an issue of sexual abuse, that during these events there was so little comment that was explicitly feminist. The image of these mothers challenging the state is one that might elsewhere cause feminists to wax lyrical and it is certainly an image of solidarity, politics and agency implicitly promoted in many a theoretical discussion of 'politics'. It is true that there was at the time some small measure of explicit support for the mothers from feminists. Andrea Dworkin, visiting the Edinburgh festival, was reported as 'enter[ing] the Sarah Payne debate by declaring that the victims of child sex abuse have the right to kill paedophiles'. Speaking of a woman who shot and killed the man who had abused her son in an American courtroom, she is quoted as saying, 'I loved that woman. It is our duty to find ways of supporting her and others like her. I have no problem with killing paedophiles.' The quotation continues, 'I'm not completely up to date about what is happening in Portsmouth but I understand people's anger. I feel sorry for the women and children in the families who have been driven out of the estate but often in these cases the men have been involved in incest on their children' (the *Guardian*, 16 August 2000). But on the whole there was only cautious support for the Paulsgrove mothers such as that from feminist journalist Ros Coward who tried to counter their representation through an understanding of their frustrations as mothers. ('New feminist' Natasha Walters in her end-of-year reflections, chose instead to remember the whole episode as a paradoxical one in which children were (ab)used in the name of resisting child abuse and murder.)

Of course the relative lack of feminist comment in media coverage may have been for a variety of reasons (quite possibly mundane reasons such as chronic discrimination within the media, or a lack of feminist journalists); but re-reading the newspaper coverage, one suspects that the difficulties of articulating a feminist reading of the actions of the parents/mothers may be due, at least in part, to two related, significant points. First, that the mothers themselves did not seem to be drawing upon previous feminist discourses or analyses of child sexual abuse, and in fact the campaign entailed some newly conservative images and articulations around child sexual abuse. Second, because although the 'women were a force to be reckoned with' (the *Mirror*, 11 August 2000: 9), to attempt to view the episode through the lens of the female figure of Antigone questioning the Good embodied in the masculine state,[11] or even simply as mothers against male sexual abusers, would be to reduce a more complex picture to only one of its significant dimensions. It is the complexities of the picture which make it difficult to prioritise the gender politics of the episode without giving attention, in particular, to how issues of 'social class' and the government of communities contextualise and cut through those politics. Moreover, certain nationalist and racialised imaginings surround the *News of the World* campaign and the parents' protests that underscore the problems of claiming it as in any way unproblematically radical, let alone feminist.

As we've seen, the mothers articulated their actions as an extension of the protection they wished, and are expected, to provide for their children, and as such, as premised upon maternal sentiment, the most defensible and most feminine of sentiments. Their words and actions, however, meant that they were repeatedly depicted as 'un-feminine', 'un-maternal', as aggressive, determined, uncompromising, tough talking and so on. The combination of symbolising both maternal attachment and the transgression of gendered norms of public behaviour, as well as their action moving them from private into public space, makes their figuration as a contemporary equivalent of Antigone's challenge to the state's attempted control of kinship relations a potentially attractive manoeuvre. Indeed, with reference to what I have argued above (pp. 112–117), one could make political capital by regarding the mothers' actions as radically illuminating the government's reliance upon kinship and the compliance of mothers. Mothers are not supposed to ask for more or better government but to continue in their role of mothering and be assured that the government's attention is on the dangers that might disrupt that idyll. By protesting that they no longer had faith in the state's handling of this danger, the mothers could be understood to represent a challenge which asserts that women cannot operate according to the logics of the state's calm diminution of the danger at stake, with the force of their particularised sentiment opposing itself to the statistical, cold-hearted, rationality of generalised knowledge. Such a rendering of events would embrace the vigilante image of the mothers, and argue against the negative imagery that depicted these women as archaic, pre-political, violent and as abusing their children by encouraging their participation in the protests.

But while a feminist reading of these events and critique of the politics of representation might pursue such a line, with some justification perhaps, it would be to ignore or cut across some other aspects of the events and their reportage. First, as I've suggested, the protesters were not articulating their fears or demands in a way that made them obviously resonant with feminist analyses. Most importantly, the mothers and protestors tended to confirm an image of the child sexual abuser that feminist analyses have sought to complicate if not displace. In the repeated use of the term 'paedophile' the mothers concurred with the wide media usage of the term that cast the men concerned within a category of the sexually aberrant. At other times termed 'monsters', 'perverts' or 'diseased', the men (and a few women) were cast as such into the realm of the abnormal, making them the dangerous individuals about whom all, excepting the liberal establishment intent on their resettlement and rehabilitation, were united in distaste and horror. In this, the parents' protests were consistently as conservative as the newspaper that believed it spoke to and for them. Indeed, in their calls for the death of those convicted of child sexual offences, they were more so. The relevance of the feminist critique of the family as an institution, or of masculinist sexualities, as pertinent to child sexual abuse had no place here as the image of the danger was clearly understood to be located outside the home in specific individuals with sexually deviant and dangerous desires. The old stereotypes recirculated as if feminist critique had had no impact. One woman on the Paulsgrove estate reportedly said: 'her seven year old son asked her "are tramps paedophiles mum?" "I had to explain the difference between dirty old men and dirty old men"' (the *Mirror*, 11 August 2000: 9).

But one mustn't allow a curious sense of feminist disappointment to cloud one's reading. After all, the mothers were reacting to a particular instance of child murder that *was*, by all available intelligence, committed by a stranger in a public space, and that had only been turned into an issue of child sexual abuse or 'paedophilia' somewhat rashly, perhaps, by the *News of the World* and other media reports. One could reasonably argue that some aspects of the feminist analysis of child sexual abuse – those that focus on the fact that perpetrators are known, that sexual abuse occurs in 'private' as opposed to 'public spaces' – would not be appropriate here, and when they did emerge – in letters to 'quality' newspapers for example – seem somewhat irrelevant, dismissive and even smug. Moreover, through their actions, if not their words, the mothers pointed to the high numbers of convicted and known sexual offenders, and the rhetoric of the newspaper campaigns – 'one for every square mile' – confirmed the feminist mantra on the issue of sexual abuse – any man, every man, anywhere. Moreover, the paradox of the printing of the photographs in the *News of the World* was, of course, that if the intention was to quell fears by locating specific individuals as dangerous, the images simultaneously demonstrated the ubiquity of child sexual abuse and the 'normality' of the abuser, in so far as they had previous lived within unsuspecting communities. Indeed, the newspaper was explicit on this point at least, printing a 'cut out and keep guide' based on one developed by the NSPCC's 'Full Stop' campaign: 'Who are the paedophiles? They can be found in all professions, all levels of society, be from any race or religion and can be a friend, relative or acquaintance. It is more rare for a paedophile to be a complete stranger' (6 August 2000: 4). Nevertheless, it would be true to say that, overall, the protests were not articulating a feminist discourse. Other aspects of NSPCC work and of feminist analysis that could have been made directly relevant, such as the feminist attention to the construction of 'normal' masculine sexuality as equating dominance with pleasure, went unarticulated on the part of the protestors, so that while the occasion of the transgression of gender norms and a challenge from mothers to the state might have seemed an opportunity for feminist glory, they were not.

Furthermore, the politics of gender that surrounded these events were very strongly entwined with a politics of socio-economic disadvantage. The mother's protests, and much of the discourse in the *News of the World* as well as that in other newspapers, presented the issue in relation to one which has not figured especially in feminist analyses – the interaction between housing policies and child sexual abuse – making the politics of its unfolding subtend a politics of social class, rarely articulated as such but consistently made relevant by references to the impact that housing policies had. Rather than a protest against patriarchy, the women were repeatedly reported as protecting their children within the contexts of housing policies that they were powerless to alter. Housing provision was relevant both in relation to the protestors' immobility and dependency upon council provision, and in relation to the resettlement of offenders, about which they felt under-consulted and ill-informed. The rhetoric of government *through, with and for* community was challenged here as the protestors indicated that their housing was neglected and the estate governed through asymmetries of power where decisions about housing sexual abusers were not consultative issues. Thus, for example, the *Mirror* reported that mothers were angry because one man who had fled to avoid a group of protesters had been 'placed by housing authorities in a flat yards from schools and a playground' (5 August 2000: 8). The *News of the World* editorial adopted the language of invasion in its reference to poor housing stock – 'Families in rundown estates react angrily against the flood of perverts rehoused into their communities' (13 August 2000: 2) – and the Member of Parliament for the Paulsgrove estate area commented: 'You don't understand what their lives are like on this estate. I do, I live among them and understand their frustration' (*News of the World*, 13 August 2000: 4). Letters to the *News of the World* from the public supported this sense of powerlessness in relation to housing policies. One woman whose child was abused wrote that, 'as if to add insult to injury the local council are going to keep his house available for his release – a house that is opposite our bedroom window' (p. 44); another that her family was having to live next door to the man who had tried to rape her daughter (p. 16).

The importance of housing provision and policies was also referred to within those arguments which characterised the protesters as a dangerous mob, peripheral to civilised society. Here, the housing estates that were presented as divided from the more 'sheltered' and 'calmer' parts of Britain, with for example a *Guardian* leader suggesting that 'liberal arguments familiar in newspapers, TV studios, parliamentary tea rooms and bishops' studies cut no ice among the boarded up stores and sub-standard housing of Paulsgrove. For them the distinction between a convicted and suspected paedophile is academic' (11 August 2000). The mothers and their housing conditions were regarded as central to these events, therefore, as central as issues of housing and overcrowding were to explaining social dangers, including child sexual abuse, a century earlier.

Rather than radical feminist, therefore, it would be easier to argue that these events were forms of radical *class* protest in which mothers were attempting to draw attention to the difficulties of their expected role as parent–protecter when the context of risk is so heavily determined by housing provision and resettlement policies.

Any attempt to read these events as radical, however, would need to pay critical attention to the sense in which the parents' protests and some of the reportage that surrounded them appealed to certain nationalistic imaginings. To give some examples: the Union Jack flag was used to present the protesters' message (*News of the World*, 9 August 2000: 17), the *News of the World* countered arguments about offenders' rights with a patriotic image of England's 'fields of wheat in high summer' becoming unsafe for a young girl to exercise her right to walk through them (23 July 2000: 6), the newspaper made repeated references to its campaign as a 'crusade', and reported proudly that a Dutch reader had written to say: 'I would be proud to be British, at last someone is fighting back' (30 July 2000: 41) as well as drawing upon the idea of communities being 'flooded' by waves of 'perverts' (13 August 2000: 2). All these instances illustrate the sense in which the issue of child sexual abuse became figured as a nation under siege, with the parents' protests described by several commentators as representing something of the *'national* psyche' or nationwide, common sentiment (e.g. in the *Guardian* leader, 11 August 2000). The solution to having the 'most vile criminal in our midst' (Chairman of the Police Federation, *News of the World*, 20 August 2000: 6) was repeatedly figured as his removal; that is, as his death – a call for his murder or for the reintroduction of capital punishment – or else territorially as 'driving him out' (the *Mirror*, 9 August 2000: 17). Moreover, the rehearsal of these images of defending the nation was not without an attendant racialisation which arguably haunts the continual references to the protesters as 'lynch mobs', the protesters' own references to 'lynching' (ibid.) and their practice of surrounding houses, chanting references to hanging as well as performing symbolic hangings (ibid.). The history of forms taken by violent white racism cannot be innocently remembered through these terms; in this sense the 'whiteness' of the protest was integral to its symbolic self-understanding.

Conclusion

Remembering the events of summer 2000 is likely to be important in the framing of future events that touch upon the issues central to it (Kitzinger, 2000), and it is with this in mind that I have presented the above comments. In particular I have been concerned to argue that the role in which the parent and especially the mother is positioned within contemporary political rationalities is an important context within which to understand the events, so that alongside any consideration of how child sexual abuse and child sexual abusers were constituted therein, there might be attention to how the mother as a risk-assessing, child-protecting figure was illuminated in all its fragility and in (some of) its political utility. The episode was not one that can be understood simply as women against the state or against men, but can be read as the mothers arguing that their role within the rationalities of contemporary government of child sexual abuse had become untenable, and it was these rationalitites that were put into a temporary legitimation crisis in which the women erupted onto the political stage only to be quickly overwhelmed with the negative media response. The ways in which the rationalities of the contemporary government of child sexual abuse were re-established drew upon these negative portrayals of the women to the extent that it was they who became the contemporary prime candidates for caricature as atavistic and anti-democratic. The re-establishment of lines of government operated, moreover, by isolating the women's demands from 'the public interest' through the discursive space that was, interestingly, opened up between public opinion and public interests by official responses. It became possible to both share the women's sentiment and to believe their demands misguided. Finally, I have argued that a feminist analysis cannot take these women as icons for feminist politics, so embroiled were their actions and discourse in reactionary, nationalist and potentially 'racist' argumentation; but I would suggest that neither can feminist theorists ignore the fact that these were women who, to a certain extent, mobilised *as* women.

Consideration of these women's action is instructive for feminist politics and analysis, I believe, on a number of counts. First, despite the gendered dimensions to their action, one might pause on the simple observation that these events did not become the site for anything one might have recognised as a feminist discourse beyond the negative point that the figure of the child abuser as a peculiarly 'psychologically disturbed' man seemed untenable; indeed, newly conservative constructions of the paedophile and child sexual abuse seemed to circulate as if there had never been a feminist body of work challenging those depictions and understandings. Second, the events underscore the importance of how we understand the contextualising factors in analysing the construction of 'child sexual abuse' and the figures that circulate in relation to it. Thus we have seen how child sexual abuse does not stand alone as a topic but draws in other aspects of political governmentality to which these women were simultaneously responding, especially parenting within a culture of 'risk assessment', modes of (access to) information and the powerless position of tenants in relation to national and local government's housing policies. Feminist analyses of child sexual abuse, therefore, need to include consideration of issues as far reaching as these (rather than confine the analysis of child sexual abuse to any single dimension). Moreover, and third, the portrayal of these mothers that emerges from the media responses – as without civilisation and as outside the political – is one that has to be understood as a credible fiction produced by the political contexts. These contexts, I have suggested, include a contemporary governmentality that promotes and requires a mode of parenting quite different from the one these mothers adopted, a 'rational' risk-assessing form of parenting that builds its possibility in turn upon the continued construction of women (and working-class motherhood in particular) as quietly passionate in such a way that, as Donzelot's argument would suggest, produces subservience to political government and its production of the familial.

Notes

1 A version of this article first appeared in *Feminist Theory*, 2002, 3, 1: 83–102.
2 For others who have approached the issue of child sexual abuse through similar Foucauldian analyses of the figures emerging at the various site(s) of its regulation, see Hacking (1992), Smart (1999), Radcliffe (2001) as well as my own work, Bell (1993).
3 In Italy, Cesaire Lombroso combined a reading of evolutionary theory with his studies of the human skull and his use of photographic portraits to present his notorious argument that criminals were atavistic, throwbacks from an earlier period, whose status as such was betrayed by their physiognomy. His photographic tables showing the faces of Italian and German criminals were initially presented in 1889 under the title 'the Anthropology of the Criminal' with the criminal's name printed underneath each of the sixty-eight portraits (see Kemp and Wallace, 2000).
4 The arguments that follow form a commentary based on reading selected newspapers from the period – the *News of the World*, for its key role, the *Mirror* as an example of a tabloid paper and the *Guardian* as an example of a more

liberal broadsheet newspaper. I have also consulted BBC news on-line archives. In the first two sections, I am not arguing that the newspapers point to this analysis, but rather that these theoretical thoughts render a certain reading of the coverage. In the third section I am presenting a reading of constructions of the mothers based on these papers' reportage.

5 Indeed, it was the perception of the high risk of re-offending sexual offenders, rather than child sexual abuse in general, that the parents' protests were about, addressed to the authorities who would not share the knowledge they had about who had offended in the past and therefore who was understood to be likely to offend in the future.

6 Although rehabilitation programmes may contain theoretical constructions of child sexual abusers, the liberal discourse does not embrace any theory in particular, but merely insists that each offender is an individual human being so that society has some duty to respond to and contain him. Re-offending becomes a crucial issue in each of these discourses, in the first for its indication of a disease that has not been, and often the implication is that it cannot be, cured, and in the second because it indicates a failure of the institutions of society to successfully police and contain these individuals.

7 This despite the fact that those child sexual offenders in the photographs and those whose homes were surrounded, were frequently reported as themselves having wives and children, and despite the numbers of incidents of men killing their partners and children, whose reportage surrounded these stories on the pages of the tabloid newspapers.

8 The techniques range from teaching children not to accept gifts from strangers to techniques that teach children the difference between different sorts of touches as well as techniques of how to create an atmosphere in which children are able to speak about unpleasant feelings or experiences.

9 Journalist Sue Carroll used the opportunity for an unnecessary comparison with protests against Section 28 when she suggested that perhaps it is time that those who had 'devoted so much time to the repeal of Section 28 [that forbids the promotion of homosexuality within local government] a crime [sic] that concerns a minority but does not strike at the heart of the average voter, might like to invest their energy into the question of how we deal with paedophiles' (26 July 2000: 9).

10 This is not to say that no such 'theoretical' accounts were expressed. In the *News of the World* an 'expert on cases of child abduction' was quoted as saying that 'once a paedophile starts to offend they have urges that don't go away. Such behaviour will have its seeds in childhood where the person will most probably have been sexually abused himself. This will start a cycle of fantasy . . .' (23 July 2000: 5). But these accounts were rather muted across the reportage, and here for example is used to argue for his incurability and dangerousness, rather than in order to understand his behaviour.

11 Although see Butler, 2000, for a complication of this oft-used image of Antigone. There is the possibility, one that I do not have time to explore here, that one could adopt Butler's re-reading of Antigone in relation to these mothers in so far as they are explicitly protesting about an issue of kinship in so far as child sexual abuse threatens the family – often from within as well as from without – and in that sense they represent an issue concerning the *limits* of kinship.

References

Beck, U. (1992) *Risk society: towards a new modernity*, London: Sage.

Bell, V. (1993) *Interrogating incest: feminism, Foucault and the law*, London: Routledge.

Bell, V. (1995) 'The spectre of incest: sexuality and/in the family', in S. Lash and M. Featherstone (eds) *Global modernities*, London: Sage, pp. 227–243.

Butler, J. (2000) *Antigone's claim: kinship between life and death*, New York: Columbia University Press.

Donzelot, J. (1979) *The policing of families: welfare versus the state*, London: Hutchinson.

Foucualt, M. (1981) *The history of sexuality vol. 1: an introduction*, Harmondsworth: Penguin.

Foucault, M. (1988) 'The dangerous individual', in L. Kritzman (ed.) *Michel Foucault: politics, philosophy, culture: interviews and other writings 1977–1984*, New York: Routledge.

Hacking, I. (1992) 'World-making by kind-making: child abuse for example', in M. Douglas and D. Hull (eds) *How classification works: Nelson Goodman among the social sciences*, Edinburgh: Edinburgh University Press, pp. 180–238.

Haug, F. (2001) 'Sexual deregulation or, the child abuser as hero in neoliberalism', *Feminist Theory* 2: 55–78.

Kemp, M. and Wallace, M. (2000) *Spectacular bodies: the art and science of the human body from Leonardo to now*, Berkeley: University of California Press.

Kitzinger, J. (2000) 'Media templates: patterns of association and the (re)construction of meaning over time', *Media, Culture and Society* 22, 1: 61–84.

Miller, P. and Rose, N. (1992) 'Political power beyond the state: problematics of government', in *The British Journal of Sociology* 43: 173–203.

Radcliffe, P. (2001) 'The conceptual practices of child and family social work: protection, risk and partnership', PhD dissertation, Goldsmiths College, University of London.

Rose, N. (1999) *Powers of freedom: reframing political thought*, Cambridge: Cambridge University Press.

Smart, C. (1999) 'The discursive construction of "child victims" of sexual abuse', *Social and Legal Studies* 8, 3: 391–409.

How we theorise and intervene in the lives of women who have experienced child sexual abuse

The 'harm' story in childhood sexual abuse

Contested understandings, disputed knowledges

Lindsay O'Dell

In this chapter I will be discussing the debates surrounding the harmfulness of child sexual abuse. The harmfulness of sexual violence (throughout the lifespan, but particularly in childhood) has formed key political axes for 'second-wave' feminist academics, practitioners and campaigners. Second-wave feminist campaigns, particularly surrounding sexual violence and child sexual abuse, are characterised by the principal focus upon action and praxis that engages with gendered bodies, gendered textual and social practices. Whilst I am not denying that these concerns remain (materially) very real – gender saturates our understandings of the social world – the position that I take within this chapter would argue that issues of power are not focused purely around the axis of gender. My approach is informed by a post-structuralist feminist practice in which there is no straightforward mapping of gender and power but intersections of gender, sexuality and ethnicity which produce a multiplicity of identity positions and inequalities without recourse to singularising ascriptions of 'identity'.

Whilst my intention is not to be seen to condone child sexual abuse or for my work to be used as a justification for arguing that child sexual abuse is not psychologically harmful, I am concerned with the highly singularised 'story' of psychological harm in which one story speaks for all women's experiences. I want to explore the ways in which a feminist-informed post-structuralist theorising can open up dichotomies: of adult/child, knowing/innocent, healthy/damaged, normal/pathological in respect to issues of child sexual abuse. I am keenly aware of the 'backlash' against both feminism and the recognition of child sexual abuse (and other forms of sexual violence). Whilst not wanting to be part of the backlash, like Gavey (and others) my concern is that, 'If we don't ask these questions about the victimizing framework, I sense that we may risk leaving a fertile gap for backlash discourse to take hold' (Gavey, 1999: 77). My concern, explicated through this chapter (and expanded throughout this volume), is that in framing child sexual abuse in terms of the psychological harmfulness and telling what is termed here 'the harm story', debate is reduced and simplified. Thus, children (and women) are treated as a singularised category regardless of their temporal, cultural positioning. Furthermore, by storying the harmfulness of child sexual abuse through a discourse of 'development', women, children and men affected by child sexual abuse are positioned as remaining a product of their past abusive experiences.

Stories

In titling this chapter the *'harm' story*, the use of 'story' is strategic and purposeful. The intention is to provide a critical distance from the mainstream understandings or 'stories' that are told about the effects of child sexual abuse. The use of the term 'story' is not to be understood as fictive or as a series of binary significations: 'fact/fiction', 'real/false' where women's accounts of past (and present) sexual abuse are either confirmed as being true or are deemed 'false'. It is not my intention to cast doubt upon women's accounts of sexual violence and I do not intend my work to be read in this way. Child sexual abuse is a powerful issue within many women's lives, the effects for many are very 'real'. My concern is with the way in which women's lives and experiences are storied. Rather, my use of the word 'story' is as a device to trouble the mainstream hegemonic stories that are accorded the role of being the singular 'truth' and the 'facts' to be known about child sexual abuse.

An overarching story within modern (Western) ontologies, epistemologies and world view is that of progress and development through time and through the use of technological 'advancement' and science. The assumption is that the world, particularly our intrapsychic world, is constructed through a series of (bio)logical steps which are linked in temporal order. Development is affected by the previous stages and which, in turn, have an impact on the following stage. This story of 'progression' and 'developmentalism' is powerful in psychological theorisation. Critical psychologists (some feminist-informed and some outwith the concerns of feminisms per se) have brought attention to the cultural and temporal locatedness of our taken for granted ideas about 'development' and more broadly 'progression' (see, for example, Morss, 1992; Stainton Rogers and Stainton Rogers, 1992; Walkerdine, 1993; Burman, 1994a for discussion of the locatedness of children's 'development', and Vandenberg, 1993's discussion of the Judaeo-Christian assumptions implicit within ascriptions of 'progression'). The overarching analytic of developmentalism has had a profound impact upon the construction of the developing child and, by implication, upon the researched effects of the sexual abuse of children. 'Development' provides a grid of intelligibility through which we make sense of child sexual abuse where sexual abuse is seen to disrupt or alter development. Thus, the sexually abused child is positioned as 'other' to the non-abused (and, by implication, 'normal') child.

Critical social scientists, including many feminists, question the notion that one discourse or story is appropriate for all times and places (Fraser and Nicholson, 1988, in Atmore, 1999). Stories are, thus, more than 'innocently descriptive' (Levine, 2000; Flax, 1992) but largely represent the mainstream understandings and ideologies about, in this instance, the effects of child sexual abuse. My contention is that such stories position those affected by abuse in particular ways and serve to construct women as victims not just of the abusive experiences at the time but throughout their lives. As with all stories, the mainstream understandings of child sexual abuse provide us with a powerful but *partial* account of sexual violence. Therefore in my work and in the work of other feminist and post-structuralist-informed critics of the mainstream accounts of child sexual abuse, 'the stakes are always political' (Atmore, 1999: 90) and shot through with issues of power, gender, sexuality and ethnicity.

The 'harm story': mainstream psychological theorisations

The mainstream discourse around child sexual abuse provides a coherent and convincing story of the professional 'discovery' of child abuse and, more specifically, child sexual abuse. It is a story of 'progress' where (psychological) science has worked to give us the 'facts' and the 'truth' about child maltreatment. Within this story child sexual abuse or incest was seen, until fairly recently (the 1950s and 1960s), as a problem of the very poor and those who lived in overcrowded conditions (see for example, La Fontaine, 1990). Before the (professional) 'discovery' of child sexual abuse, the wrongfulness of the acts was seen within the context of taboo and, latterly, a legal violation (see Bell, 1993 and Armstrong, 1994's discussion of this). Sex researchers such as Kinsey and his colleagues added (pseudo) scientific weight to the notion that child sexual activity was at worst an everyday childhood issue and at best good training for girls to understand their adult married role (Kinsey, *et al.*, 1953, in O'Dell, 1997). In their study of the sexual behaviour of women, the researchers conclude that there is 'some evidence [that] the pre-adolescent contacts had provided emotional satisfactions which had conditioned the female for the acceptance of later sexual activities' (Kinsey, *et al.*, 1953: 15).

The professional, medical and psychological discovery of the 'truth' about child abuse and child sexual abuse begins with the work of Kempe and his colleagues in the 1960s and has led to a widespread recognition of the psychological harmfulness of child sexual abuse. Constructing the effects of child sexual abuse as a pathological disorder enables and warrants medical and psychological intervention, as Weir (1992: 394) suggests, in a '*subtly coercive and all-pervasive*' way. The aetiology of the 'problem', the symptomology and the possible 'cures', are situated within a psycho-medical framework. The lists of 'symptoms' of child sexual abuse are in almost every article or book written on the subject, together with the author's opinions on 'cures' for the disorders, or a commentary on the 'healing process' (such as Waterman, *et al.*, 1994; see also O'Dell, 1997 for a critique of such conventions). The notion that child sexual abuse is a form of pathology is evident in much of the child abuse literature, in traditional research, incest is 'a disease whose carrier is the parent and whose victim is the child' (Kempe and Kempe, 1978: 6). It is also a theme evident in some feminist literature: 'incest represents a common pattern of traditional female socialisation carried to a pathological extreme' (Herman and Hirschman, 1981: 125).

Feminist contestations

Feminist and feminist-informed critics such as MacLeod and Saraga (1988) have argued that drawing upon the mainstream psychological (pseudo) scientific research into the harmfulness of child sexual abuse serves to warrant feminist political claims by scientifically demonstrating the damaging nature of male dominance. For example, feminist action has been highly successful in changing rape laws (Gavey, 1999; Lamb, 1999). However, whilst such second-wave feminist action strategically draws upon psychological science in order to challenge the order of things, particularly the organisation of society and understandings of gender (see, for example, Dominelli, 1986; Burman *et al.*, 1998), in doing so the dominant psycho-medical construction of harm is reified (Armstrong, 1994) and the harm story retold. Furthermore, Armstrong (ibid.) and Kitzinger (1992) argue that second-wave feminist concerns have been co-opted into mainstream understandings of child sexual abuse, thus the political aspect of such theorising has been marginalised and silenced. Lamb notes that 'I am not the first to have been dismayed at how abuse has become apolitical' (Lamb, 1999: 131), where the language of feminism, choice, power and liberation has become caught up in and co-opted by therapeutic language and practices.

Bell (1993) argues that the 'psy-disciplines' have been instrumental in transfiguring the context of debate about child sexual abuse from a legal and moral arena to a strongly psychologised and medicalised inscription of the causes and harmfulness of abuse. The 'old powers' of law and medicine are increasingly reliant upon psychological knowledge to warrant action. For example, adult 'survivors' of child sexual abuse have used the law to gain financial redress from their abusers (see also Gavey, this volume). Such cases *require* a demonstration of sustained, *long-term* psychological harm caused by child sexual abuse in order that a woman's claims be heard and taken seriously; 'For abuse to *count*, the suffering can never go away' (Lamb, 1999: 113). A similar reliance upon psychological knowledge and expertise is inscribed in the UK within the Children Act

(1989) which sets in law the notion of 'significant harm' as psychologised, observable and demonstrable harmfulness of child abuse. Furthermore, implicit within this construction of 'harm' is the notion of development and the lack of appropriate development for those sexually abused as children. Thus 'development' has become reified as the mechanism through which 'professionals' can understand and act for abused children.

A textual analysis

The analysis presented in this chapter is a macro discourse analysis of texts (see, for example, Stenner, 1993; Curt, 1994), in which the analysis is drawn from the assumption that discourses are explanations or representations available within specific temporal, cultural contexts, in which discourse can be talk, text, social and textual practice or representations of shared meanings. My analysis focuses upon the overarching textual practices and implicit understandings that are drawn upon by the speakers in my study.

The participants in my study were professionals who worked with children or adults who had a history of child sexual abuse, and women (and men) who identified themselves as adult 'survivors' of child sexual abuse. The use of stories (an approach termed 'seeded thematics' by Stenner, 1993) was employed because it provides an indirect way of encouraging participants to talk about issues without requiring them to talk about their own experiences – whether this was a survivor talking about their childhood or a professional talking about their professional practice. Each participant was given a series of fictitious scenarios, each of which described a case of child sexual abuse. The scenarios altered in terms of factors that are identified within existing literature as pertinent issues such as age, gender and ethnicity of the child, kinds of abusive experiences, familial (and others) reactions to disclosure. Participants were invited to discuss the scenarios and think about what would be the best and worst outcome for the child at the time and in the future.

I was interested in the ways in which harm was storied, particularly in the notion of 'development' and developmentalism as it constitutes a grid of intelligibility through which the effects of child sexual abuse become understood. Below I will illustrate how an overarching analytic of developmentalism has fed into the stories told about the harmfulness of child sexual abuse. The 'harm story' positions 'survivors' of child sexual abuse as qualitatively different to other, non-abused children (seen, by implication, to be 'normal' children). As such, sexually abused children are storied as 'other', as damaged and having lost the opportunity of experiencing (normal) childhood. I will also argue through my analysis that in telling the 'harm story', singularised assumptions about gender, sexuality and ethnicity are drawn upon and implicitly reified.

The harm story and 'development'

The notion of the harm story draws upon the concept of developmentalism: that development is a series of linear stages in which childhood is causally related to later life and, for most children, change with time is fundamentally progressive (Morss, 1990). The concept of the child as a developing organism is central to understandings of childhood and child sexual abuse. Childhood is constructed as an immature state in which the child lacks skills such as cognitive ability and knowledge needed to operate adequately in the (adult) world. This is evident in definitions of child sexual abuse where the child is seen to be unable to 'fully comprehend' the experiences. The British Psychological Society (1989) Psychologists and Child Sexual Abuse: Report of the Working Party of the Professional Affairs Board of the BPS has drawn on Schecter and Roberge's 1976 definition which specifically includes the notion of developmentalism; 'the involvement of dependent, *developmentally immature* children and adolescents in sexually abusive activities they do *not fully comprehend* to which they are unable to give informed consent or that violate the social taboos of family roles' (emphases added). Thus the notion of developmental 'immaturity' is implicit within such understandings of child sexual abuse. Within the mainstream definitions there is little, if any, consideration of the relative power differentials of children and adults. Furthermore, the assumption of progression and development sets up a number of implications for those affected by child sexual abuse. First, that child sexual abuse disrupts the usual, 'normal' developmental trajectory and, as such, is storied as a loss for the child at the time and for the rest of her life. Second that childhood is viewed as qualitatively different from adulthood and is held to be 'other'.

Within a developmentalist discourse, the child's perceived lack of skills feeds into explanations of why younger children are often seen to be at most risk of harm from child sexual abuse. Children are assumed to lack the developmental skills necessary to cope. This is drawn upon by *J* (a paediatrician) to explain why younger children may not be able to deal with abuse: 'She's going to be left with the memory of what he'd done, the fact that he'd hurt her. She's only seven, *she may not have known very much about what was going on*' (emphasis added).

Early childhood is seen as vitally important when development is constructed as a process of building up skills and proficiencies. This is a common theme within developmental psychology as a discipline; in its theorising and in developmental psychology texts (see, for example, Burman's critique of the discipline of developmental psychology, 1994b). The assumption is that if the 'foundations' of development are assumed to be faulty then the subsequent growth is also problematic. Both *J* and another participant, *A* (a counsellor who works with sexually abused children and their families), demonstrate the notion of progression:

It's just to me if you're going to grow up emotionally sound, as you might say, you need good experiences early on ... Good building blocks that you add together and at the end of the day it makes you feel a secure adult.

(J)

if that [development] gets interfered with before the age of two, and it always gets interfered with a sexually abused child, in my experience, then it seems to be much more difficult to move, to shift, to do anything about ... That's all going to be, I was going to say destroyed, but that's not the word, er is going to be destroyed so much then in my mind that is going to make a lot of difference to the damage that's done to the child.

(A)

The notion of the child as a developing organism is a central part of the storying of the effects of child sexual abuse. The construction of development as a building up of competencies and skills further positions the sexually abused child as damaged and potentially damaged through life.

Harm as loss

Viewed through the lens of 'development', the effects of child sexual abuse are storied as a loss. Child sexual abuse is seen to cause a loss of 'normal' childhood activities and possibly the cause of a loss of life experiences in adulthood. The issue of loss is evident in academic and survivors' literature (see, for example, Hall and Lloyd, 1989). The loss of 'normal' development was seen by some of the therapists in my study as a key therapeutic issue. *AC* (a drama therapist) was asked what the client would be grieving for:

– Grieving for the loss.
– *The loss of what?*
– The loss of childhood, the loss of innocence, the loss of the time often I mean.

AC further illustrates that loss is often irredeemable:

– *Do you think that it is possible to regain the losses?*
– No. Some of them are lost. Some of them are absolutely lost. If a woman has not been able to have children she has lost opportunity. That's a fundamental loss.

Whilst loss may be a key aspect of experiencing the after effects of child sexual abuse for many, it remains a potentially divisive concept. The storying of loss of innocence and childhood feeds into a broader cultural understanding of children as developmentally immature and the conflation of innocence (produced through the lens of the 'developing' child) and sexual naiveté. Furthermore, by constructing childhood as a time of innocence, children who have been sexually abused are stigmatised for the very loss of their 'innocence' (Kitzinger, 1992).

Sexually abused children as a marked category

As already stated, the storying of the effects of child sexual abuse constructs survivors as qualitatively different to other, by implication 'normal', children and adults. *AP* (a guardian *ad litem*: an appointed legal representative for children) articulates the otherness of sexually abused children when she discusses the 'difference' of sexually abused children she has worked with: 'In disturbed behaviour, they can't learn, they have no concentration, there is something quite different about them, they don't have relationships, because their family life bears no resemblance to their peers.'

The constructed difference between non-abused children and 'others' positions sexually abused children as pathological and problematic. Furthermore it marks and makes visible the sexually abused child. *AP* exemplifies this in her reflection of her experiences in professional practice:

> in a class would be a child that anybody who works with children would pick out as being abused. You only have to look at their skin, the way they sit, everything about them screams that they have been deprived in some way.

Similarly, *AC* (a drama therapist) articulates the visibility of sexually abused children: 'they're lonely, vulnerable children and that abusers seem to be able to spot these children, possibly because they themselves were lonely children.'

The overarching analytic of developmentalism provides a context through which harm is understood. Conceptualising 'development' as a continual, coherent (bio)logical process in which past events feed into present (and future) functioning positions the sexually abused child/adult as highly vulnerable. The construction of the 'developing child' further contributes to the otherness and vulnerability of sexually abused children as children *and* as they grow into adulthood. Particular life events are seen to trigger the effects of the abusive experiences: 'We've developed the notion that the resolution doesn't happen all at once. It has to be worked on at various stages in one's life' (*AL*).

The notion that the effects of child sexual abuse can recur much later in life was a common understanding by both the professionals and survivors who contributed to my study. For example, *AL* (a social worker) and *AP* (a guardian *ad litem*):

> the message we give is that it's not like you've got a disease and you're cured – it's not the model. It's that it's an experience that can be troublesome, if you work on it until you feel OK about it, but it's part of you, it's part of your history and may come to the fore again.
>
> (*AL*)

> when your own daughter reaches the age of seven then in fact you remember through seeing your own child.
>
> (*AP*)

Thus, harm is a series of ongoing problems that can be reactivated by life events and developmental status. For example, in *AL*'s and *J*'s discussion:

> Yes. So like if Alex enters into a relationship whatever that may be and the plan is for that to be a long one, that commitment raises these issues again in some way so there may be a need then to spend some time working on that so he's clear what he brings to the relationship and what he wants from it, and then he had a child. It may resurrect things as the child gets old enough, getting into sexual behaviour in some way.
>
> (*AL*)

> I think that she needed more help as she went through childhood, preadolescence, adolescence, right up into adulthood, which is the way we see therapy at the moment.
>
> (*J*)

Within the 'harm story' the harm caused by child sexual abuse will always warrant attention and 'would always pop up again or the effects of it will come out' (*TH* social worker). The presence of harm throughout life can be seen to compound the original damage: 'I think that if things are left unresolved then the damage may never end' (*TH* social worker); 'I am always worried that although I feel fine now something is going to trigger it off again' (*SB* survivor).

Those affected by child sexual abuse are positioned and storied as in need of help or (more pervasively) potentially in need of help throughout their lives. Invulnerability can be conceptualised as a developmental task where non-abused children grow/develop from vulnerability to invulnerability. However, for sexually abused children, 'that vulnerability just grows' (*AL* a psychotherapist).

Within mainstream understandings of the effects of child sexual abuse there is a clear expectation of the development of negative symptoms. Furthermore it can be argued that the mainstream harm story actively *produces* victims (O'Dell, 1997; Lamb, 1999). 'Victims' are always positioned as suffering even if the woman concerned does not position herself in such a way (see Lamb's discussion of this). The emphasis on suffering ignores alternatives available to those affected.

Contested understandings: gendered, (hetero)sexualised and 'raced' subjectivities

The harm story is presented as a universal story in which all those affected by child sexual abuse are damaged and positioned as vulnerable throughout life. It stories a symptomology of sexual abuse which documents and sets up a taxonomy of psychological harmfulness. The mainstream research endeavour in constructing symptomologies of the harmfulness of child sexual abuse serves to map the abnormal, the damaged, and implicitly reifies what is taken to be normal and well adjusted (see Rose, 1990; Parton, 1991; Reavey and Warner, 2001). Where the universality of harm is questioned, it is done in terms of simplistic dichotomies: long-term and short-term effects, etc., implicit within which are assumptions about the singularity of, for example, the 'child'. However the 'story' is a highly partial one and one which is gendered, heterosexualised and 'raced'. Whilst assuming to story every child's experiences of child sexual abuse, issues of gender, sexuality, ethnicity and culture are either simplified or rendered invisible. In the following section I will examine how gender, (hetero)sexuality and ethnicity are enmeshed within understandings of child sexual abuse and the mainstream harm story.

Regulation of (hetero)sexuality and gender

A brief reading of the research literature about the effects of sexual abuse gives a clear story of what a good/normal woman should be.

(Warner, 1996a: 47)

Feminist commentators have been instrumental in challenging the assumed gender neutrality of mainstream understandings of child sexual abuse. Gender differences are powerfully regulated and enmeshed within ideas about the harmfulness of child sexual abuse (Levett, 1994). The portrayal of women who have been sexually abused as the vulnerable victim reinforces the ideology of passive and submissive women and girls whose sexuality is defined with reference (and deference) to men's (Dominelli, 1986; Lamb, 1999). The gendered nature of child sexual abuse was clearly articulated by participants in my study:

I think women tend to internalise their violence and direct it against themselves but you can imagine Alex externalising his violence and either attacking men and women, erm ... There are probably a lot of male survivors in the criminal justice system erm having harmed someone else whereas women tend to harm themselves.

(AC)

girls are socialised. They tend to go more in a victim mode which means they're quieter and they are unlikely to act out.

(A)

The dominant construction of harm serves to regulate sexuality and 'appropriate' relationships, in which 'appropriate' is constituted through and within the 'heterosexual matrix' (Butler, 1990). This was evident in discussions with my participants: 'She was bound to be damaged, in fact my guess would be that what she would do would be she would find herself *unable to have relationships with men. (A*, emphasis added); 'I think her ability to form positive relationships with boys could be seriously damaged' (*TH*).

Within the harm story, women who have been sexually abused, like children, are not seen as capable of making up their own minds. Debates around 'false memory syndrome' also highlight the conflation of women and children's minds and the notion that women are not capable of knowing their mind (or memories). Thus, decisions to be a lesbian, celibate or promiscuous are seen to be outside the realm of individual choice (see Kitzinger's discussion of this, 1992). Whichever variant of 'abnormal' sexuality, it is seen as a symptom of a 'problem' of child sexual abuse and not a deliberate, informed decision. 'Homosexual' relationships were viewed in terms of pathology in which lesbianism and homosexuality is a problem that is 'transmitted' by sexual abuse: 'I had one little boy actually burst into tears and say "that means I'm a poof now" and so it does affect how they feel about themselves and their sexuality' (*J*).

A seemingly more acceptable assumption is that of homosexuality as a coping mechanism: 'if you had a coping mechanism which is going into a nunnery or becoming a political lesbian and you have a perfectly happy life doing that well so what?' (*A*).

However, implicit within both of these considerations of lesbianism and homosexuality is the assumption that it represents a deviation from the 'normal' development of (hetero)sexuality. In none of my interviews was homosexuality raised as a deliberate life decision or heterosexuality discussed as an implication or effect of child sexual abuse. The harm story serves to naturalise heterosexuality and produce understandings of homosexuality as a deviation and hangover from previous trauma.

I have used the extracts above to provide an analysis and commentary on the gendered assumptions inherent within the harm story. As a feminist-informed commentator, I am keen to highlight the gendered nature of child sexual abuse. However, I do not want to draw upon 'gender' and 'sexuality' as if these concepts are singular, straightforward and untroublesome. Issues of gender and sexuality may become highly relevant or subsumed within the context of local meanings and situations. Women's 'identity' and experiences are multiplicitous; fragmented with issues of gender and sexuality but also culture, ethnicity, geographical location and age. The harm story singularises and elides over such multiplicity in assuming that there is one story of the effects of child sexual abuse. In the following section I want to examine issues of gender, ethnicity and culture to argue that child sexual abuse is not singular but multiplicitous.

Regulation/invisibility of ethnicity

The notion of a universal harm story renders invisible particular kinds of children and locations of children outside of the (over)developed world. Children from outside of Western Europe and North America are often positioned as standing outside of the category of 'child' and often are not counted as 'victims' of child sexual abuse in the same way as their Western counterparts (see Holland, 1991; Burman, 1994a). Where ethnicity and culture are raised as issues in research they are often treated in highly simplistic ways where ethnicity translates as an additional 'independent variable' (such as in the work of Wyatt, 1990 and McGruder-Johnson, et al., 2000).

Within my textual analysis 'cultural issues' often viewed as 'cultural *problems*', were only raised by participants in relation to discussions about children from 'minority' ethnic groups. As such it was expressed in terms of additional problems for the child. In discussions of a fictitious case study of a girl called Pallavi many of my interview participants focused upon ethnicity rather than issues of child sexual abuse. AW (a social worker) commented that: 'the name suggests that there maybe some kind of cultural problems, the importance of virginity and those sorts of things.'

Issues of religion and virginity were raised only in relation to the story of Pallavi (although I used another nine fictitious case studies, the majority of which had more European/Western sounding names). In the case study, Pallavi was sexually abused by her uncle, described as a visitor. Where participants discussed this case, the implication was that 'we've got some cultural things because he's a visitor' (AW social worker). For most participants who commented on the story they assumed that 'visitor' meant visitor from the Indian subcontinent rather than from elsewhere in the UK. A drama therapist (AC) in his discussion of Pallavi illustrates that child sexual abuse for children of minority ethnic groups is subsumed within the overarching problematic issue – that of 'otherness' and minority ethnic grouping:

> Then that would actually become a cultural issue. She might actually … I'm a psychological dramatist – we might end up doing drama where she was talking to a Mullah about honour and family honour and dishonour and so on, and *she might end up angry with her religion and the culture* (emphasis added).

'Some kind of cultural problems' become the salient focus of concern for children from 'minority' groups. It serves to translate the problems faced by such children from issues of child sexual abuse into 'problems of culture'. Blame is located within 'culture' rather than with individual abusers. Additionally it serves to detract attention from scrutinising the complex and difficult impaction of ethnicity, culture, racism (and other forms of oppression) and child sexual abuse. The operationalisation of ethnicity and culture in terms of 'minority' groups and children serves to reify the majority culture and naturalises 'whiteness' as the norm.

Unsurprisingly, the 'otherness' of Black and Asian children was articulated predominantly by white, middle-class professionals in my research. However, for two Asian men who agreed to take part in my study, child sexual abuse was, something that was 'other' to their culture. They withdrew from the study because both felt that they had nothing to contribute to discussions. This is obviously not a simplistic ethnic/cultural divide. Black and Asian women researchers have noted the widespread denial of men within their own cultures. Patel (1991) encountered widespread denial (particularly amongst Asian men) when conducting her study on Asian cultures and attitudes to child sexual abuse. In addition, Wilson (1993) and others have noted similar issues in relation to African–Caribbean families, particularly African–Caribbean men. Both Patel and Wilson (amongst others) point to the inherent difficulties in dealing with such sensitive issues as child sexual abuse and rape in the face of institutional (and individual) racism and cultural denial.

(In)conclusion: disputed knowledges, post-structuralist contestations

The dominant construction of the harmfulness of child sexual abuse operates on the assumption that it is a universal phenomenon experienced equally by all children in the world and treatable by the same, or similar, interventions. The 'harm story' has been criticised for being an individualising, totalising, singularising and deterministic account which obscures political aspects of abuse (and the location of children throughout the world). The reduction of such a complex issue forecloses debate and sidesteps the constructedness of the categories of 'child', 'adult', 'gender', 'sexuality' and culture. The material conditions of children throughout the world make the ascription of a singular category of 'child' (at best) problematic. Furthermore gender needs to be explored in relation to 'race' particularly in contexts of colonialism where the intersection of 'gender, class, race and sexuality [in ways which] challenge any simple rendering of women into a binary of colonized/colonizing' (Kosambi and Haggis, 2000: 4).

The reliance upon the harm story, a psychologised construction of child sexual abuse, risks and often requires that feminist activists get caught up in taxonomies or symptomologies which seek to demonstrate exactly how and why child sexual abuse is harmful. Whilst second-wave feminism is a highly powerful analytic and practice through which child sexual abuse can be made visible and taken seriously, it sets up particular conditions for the ways in which women and men are positioned with regard to abuse. Drawing upon psychological science (and implicitly the notion of developmentalism) to demonstrate the harmfulness of child sexual abuse to both the developing child and to the 'damaged' adult draws activists into positioning those affected by child sexual abuse in problematic ways (O'Dell and Reavey, 2001). Furthermore, it serves to reify the truth-making of psychological science and sediments singularised understandings of 'the child', gender, (hetero)sexuality and ethnicity.

Armstrong argues that 'The real answer ... lies less in looking on sexual abuse as a psychological event than as a political one' (1994: 43). For some, this may mean a re-energised 'second-wave' feminist politics in which the harmfulness of sexual violence is at the 'cradle' of political action. Feminist political action has included the campaigning and lobbying of the New Zealand government embassy in London during the extradition of Elizabeth Morgan from New Zealand to the United States. (Elizabeth Morgan illegally took her daughter from her home in the United States and went into hiding in New Zealand to avoid her daughter 'Hilary' being legally required to see her father who she accused of sexually abusing her. Elizabeth Morgan is the only woman in the United States to be imprisoned for such action, see Armstrong, 1996 and Groner, 1991). However, from a post-structuralist-informed position, a political practice must be critical of the deployment of 'innocent' knowledge in relation to the harmfulness of child sexual abuse. It requires a critical examination of the textual production of subjectivity and scrutiny of the notion of psychologically 'harmed' and 'damaged' selves as a result of abuse. Such a stance challenges the taken for granted assumptions of a modernist view of 'self' where identity is seen as 'separate, stable and additive' (Burman, 1998: 3) which 'follows unproblematically from experience' (Lather, 1990: 76). There is a need, then, to challenge the mainstream research enterprise that abstracts and reifies identity and social categorisations. We need to step outside the modernist endeavour of taxonomies and look at the textual and academic production of such knowledge: what does it enable and what subjectivities are produced as a result? Although contesting the work on the harmfulness of child sexual abuse is a problematic position to take, we need (as critical commentators) to stand outside the realm of science (often drawn upon by second-wave feminist academics and campaigners) to examine the wrongfulness of child sexual abuse in ways that examine issues of power, the construction of the 'developing child', identity and morality.

A post-structuralist-informed feminist practice could involve the mobilisation of a series of practices (including both second-wave feminist science and post-structuralist analytics) for strategic uses within specific geopolitical contexts. Skeggs (2000) stresses that feminism is a stance, a strategy, and can be represented by different historical–temporal moves at the same time where feminists may be both critiquing and claiming particular concepts. Furthermore, it is important that in developing feminist-informed post-structuralist debates concerning the limitations of second-wave feminist theorisations around sexual abuse, the work of such campaigners are acknowledged. It is only because of the work of earlier feminist academics and campaigners that we can take the debates and subject them to critical scrutiny. Furthermore, it is essential to recognise that, whilst child sexual abuse has been the focus of widespread media attention in the West (particularly North America and the UK), this is not a worldwide recognition. Second-wave feminist campaigns are highly relevant and necessary in some geographical and temporal locations to promote the recognition of child sexual abuse.

References

Armstrong, L. (1994) *Rocking the cradle of sexual politics: what happened when women said incest*, New York: Addison-Wesley.

Atmore, C. (1999) 'Sexual abuse and troubled feminism: a reply to Camille Guy', *Feminist Review* 61: 83–96.

Bell, V. (1993) *Interrogating incest: feminism, Foucault and the law*, London: Routledge.

Burman, E. (1994a) 'The abnormal distribution of development: policies for southern women and children', *Gender, Place and Culture* 2, 1: 21–37.

Burman, E. (1994b) *Deconstructing developmental psychology*, London: Routledge.

Burman, E. (1998) *Deconstructing feminist psychology*, London: Sage.

Butler, J. (1990) *Gender trouble: feminism and the subversion of identity*, New York, London: Routledge.

Curt, B.C. (1994) *Textuality and tectonics: troubling social and psychological Science*, Buckingham: Open University Press.

Dominelli, L. (1986) 'Father–daughter incest', *Critical Social Policy* 16: 8–22.

Flax, J. (1992) 'The end of innocence', in J. Butler and J.W. Scott (eds) *Feminists theorise the political*, London: Routledge, pp. 440–458.

Gavey, N. (1999) '"I wasn't raped but ...": revisiting definitional problems in sexual victimization', in S. Lamb (ed.) *New versions of victims: feminist struggle with the concept*, New York and London: New York University Press, pp. 57–81.

Groner, J. (1991) *Hilary's trial: the Elizabeth Morgan case: a child's ordeal in America's legal system*, USA: Simon and Shuster.

Hall, L. and Lloyd, S. (1989) *Surviving child sexual abuse: a handbook for helping women challenge their past*, Basingstoke: Falmer Press.

Herman, J. and Hershman, L. (1981) *Father–daughter incest*, Cambridge and London: Harvard University Press.

Holland, P. (1991) *What is a child? Popular images of childhood*, London: Virago.

Kempe, R.S. and Kempe, C.H. (1978) *Child abuse*, London: Fontana/Open Books.

Kinsey, A.C., Pomeroy, W.B., Martin, C.E. and Gebhard, P.H. (1953) *Sexual behaviour in the human female*, Philadelphia and London: W.B. Saunders and Co.

Kitzinger, J. (1992) 'Sexual violence and compulsory heterosexuality', *Feminism and Psychology* 2, 3: 399–418.

Kosambi, M. and Haggis, J. (2000) 'Reconstructing femininities: colonial intersections of gender, race, religion and class', *Feminist Review* 65: 1–4.

La Fontaine, J. (1990) *Child sexual abuse*, Cambridge: Polity Press.

Lamb, S. (1999) 'Constructing the victim: popular images and lasting labels', in S. Lamb (ed.) *New versions of victims: feminist struggle with the concept*, New York and London: New York University Press, pp. 108–138.

Lather, P. (1990) 'Postmodernism and the human sciences', *The Humanist Sciences* 18, Spring: 64–84.

Levett, A. (1994) 'Discourses of child sexual abuse: regimes of power', in G. Lopez and J.L. Linaza (eds) *Psicologia, Discurso y Poder: Metodologias cualitavas perspectives critical*, Madrid: Visor.

Levine, P. (2000) 'Orientalist sociology and the creation of colonial sexualities', *Feminist Review* 65: 6–14.

McGruder-Johnson, A.K., Davidson, E.S., Gleaves, D.H., Stock, W. and Finch, J.F. (2000) 'Interpersonal violence and posttraumatic symptomology: the effects of ethnicity, gender, and exposure to violent events', *Journal of Interpersonal Violence* 15, 2: 205–221.

MacLeod, M. and Saraga, E. (1988) 'Challenging the orthodoxy: towards feminist theory and practice', *Feminist Review* 28: 16–55.

Morss, J.R. (1990) *The biologising of childhood: developmental psychology and the Darwinian myth*, Hove, Sussex: Lawrence Erlbaum.

Morss, J.R. (1992) 'Making waves, deconstruction and developmental psychology', *Theory and Psychology* 2, 4: 445–465.

O'Dell, L. (1997) 'Child sexual abuse and the academic construction of symptomologies', *Feminism and Psychology* 7: 334–337.

O'Dell, L. and Reavey, P. (2001) 'Listening and speaking: the lost and found voices of women survivors of sexual violence', *Psychology of Women Section Review* 3: 4–14.

Parton, N. (1991) *Governing the family: child care, child protection and the state*, Basingstoke, Macmillan Education Ltd.

Patel, D. (1991) 'Asian women's experiences of child sexual abuse: an initial project', unpublished project, University of East London.

Reavey, P. and Warner, S. (2001) 'Curing women: child sexual abuse, therapy and the construction of femininity', *International Journal of Critical Psychology, Special Issue on Sex and Sexualities* 3: 49–71.

Rose, N. (1990) *Governing the soul: the shaping of the private life*, London: Routledge.

Schecter, M.D. and Roberge, L. (1976) in the British Psychological Society (1989) *Psychologists and Child Sexual Abuse: Report of Working Party of the Professional Affairs Board of the B.P.S.*

Skeggs, S.B. (2000) in Alldred, P., Dennison, S., Azim, F., *et al.* (2000) 'Feminism 2000: One Step beyond?', *Feminist Review* 64: 113–138.

Stainton Rogers, R. and Stainton Rogers, W. (1992) *Stories of childhood: shifting agendas of child concern*, Hemel Hempstead: Harvester Wheatsheaf.

Stenner, P. (1993) 'Discoursing jealousy', in E. Burman and I. Parker (eds) *Discourse analytic research: repertoires and readings of texts in action*, London: Routledge, pp. 114–132.

Vandenberg, B. (1993) Developmental psychology, God and the good, *Theory and Psychology* 3, 2: 191–205.

Walkerdine, V. (1993) 'Beyond developmentalism', *Theory and Psychology* 3, 4: 451–469.

Warner, S. (1996) 'Constructing femininity: models of child sexual abuse and the production of "woman"', in E. Burman, P. Alldred, C. Bewley, *et al.*, *Challenging women: psychology's exclusions, feminist possibilities*, Buckingham: Open University Press, pp. 36–53.

Waterman, J., Kelly, R.J., Oliveri, M.K. and McCord, J. (1994) *Behind the playground walls: sexual abuse in preschools*, New York: The Guildford Press.

Weir, R.I. (1992) 'An experimental course of lectures on moral treatment for mentally ill people', *Journal of Advanced Nursing* 17: 390–395.

Wilson, M. (1993) *Crossing the boundary: Black women survivors of child sexual abuse*, London: Virago.

Wyatt, G.E. (1990) 'The aftermath of child sexual abuse of African American and white American women: the victim's experience', *Journal of Family Violence* 5, 1: 61–81.

Chapter 9

When past meets present to produce a sexual 'other'

Examining professional and everyday narratives of child sexual abuse and sexuality

Paula Reavey

> What we should be able to learn from ... is something of the enormity of the work to be done in making sense of the past as it is lived in the present.
>
> (Segal, 1999: 143)

Introduction

When trying to make sense of our adult sexual identities and the sexual choices we make, psychological discourses often invite us to examine how our past histories weave themselves into our present desires. In particular, those past histories that are sexually abusive are positioned at the forefront of psychological and therapeutic concerns over present adult sexual 'problems' and pathologies (Hacking, 1995).

The literature on child sexual abuse, for example, suggests how 'survivors' are compelled to repeat past abuses in the present context of their sexual encounters and relationships (Jehu, 1989). However, what is noticeable is the gendered production of these types of stories and how they rely on certain assumptions about gender relations and the possession of power – although this is rarely sign-posted in the literature (Haaken, 1999). In many of these texts, it is clear that women become further 'victims' of abuse, as opposed to men with a history of abuse who are seen to be in danger of victimising others. The form of dis/order for women, is the re-enactment of passivity and powerlessness, which clearly are culturally perceived feminised sexual traits, resting on straightforward dichotomies of male (abuser) and female (abused) behaviour (Hare-Mustin and Marecek, 1994: 16).

Rather than accepting these explanations as the only viable 'truth', I think it has been made possible to tell stories about women survivors' lives, where past and present are connected in a literal manner because of the way in which trauma, storytelling practices and gender are constructed in professional and everyday cultural discourses. What is further confused is that many of these 'symptoms' are associated with women generally (irrational, powerless, unreasonable – see Warner, 1996a).

It is my aim in this chapter to explore some of these narratives as they appear in a variety of genres, including therapeutic, self-help and survivor accounts of the effects of abuse on women's sexualities and the production of their identities. The source of this material includes an assortment of already published literature in the field as well as empirical data based on interviews I have conducted with professionals/therapists and survivors (Reavey, 1998). Hence, my focus is on the narratives themselves, and the discursive effects of participants framing understanding of survival in this way, rather than the individuals who use them. A further aim is to cast a critical eye over the discourses that make these texts appear convincing and 'obvious' to the reader. Thus, I present a feminist-post-structuralist reading of the ways in which women survivors are written into not only narratives of abuse, but also the normative representations of sexual choices that take for granted certain heterosexual scripts as guides for behaviour.

Some of the questions that guide these readings are: how are women, as sexual subjects, constituted by discourses of child sexual abuse and by culturally available representations of femininity and heterosexuality? My interest lies in the claims made for and about women survivors in order to explore the identities that are produced and the corresponding associations that arise. As Jeanne Marecek (1999: 159) notes, '[D]escriptions are never just descriptions; they are also explanations': how, then, do these theoretical, political and common-sense explanations hold together as reasonable discourses on women's sexualities?

Inevitably, the form my questioning takes is informed by my theoretical and political approach, that of feminist post-structuralism. Central to this approach is the role that language has in constituting social reality. In this sense, language shapes how we see and think as well as how we express and experience private thoughts. Language and our subsequent discursive practices are seen to be products of historically and culturally produced exchanges between speakers and in the dominant cultural texts (Potter and Wetherell, 1987; Edwards, 1997). Thus, meaning is never fixed once and for all but is shifting and subject to social change. Child sexual abuse and subjectivity are viewed, then, not as fixed 'truths' waiting to be discovered but as phenomena laced and constructed in culturally created and gendered meanings (Haaken, 1998; O'Dell and Reavey, 2001: Reavey and Warner, 2001).

Professional and everyday interpretations: the looping effects of culturally ingrained narratives

Out of the proliferation of women's stories of abuse in the 1980s and 1990s came a revised, yet more psychological language for understanding women's distress and men's culpability, a language that was further removed from the field of women's political activism and closer to the language of mental health and illness (Armstrong, 1994). Wide cultural discourses have tended to embrace individualised interpretations of those who abuse as well as the 'victims' of such abuse. As many writers have noted, child sexual abuse became a way to discuss symptoms of trauma and mental disorder, rather than feminist politics or the social inequalities that exist between men, women and children (Alcoff and Gray, 1993; Choi and Nicolson, 1996).

Part of the reason for my examination here of both professional (psychological/therapeutic) and everyday (self-help/autobiographical) discourses on child sexual abuse, women and sexuality was the wish to not render categorically 'distinct' the stories that 'experts' and 'women' tell (Soyland, 1995). Psychological, therapeutic, self-help and personal stories are all culturally situated narratives, and there is inevitable overlap between them.

This 'overlap' is what Ian Hacking refers to as the 'looping effect of human kinds' where both professional knowledge has come to account for everyday practices and vice versa (especially in the psy-disciplines). Consequently, the boundaries between professional and everyday discourses have become blurred and intertwined (see also Rose, 1990; Reavey, 1998).

Although in clinical psychology and in some therapeutic discourses in the UK the ideal portrayal is one of scientist–practitioner, this position has been severely criticised for failing to acknowledge a litany of cultural assumptions (regarding race, gender, class and able-bodiedness) that underpin both clinical diagnosis and therapeutic theory and practice (Parker et al., 1995; Boyle, 1997; Harper, 1999). According to these critics, 'truth' is always negotiated within a cultural space. Furthermore, it has long been acknowledged by many therapists that their work is necessarily eclectic (Norcross et al., 1995), drawing upon a number of humanistic, practical and cultural interpretations of personal distress. This very 'admission' indicates that the discursive space in which both personal and therapeutic narratives can operate and be negotiated is open to a number of interpretations as well as influences by the therapist (O'Hanlon, 1992). It is these interpretations surrounding gender and sexuality that I wish to explore in the following analysis in order to situate their origins and implications for making sense of women survivors' sexualities and identities.

Analysing texts

Discourse analysis is represented by a number of approaches for working with language. An important aspect of discourse analysis is how 'objects' (female survival and sexuality) get talked about and constructed in a given context (in this case, therapeutic, self-help and personal narratives). The following analysis is based on interviews conducted in the UK and a reading of some popular self-help texts. Ten semi-structured interviews were conducted with professionals across the UK public and private sector (psychiatrists, counsellors, sex therapists, clinical psychologists and psychoanalytic psychotherapists). None of these therapists identified as feminist therapists and all had seen male and female clients who had been sexually abused in childhood. Myself and a co-researcher (see Fuller, 2000) conducted a further ten interviews with women who described themselves as 'survivors' of child sexual abuse. Finally, an analysis of four of the most popular self-help texts available to survivors of child sexual abuse was also carried out, including *The Courage to Heal* (Bass and Davis, 1988), *Reach for the Rainbow* (Finney, 1990), *Hope for Adult Survivors of Incest* (Poston and Lison, 1989) and *Secret Survivors: Uncovering Incest and its Effects in Women* (Blume, 1990).

My main concern across all of these studies was to ask questions about how women's sexuality was viewed in relation to past experiences of child sexual abuse and how associations between past and present (sexual) lives were constructed in these professional and everyday accounts. Often, such discourses are represented as 'innocent forms of knowledge', there only to neutrally 'report' what they see and what the truth 'appears' to be (Flux, 1992). In the case of abuse survival, the analysis examines not only how sense was made of past experiences of child sexual abuse but also how the identities of the survivor are 'produced' by particular discourses that describe her as a woman, survivor, agentic sexual being and responsible adult. A further analytical focus was the narrative frameworks that made these representations of women's sexuality appear plausible and, at the same time, reasonable or even true. However, in feminist post-structuralism, 'truth' is a contested territory, even when referring to a subject's account of his or her experience. As Joan Scott writes:

> When the evidence is offered as the evidence of 'experience', the claim for referentiality is further buttressed – what could be truer, after all, than a subject's own account of what he or she has lived through? It is precisely this kind of appeal to experience as uncontestable evidence ... as a foundation upon which analysis is based that weaken the critical thrust of histories of difference ... they take as self-evident the identities of those whose experience is being documented and thus naturalize their difference.
>
> (1992: 24)

In discourses of child sexual abuse, it is the gendered fictions that constitute the sexual identities of survivors that often remain hidden, and in the following analysis I investigate these in more detail. The analysis is not intended to speak for 'all' women or produce a unitary version of womanhood. Instead, the intention is to highlight how gendered identifications operate in relation to discourses of survival and the subsequent versions of woman being produced through these accounts. Moreover, I wish to illuminate some of the connections between individual sexual identities and wider narratives of gender and heterosexuality by making, (1) Wider power issues more visible and expanding the analysis of the 'individual survivor' to incorporate the socially situated nature of sexual difficulties; and (2) acknowledging the wider problematics of women survivors' sexuality in the context of heterosexuality.

The purpose here is not to use these textual examples as a way of generalising about all therapists, survivors and self-help texts, but to highlight how some interpretations of women survivors' sexuality are problematic. The material also focuses on heterosexual women, as the therapists and survivors in these studies spoke mainly of heterosexuality in relation to women survivors and because the self-help literature contained no 'specialised' sections on alternative sexual orientations.

In the following analysis, I present four dominant themes which address how women's survival and gender relations were constructed in the texts:

1   abused women as 'other' in discourses of gender and womanhood.
2   women's sexual choices and discourses of re-enactment and re-victimisation.
3   normative femininity and the problematics of sexual choices.
4   masculine subjectivity and the context of heterosexuality.

Abused women as 'other' in discourses of gender and womanhood

In professional and everyday discourses, statements about abused people 'often rest on the discursive frameworks of non-abused people' (Miltenburg and Singer, 2000: 517). In other words, when we talk about abused men and women, we are assuming that non-abused people have been allowed to follow a 'normal' developmental path to a healthy sexuality. Circulating in much of the therapeutic and self-help literature in contemporary writings on women survivors (and in the literature on sexuality in general – see Plummer, 1995) are discourses of 'choice', 'personal power' and 'healing' which all survivors have a right to (see Kitzinger, 1992).

It is often assumed that the global context of sexuality can offer non-abused individuals access to choice – a *liberal ideology* that is also the focus of much post-feminist writings on sexuality. Certainly, contemporary discourses of sexuality in general are largely defined according to liberal standards of self-fulfilment, such as 'choice' which equates with the so-called free market of desire (Plummer, 1995).

By framing our understanding of sexuality within the rhetoric of liberalism, however, it is easier to isolate the survivors' difficulties and locate them internally.

In positioning the survivor as separate from the norm, outside the 'healthy' developmental path of non-abused individuals, it is easier to locate their 'symptoms' and make secure an identity for them as 'other' to women who supposedly develop within a notion of naturalised femininity (O'Dell, 1997; Haaken, 1998; Miltenburg and Singer, 2000; Reavey and Warner, 2001):

> The most fundamental reason adult women survivors of incest feel that there is something wrong with their sex lives is that they are speaking a language different from everyone else's ...
>
> (Poston and Lison, 1989: 175)

Such individualistic depictions, however, fail to acknowledge the various hierarchies under which development takes place, one of which is gender. Consequently, in situating abused women as distinct from non-abused women who were, theoretically, 'left' to develop their sexuality in a normal and natural way, the problems they potentially face are categorised as individual problems:

> 'I don't know what normal is ... I think other women who haven't been through what I have *do* ... I think there must be something *about me*' (Survivor no. 4); They [survivors] will use their sexuality in quite a different way from other women, they have a very different attitude towards men as a result ... disturbed (sex therapist).

Thus, when survivors face problems with their sexuality, they are advised to seek more 'correct' ways of thinking about sex:

> Think about the information and attitudes you picked up about being female and remember where you learnt them. Share these with some women friends to help you sort out your underlying beliefs about yourself as a female. Revise those rules and attitudes that you disagree with and that hold you back from living your life and sexuality to the fullest.
>
> (Kunzman, 1990: 41)

One of the aims of our therapy is to get women to acknowledge that the context of sex is safe ... it's getting them to recognise that the way they think is linked to what happened in the past.

> (Cognitive-behavioural therapist)

Here it is suggested that 'other' women hold 'liberating' ideas about being female and that survivors can be 'taught', using their 'inner power', to correct their thinking about sex and men. However, the problem with this approach is that the threat of sexual violence or a lack of trust is globally endorsed as something which only certain individuals (i.e. abuse victims) experience or are fearful of. This is nowhere more apparent than in one of the self-help texts which has been written by therapists, one of whom is a survivor and one who is not. Their analysis of the difference in perception of survivors and non-survivors is spelt out via the embodiment of each therapist in the contrasting positions:

> women who are not incest survivors, such as Karen Lison, the co-author of this book, think that this feminist reading of the power differential with which survivors can associate their feelings is a misreading of a harmless sexual message system.
>
> (Poston and Lison, 1989: 182)

Although this particular book (see also Bass and Davis, 1988) does include a feminist reading of generalised power dynamics in relation to sexuality, the differences in the two women's perceptions are located in their personal life histories. In problematising these narratives, I am not suggesting that some survivors of child sexual abuse do not experience difficulties with their sexuality or that they do not feel vulnerable or hurt. What is problematic is how these accounts suggest that struggles for meaning over gender and sexuality are confined only to the abuses of an individual's past, rather than the operations of power in the present lives of all men and women. I would suggest that separating 'abused' from 'non-abused' women could serve to personalise problems that survivors have with sexuality. Furthermore, such discourses fail to acknowledge that the general climate for heterosexual women is frequently difficult and troubling when it comes to negotiating choices and balancing power relations (see Gavey, 1992).

It is also clear from the examples that follow that even though women survivors are viewed as separate from the norm, they are certainly judged against the standards required from normative prescriptions of gender and (hetero)sexuality. Moreover, is it right to assume that 'non-abused' women do not struggle to negotiate their sexualities in a healthy way and that their personal narratives are saturated with various experiences of both feminine vulnerabilities *as well as* choice and agency? By assuming that the world of sexuality is a 'liberating' and 'choice saturated' territory, many of the problems survivors face can only be explained according to 'their' own personal vulnerabilities, reinforcing the idea that survivors can change (or should change) their sexual functioning by changing themselves, by reclaiming their sexuality through individual healing and being liberated by their 'choices'. But what do these accounts obscure? I am not suggesting that women do not have choices with regards to their sexuality, but that the territory of sexuality is often far from liberal or neutral for many women, as many empirical accounts from 'ordinary' heterosexual women in the literature have indicated (see Gavey, 1992, 1996; Holland *et al.*, 1994, 1998). Moreover, if we see sexual desire and the subsequent relations we form only as a 'choice', how do we account for women who have had seemingly 'normal', 'safe' and supportive histories making 'bad' choices in their adult relationships?

Women's sexual choices: discourses of re-enactment and re-victimisation

> When I was raped as an adult, and I took it to court, they were more interested in the fact that I had been sexually abused as a child, as if that was the reason why these things had happened to me.
>
> (Survivor no. 8)

There is a widespread notion in the professional, self-help and autobiographical literature on child sexual abuse that some abused women re-enact many aspects of their abuse. This narrative depicts women survivors as passively and irrationally 'choosing' further abuse (Kitzinger, 1992; O'Dell, 1997; Warner, 1997), such as relationships with violent men, prostitution and so on. The survivor's behaviour, therefore, can be viewed as a self-fulfilling prophecy as she transfers her victimhood through time and other people: this portrayal can feed a crude psychoanalytic reading that focuses only upon the faults of the woman's 'mental apparatus' (Kitzinger, 1992; Reavey and Gough, 2000).

For example, the following accounts appear to be plausible because of their depiction of the 'visible' victim and hidden (and even passive) perpetrator and the unitary reliance on the identity characteristics of the female victim/survivor.

> By such demeanour a woman survivor is giving out another signal loud and clear, and that is, 'I am not looking at you because I am afraid'. Her body language broadcasts a message that she is a helpless victim, frightened even to exchange glances with a man.
>
> (Poston and Lison, 1989: 169)

> Until she deals with the memories of her past, she can expect the acts which terrorised her to be repeated.
>
> (Finney, 1989: 39)

> I don't think they consciously seek out abuse ... but it often feels that they're drawing out from men what they've always been used to ...
>
> (Clinical psychologist)

and the rape ... I don't know whether it was unconsciously inviting them in, giving them signs and cues, do you know what I mean? I'd already said no I don't want to, but he would never be able to understand where I'm coming from ... and basically I'd led him on, so I deserved it ... and I ... I don't know whether I was unconsciously inviting them in.

(Survivor no. 3)

These seemingly monolithic and straightforward explanations of re-victimisations offer little attempt to contextualise the occurrence of sexual violence, citing the reason for re-victimisation in the woman's behaviour, her visible vulnerability and unconscious 'choice' of partner (Lamb, 1996, 1999). While these readings of women's choices proliferate in the literature, scant attention has been paid to providing adequate justifications for these types of readings. As Warner (1996) has noted, it is hard to imagine that on women's list of desirable male assets, rapist, batterer and emotional abuser is amongst them.

When assessing the behaviour of abuse survivors in the present, the tendency in professional and everyday discourses is to opt for less ambivalent, and therefore less complex currents of sexuality, situating conflict in the site of abuse only (Haaken, 1998). Instead of perceiving sexual threat as a realistic prospect for all women, survivors are given instructions on how to 'correct' their attitudes towards men. As Jenny Kitzinger notes, correction of the self means that:

... [T]he threat of male violence can be transcended by the woman who has the correct attitude, good role models or effective assertive techniques ... [i]nstead of talking of demands ... many women now talk of 'rights' as if each individual already has them and need only claim them.

(1992: 410)

Such individualised depictions of sexual threat once again invites focus on the individual and her erroneous perceptions and damaged character. They also mirror the tendency in 'everyday' attitudes towards women who are raped, where characterological blame is more frequently attributed to women than men. This cultural tendency invites women's characters and personality types to be scrutinised, rather than the contexts of the victimisation itself or the behaviours involved (see Anderson, 1999). For example, the above extract from a survivor's account indicates how, even when a woman starts off believing she has said 'no' firmly, she still ultimately doubts herself and questions only her own motives – as was the case for the majority of women in these studies (see Reavey and Gough, 2000). In such cases, the survivor is constructed as the *source* of the issue, as she does not behave as 'normal' women behave and the choice to lead a healthy sexual life rests on her individual ability to 'change'. She must, therefore, engage in a process of self-discipline in order to save herself from further attack.

What is also troubling about such accounts is the tendency to overlook the similarities between survivors and many women in the context of heterosexuality; for example, their struggles over agency, the difficulties in achieving autonomy in sexual encounters, the compromise of choices in order to 'be feminine' and the complexity of saying yes and no to sex, when we are not always heard or our desires always listened to. These are cultural struggles that are found in many 'non-abused' women's experiences of heterosexual sex (Gavey, 1992) and it is this recognition that needs to be made in order for a more culturally sensitive understanding of survivors' sexuality to be achieved. If child sexual abuse continues to act as a causal narrative in accounts of sexual violence and problematic sexual relations in adult life, the very organisation of heterosexuality remains unexamined, and men and women's subject positions are 'naturalised' (Butler, 1993) within a regulatory notion of heteronormativity. This can lead to a narrow focus on the recovery of 'different' and 'damaged' women, without sufficient attention to the situations that give rise to sexual attacks (Warner, 1997).

Normative femininity and the problematics of sexual choices

> sexual abuse assumes priority as a causal factor in female disturbances because it symbolizes dilemmas more common to women: specifically, vulnerability to masculine invasions and subjugations to male assertions of sexual entitlement.
>
> (Haaken, 1999: 17–18)

> Q. You said something about not being quite sure what 'women' are supposed to be like, can you explain what you mean by this?
>
> A. Women? Like ten year old girls ... like the kind of fable thing that existed, you know, but where no-one's quite sure what they are.
>
> (Survivor no. 5)

Much of the psychological research into the long-term effects of child sexual abuse is conducted using women as participants or 'subjects'. However, the way in which 'gender' and 'heterosexuality' is constructed by this research and practice is rarely acknowledged, leaving the reader to assume that abused women experience their sexuality in *categorically* different ways from non-abused women. However, not all women's experiences are the same, and certainly even abuse survivors have diverse stories to tell (from varying positions of race, class, religiosity, sexual orientation) that shape their interpretations of their sexuality (see Wilson, 1994; Warner, 1996; Haaken, 1999; O'Dell and Reavey, 2001). In the therapists' and survivors' accounts, many of the participants talked explicitly about the effects of child sexual abuse in 'gender neutral' (as in 'effects' are seen to be the same for women and men) terms. However, a closer reading reveals that women's subsequent choices are often theorised in highly gendered ways. For example, many of the participants in the studies mentioned here acknowledged the role of gender in the formation of their ideas of sexuality and choice, and spoke of how seeming ideals of femininity placed severe limits on women's abilities to make positive choices regarding their sexuality. For many of the therapists and survivors, femininity was viewed negatively; as fragile, more complex and ambivalent, and as a more malleable starting point for sexual expression to take place. Furthermore, several ways of constructing femininity were deployed that potrayed femininity as a less stable position from which to express sexuality. The following extracts indicate how women's sexual expression was seen as *inherently* more prone to damage through past experiences of child sexual abuse:

> Q. ... you mentioned that at some point women can have a more fragile expression, can you explain that a bit more?
>
> A. ... it seems that women tend to, women's sexuality seems to be more easily affected or influenced by things, whether it's attitudes, parental attitudes, or parents with the child, the way we learn about sexuality, it seems to be very easily knocked off course and influenced by things, because of the way they respond sexually, maybe partly to do with physiology, and the way women are made, and so, um so basically they seem to be affected differently to men.
>
> (Psychoanalytic psychotherapist)

or through an internalisation of society's treatment of women, leading to a state of immobility and inhibition:

> and the problem is men's awful innate aggressive drive which is very much tied up with their sexual drive and I think women who have been abused suffer more because of the way in which society is set up, they're much more likely to have blanket inhibitions on their sexual experiences, or sexual feelings and so on, um ... and that can make them very inhibited people sexually, very inhibited ... no, sexual liberation hasn't really happened.
>
> (Psychiatrist)

In the following extracts, the role women play in order to be perceived as normal (according to male standards) inevitably leads to their vulnerability. However, powerlessness cannot simply be seen as generated through intra-psychic struggles when dealing with abuse issues, as it is also produced through the culturally available depictions of femininity:

> I envy women who can be feminine ... weak, I envy women like that who can laugh at things ... men like to be around them because it makes them feel masculine, because they can pick up the woman and dust her down and sort her out because she's sweet and feminine and petite and tiny and vulnerable and I envy women like that because I think they are playing, not necessarily a game but I think they are playing on their sexuality, playing on their gender.
>
> (Survivor no. 10)

> [...] it's always the feeling at the back of my head, you know, nice girls don't do that sort of thing, they don't argue, they are quiet, and they put up with things and that's how it should be ... because I see my femininity as very much stemming from masculine ideas as to what women should be, you are feminine if you fit in with what your bloke sees as feminine.
>
> (Survivor no. 8)

In accounts such as these it is difficult to extract any notion of choice as positive. This is because female sexuality is typically associated with a position of passivity. Similarly, it is clear that normative femininity also functions as a common way through which women survivors are judged, not just by others, but also in the ways in which they attempt to discipline themselves (Warner, 1996). The invitation to judge themselves negatively is especially apparent when women are seen to 'choose' to have sex that is outside of the boundaries of normative ideals of femininity, because of the ambiguous and derogatory meanings that can be associated with women's sexual agency within the confines of heteronormativity.

> [A]s a woman ... [you] realise that the issue of abuse is much more complex ... I want women to say, the child had no choice in it ... when you're an adult, you are making choices, as a child you might not have, but you are when you're adolescent and adult women know this, and read about this, and so ... what's to stop them sort of thinking, well she was a bit, she was a bit of a slut really, something to do with, perhaps she was like that from early on, do you know what I mean? I mean I know that people used to think that I was a slag [laughs] [P yeah] if they'd have known my past then I think they [women]

wouldn't have thought 'Oh dear what a shame, that's why she's doing that'. They'd have thought, 'What a slag, she was like it as a kid' ... it sounds horrendous.

(Survivor no. 3)

I would suggest that the difficulty in seeing women as active agents in their sexual encounters is a pervasive story in women's accounts of their sexuality generally (Segal, 1992; Holland *et al.*, 1994). But, in the abuse literature, such issues are rarely sign-posted with reference to how these difficulties are culturally situated. Accessing successful adult relationships is not, therefore (as some of the therapists and self-help texts suggested) a simple matter of abused women 'correcting' their thoughts on what it means to be a 'healthy' woman because it may be the case that femininity in general is perceived to be symbolic of all that is frightening and 'guilt-ridden' about sexuality (Warner, 1996).

In order to understand the problems survivors face in interpreting their sexuality it is, therefore, important to grasp how sense is made of the wider landscape of sexual encounters which normatively prescribes how women should behave and where gendered inequalities reside. This entails a closer look at how not only femininity is defined, but how masculinity enters into the sexual equation when talk of survival is conducted (Reavey, 1998). Masculinity, for example, is often depicted as the gate-keeper of all that is powerful within the context of heterosexuality. Such a depiction reiterates the notion of masculine authority and female deference in culture generally, a position which was of significance in these studies when talk of power issues in sexuality arose.

Masculine subjectivity and the context of heterosexuality

In feminist discourses of women's sexuality, it is acknowledged that women and girls have less access to the more agentic sexual narratives (Segal, 1999). Women's personal narratives are so culturally infused with reference and deference to a powerful masculine 'other' that the threat of potential control, power and violence over their sexuality is, at times, perceived to be inescapable (Gagne, 1992; Levett, 1995). Unsurprisingly this position was reproduced in some of the therapists' accounts; however, it occurred in a way that suggested women should accept, or come to terms with their lack of power, because they choose it:

Q. What do you *mean?* by them needing a man with authority?

A. Well, I think they might go for a mild, kind, loving man, but may be somebody who isn't strong enough to trust to say, um, I don't want you to do that, that isn't right. Um, [pause] you know, you need some-body who's powerful but to use their power well, I think they can be attracted to somebody who's mild, that they're not maybe strong enough or firm enough.

(Psycho-sexual counsellor)

Often it's the men and the power, and the dominance, aggression out, which a lot of men have, and it comes out sexually ... but I think that they [abuse survivors] are drawing out of that man what they've always been used to.

(Psychiatrist)

Because the history seems to be that you choose a partner that doesn't understand, or isn't there for you ... well a survivor can pick a rescuer, so a man that needs to rescue this woman ... quite a traditional role really.

(Counsellor)

Women survivors are restricted in their ability to be seen as active agents as their 'choices' are already limited by an often automatic reference to masculine power and control (Hollway, 1995; Levett, 1995; Gavey, 1996; Holland *et al.*, 1998). This is also tied in with the way in which femininity is produced within these accounts, which inevitably reinforces a traditional heterosexual script that women should, to a certain extent, even find this position of powerlessness desirable.

Such expectations surrounding women's position as deferential to men's were especially pertinent when some of the therapists were dis-cussing the cultural idea that achieving penetration and providing for men's sexual needs was part of a normal heterosexual performance, as the following extracts indicate:

A. They [survivors of child sexual abuse] may be very much more needing to control, not let themselves go, making sure that there's a safe, longing for quite unrealistically, a man without any force, when in fact what they do need is a man with force, because they end up getting a man without any power, and then that isn't going to work for them because they need a powerful man, and one with authority, but it needs to be a good authority, not a manipulative and abusing one. If that makes any sense?

(Sex therapist)

Men, I think, have an innate need for penetration, to exercise control over women which victims of abuse have trouble with.

(Psychiatrist)

Penetration is part of most people's everyday sexual experience and survivors have to deal with the fact that that will be expected and that they have at some point to release their control over the sexual act.

(Clinical psychologist)

This rather uncritical take on the legitimacy of male power and the 'unrealistic' expectations of women survivors who think that they can take control of the sexual situation was not shared by all of the therapists. Others saw the focus on penetration as potentially confusing for survivors yet prescribed by the normative expectations of heterosexual sex:

[S]ometimes, a lot of the time, it's not, they're trying to have a normal life so they can't have sex and the partner can't penetrate, that's something we immediately look for, whose goals ... so their sexuality, if you like is very confused as to what they want and what their partner wants ... and by definition the only thing they can give a man is penetrative sex.

(Counsellor)

Rather than accepting the inevitability of male power and control as innately aggressive within heterosexual relationships, more liberating stories of women's desire and expressions of sexuality should be promoted in therapy as well as in everyday life. Otherwise, we contribute to existing power relations rather than creating the means to challenge them.

Conclusions

I have argued that culturally defined representations of femininity and the context of heterosexuality offer a significant discursive space in which to read the subjectivities of abuse survivors and challenge the normative prescriptions on which they are based. This involved exploring how past abuse was seen to be situated in present day sexual lives, wherein deeply ingrained cultural narratives of gendered power relations and binaries were brought into being. For example, there were numerous references to positions of power in a variety of different contexts of survival representations of the power-ful (men) and power-less (women) and how such positions were (culturally) deemed to be un/desirable (in positive and negative terms). These discourses had implications in terms of the ways in which responsibility and unconscious motivations were framed whilst the social production of such narratives often remained hidden. For example, the centralising narrative of re-enactment obscured the social context of rape and the problematics of heterosexuality.

Furthermore, 'choice' was utilised in organising accounts of the past (where women made bad choices) and the present (where women can be freed up to make good choices) which often prevented a more socially located reading of the wider problematics of agency among women more generally. According to a feminist post-structuralist reading, choices are, therefore, never complete and always partial. In this way, they can be read for what they are doing in relation to a personal narrative and not what they essentially 'reveal' about a person. However, central to my analysis has also been an engagement with the 'politics' of survivorship and sexuality in order to thrust the politics of survival back into personalised readings of the 'effects'.

Linking past with present, is far from straightforward and entails looking beyond individual experiences of abuse in order to render visible a whole host of power struggles and normative constraints on all sexual subjectivities. Although I agree that psychological investigations into the 'unconscious', and the 'mind' are useful at certain times when engaging with women who have been abused (see Warner, this volume), I would question the way in which such metaphors become set up as internalised states. As this chapter demonstrates, there is a need to understand not only past experiences of abuse, but to situate individualised narratives in the social production of abuse, femininity and heterosexuality. In this way, the identificatory practices associated with them can enable a greater understanding of the social production of women who have been abused and militate against an overarching focus on individualised 'choices' and personal responsibility.

Acknowledgements

I would like to thank Nicola Gavey, Katherine Johnson and Val Gillies for their helpful comments on earlier drafts of the chapter.

References

Alcoff, L. and Gray, L. (1993) 'Survivor discourse: transgression or recuperation?', *Signs* 18: 260–290.

Anderson, I. (1999) 'Characterological and behavioural blame in conversations about female and male rape', *Journal of Language and Social Psychology* 18: 377–394.

Armstrong, L. (1994) *Rocking the cradle of sexual politics. What happened when women said incest?* London: The Women's Press.

Bass, E. and Davis, L. (1988) *The courage to heal: women's guide to survival*, Bolton: Cedar Press.

Blume, E. (1990) *Secret survivors: uncovering incest and its effects in women*, New York: Ballantine Books.

Boyle, M. (1997) 'Clinical psychology: theory making gender visible in clinical psychology', *Feminism and Psychology* 7: 231–238.

Butler, J. (1993) Bodies that matter: on the discourse limits of 'sex', New York and London: Routledge.

Choi, P. and Nicolson, P. (1996) *Female sexuality*, London: Sage.

Edwards, D. (1997) *Discourse and cognition*, London: Sage.

Finney, L.D. (1990) *Reach for the rainbow: advanced healing for survivors of sexual abuse*, Park City: Changes Publishing.

Flux, J. (1992) 'The end of innocence', in J. Butler and J.W. Scott. (eds) *Feminists theorize the political*, London: Routledge.

Fuller, J. (2000) 'Examining partner choice for women survivors of child sexual abuse', unpublished dissertation, South Bank University.

Gagne, P.L. (1992) 'Appalachian women: violence and social control', *Journal of Contemporary Ethnography* 20: 387–415.

Gavey, N. (1992) 'Technologies and effects of heterosexual coercion', in C. Kitzinger and S. Wilkinson (eds) *Feminism and psychology: special issue on heterosexuality* 2, 3: 325–353.

Gavey, N. (1996) 'Women's desire and sexual violence discourse', in S. Wilkinson (ed.) *Feminist social psychologies: international perspectives*, Buckingham: Open University Press.

Haaken, J. (1998) *Pillars of salt: gender, memory and the perils of looking back*, London: Free Association Press.

Haaken, J. (1999) 'Heretical texts: *The courage to heal* and the incest survivor movement', in S. Lamb (ed.) *New versions of victims: feminists struggle with the concept*, New York: New York University Press.

Hacking, I. (1995) *Rewriting the soul: multiple personality and the sciences of memory*, Princeton: Princeton University Press.

Hare-Mustin, R. and Marecek, J. (1994) 'Feminism and post-modernism: dilemmas and points of resistance', *Dulwich Centre Newsletter* 4: 13–19.

Harper, D. (1999) 'Tablet talk and depot discourse: discourse analysis and psychiatric medication', in C. Willig (ed.) *Applied discourse analysis*, Buckingham: Open University Press.

Holland, J., Ramazonoglu, C., Sharpe, S. and Thomson, R. (1994) 'Power and desire: the embodiment of female sexuality', *Feminist Review* 46: 20–38.

Holland, J., Ramazanoglu, C., Sharpe, S. and Thomson, R. (1998) *The male in the head: young people, heterosexuality and power*, London: Tufnell Park Press.

Hollway, W. (1995) 'Feminist discourses and women's heterosexual desire', in S. Wilkinson and C. Kitzinger (eds) *Feminism and discourse: psychological perspectives*, London: Sage.

Jehu, D. (1989) 'Sexual dysfunction among women clients who were sexually abused in childhood', *Behavioural Psychotherapy* 17: 53–70.

Kitzinger, J. (1992) 'Sexual violence and compulsory heterosexuality', in C. Kitzinger and S. Wilkinson (eds) *Feminism and psychology: special issue on heterosexuality*, London: Sage.

Kunzman, K.A. (1990) *The healing way: adult recovery from childhood sexual abuse*, London: Harper Row.

Lamb, S. (1996) *The trouble with blame: victims, perpetrators, and responsibility*, Cambridge: Harvard University Press.

Lamb, S. (1999) 'Constructing the victim: popular images and lasting labels', in S.

Lamb (ed.) *New versions of victims: feminists struggle with the concept*, New York: New York University Press.

Levett, A. (1995) 'Stigmatic factors in sexual abuse and the violence of representation', *Psychology in Society* 20: 4–12.

Maracek, J. (1999) 'Trauma talk in feminist clinical practice', in S. Lamb (ed.) *New versions of victims: feminists struggle with the concept*, New York: New York University Press.

Miltenburg, R. and Singer, E. (2000) 'A concept becomes a passion: moral commitment and the affective development of the survivors of child abuse', *Theory and Psychology* 10: 503–526.

Norcross, J., Brust, A. and Dryden, W. (1995) 'British clinical psychologists: a national survey of the BPS clinical division', *Clinical Psychology Forum* 40: 19–24.

O'Dell, L. (1997) 'Child sexual abuse and the academic construction of symptomatologies', *Feminism and Psychology* 7, 3: 334–339.

O'Dell, L. and Reavey, P. (2001) 'Listening and speaking: the lost and found voices of survivors of sexual violence', *Psychology of Women Section Review* 3: 4–14.

O'Hanlon, W.H. (1992) 'History becomes her story: collaborative solution-oriented therapy of the after-effects of sexual abuse', in S. McNamee and K.J. Gergen (eds) *Therapy as Social Construction*, London: Sage.

Parker, I., Georgaca, D.H., Harper, D., McLaughlin, T. and Stowell-Smith, M. (1995) *Deconstructing psychopathology*, London: Sage.

Plummer, K. (1995) *Telling sexual stories: power, change and social worlds*, London: Routledge.

Poston, C. and Lison, K. (1989) *Hope for adult survivors of incest*, Boston: Little Brown and Company.

Potter, J. and Wetherell, M. (1987) *Discourse and social psychology: beyond attitudes and behaviour*, London: Sage.

Reavey, P. (1998) 'Child sexual abuse: professional and everyday constructions of women and sexuality', unpublished PhD thesis, Sheffield Hallam University.

Reavey, P. and Gough, B. (2000) 'Dis/locating blame: survivors' constructions of self and sexual abuse', *Sexualities* 3, 3: 325–346.

Reavey, P. and Warner, S. (2001) 'Curing women: child sexual abuse, therapy and the construction of femininity', *International Journal of Critical Psychology, Special Issue on Sex and Sexualities* 3: 49–71.

Rose, N. (1999) *Governing the soul: the shaping of the private self*, London: Free Association Books.

Scott, J.W. (1992) 'Experience', in J. Butler and J.W. Scott (eds) *Feminists theorize the political*, New York: Routledge.

Segal, L. (1992) 'Sexual uncertainty, or why the clitoris is not enough', in H. Crowley and S. Himmelweit (eds) *Knowing women: feminism and knowledge*, Cambridge: Polity Press.

Segal, L. (1999) *Why feminism?* Cambridge: Polity Press.

Soyland, A.J. (1995) 'Analysing therapeutic and professional discourse', in J. Siegfried (ed.) *Therapeutic and everyday discourse as behaviour change: towards a micro-analysis in psychotherapy process research*, Norwood: Ablex Publishing Corporation.

Warner, S. (1996) 'Constructing femininity: models of child sexual abuse and the production of "woman"', in E. Burman, P. Alldred, C. Bewley, *et al.* (1996) *Challenging women: psychology's exclusions, feminist possibilities*, Buckingham: Open University Press.

Warner, S. (1997) Review article, of Davies, M. *Healing Sylvia*, S. Orr's *No right way* and P. Reder *et al.*'s *Beyond blame, feminism and psychology* 3: 377–383.

Wilson, T. (1994) 'Silences, absences and fragmentation', in L. Doyal, J. Naidoo and T. Wilton (eds) *AIDS: setting a feminist agenda*, London: Taylor and Francis.

Chapter 10

Diagnosing distress and reproducing disorder

Women, child sexual abuse and 'borderline personality disorder'

Sam Warner and Tracy Wilkins

Introduction

Many women who report histories of childhood sexual abuse negotiate their adulthood with few discernible negative effects. Some women, however, are so traumatised by their early experiences of abuse that their ability to negotiate adulthood is severely compromised.

Some of these women may develop so-called serious mental health problems. Indeed, whilst childhood sexual abuse does not necessarily have a debilitating effect on mental health, many people who experience mental health problems also report histories of childhood sexual abuse (Herman, 1993). It is unsurprising, therefore, that mental health services contain considerable numbers of women who report histories of childhood sexual abuse. The behaviour of some of these women may be considered to be so abnormal, or so out of control, that community-based services are not thought able to contain them (Warner, 1996a, b, 2000a, b, c). They may then be directed into secure mental health services. A minority of these women may be deemed to be so problematic that they require detention within hospitals of *maximum* security or 'special' hospitals as they are referred to in the UK. This chapter is about these women: women that seem so unreasonable and so extreme that they cannot be contained elsewhere.

There are many reasons (other than childhood trauma) given to warrant women's compulsory detention within secure mental health systems (Warner, 1999). However, over recent years child sexual abuse has emerged as a significant narrative in the lives of such women (Warner, 1996a, b; see also WISH, 1999), just as it has more generally emerged as a significant social story in Western cultures (Plummer, 1995). Concomitantly, there has been a significant increase in the number of women, detained in special hospitals, who are diagnosed as having a borderline personality disorder (WISH, ibid.). In this chapter, we draw on research conducted in a British special hospital to explore some of the intersections between women (patients), the diagnosis of borderline personality disorder and experiences of child sexual abuse. We draw on post-structuralism and feminism to critically examine some of the unacknowledged assumptions implicated in these narratives in order to explicate the ways in which women's placement and treatment in special hospitals is achieved and regulated. Both post-structuralist theory and feminist politics provide frameworks that can be used to explore the discursive mechanisms that fashion and preserve social structural hierarchies as if they represent a natural social order. Our aim in this chapter is to utilise these frameworks to elaborate the discursive construction of compulsory mental health services in order to explicate the role the medical model plays in the mediation of secure psychiatric care of women. We do this by interrogating the ways in which women, borderline personality disorder and child sexual abuse are spoken about. The quotes, except where otherwise stated, are taken from interviews conducted by the second author with patients and members of staff at a British special hospital.

We begin by explicating the role diagnosis plays in the maintenance of medical hegemony and examine the regulatory effects of current conceptualisations of borderline personality disorder. We argue that borderline personality disorder relies on and reproduces normative assumptions about gender. We demonstrate how narratives about child sexual abuse are used to justify the category of borderline personality disorder, yet remain hidden, and therefore unexplored. We consider the ways in which the Mental Health Act (1983) is implicated in the disposal of women diagnosed as having borderline personality disorder and demonstrate that a recognition of the social foundations of mental distress has not led to more progressive approaches to mental health care. Specifically, we explicate the ways in which narratives about the 'effects' of child sexual abuse can be mobilised to pathologise women and obscure the role of current institutional shortcomings in the maintenance of so-called personality disorder. We argue that workers must reflect on their own investments in current psychiatric hierarchies if services are to do more than simply re-enact abusive relationships. We conclude that a more social and provisional understanding of current categorical practices is necessitated if we are to expose their fictionality and, in so doing, restrict their regulatory effects.

Creating the category: the medical model and the art of diagnosis

From the perspective of scientific medicine, mental disorder can be understood as being a fixed and internal property of individuals which can be deciphered through tracking causality and interpreting symptoms (Madigan, 1999). Diagnosis, therefore, holds a central place within the practice of scientific medicine because it represents *the* mechanism through which (mental) abnormality can be recognised, named and fixed.

Diagnosis translates individual experience into internalised disorder through categorising 'some forms of human misery as medical problems' (Kleinman, 1988: 7). Whilst diagnosis necessarily relies on interpretation, the ways in which human misery is discursively regulated through the structuring effects of categorisation remains hidden. This is because opinion is presented as truth; such truths subjugate other knowledge; and their ready availability further confirms their veracity (Warner, 1996a). Hence, the practice of diagnosis does not simply reveal 'facts' about human misery, but rather is implicated in the social production of what counts as the 'truth' about human misery (cf. Foucault, 1992). With over four hundred possible ways to be considered miserable/abnormal (Caplan, 1995), psychiatry rarely has difficulty in force-fitting individuals into its many predetermined narratives of distress (see the *Diagnostic and Statistical Manual of Mental Disorders, Fourth Revision*, DSM IV, American Psychiatric Association, 1995).

Diagnostic manuals are, therefore, instrumental in structuring the landscape of misery, and thereby regulating the boundaries of normality. Certain assumptions are implicated in the production of diagnostic manuals, such as DSM IV. Fundamental to the production of diagnostic manuals is the assumption that disorders of the mind are functionally distinct and that clusters of (psycho)pathology can be determined because they are relatively stable over time. The art of diagnosis, then, is to locate the best (general) narratives of psychopathology for describing (individual) expressions of distress. Categorisation, then (amongst other things) requires a belief in, and the ability to objectively define, 'sameness' in people. In terms of mental (ill)health this is understood as 'the tendency of people to do the same painful things, feel the same unpleasant feelings, and establish the same self-destructive relationships, over and over and over' (Mitchell, 1988: 26). Diagnostic categorisation, therefore, provides a means of simplifying complex human behaviour. As a female psychologist stated: 'It is easier to stick one label on all of that sort of stuff, and for us to feel that we've got some kind of handle on it, without having to go down to the complexity of it.'

Since it is not possible to process more than a small part of the information available in any social situation, labels are perceived as a means of organising input and also for determining what further information will be salient (Langer and Abelson, 1974). Unfortunately, this can result in a circular process by which clinicians seek information to confirm their hypothesis, and by doing so, fail to explore other relevant issues. As one male senior manager argued:

I think the problem with very complex situations is you give them one label and therefore approach it in one way, you're likely to not treat a secondary [issue] or ignore the other things. I think it's questionable how well the sort of conceptual frameworks are designed. I just wonder if they get it right sometimes, and therefore single labels in those things are pretty unhelpful.

Hence, as Becker (1997: 48) suggests, 'many clinicians often find what they expect to find, not necessarily what is "out there" to find'. Yet, when faced with the complexity of human behaviour, diagnosis can function as a problematic, but inevitable strategy for sifting information:

> I've wavered over the years from a view that diagnosis is an over simplification and medicalisation, and not that useful, whilst tending to still categorise. There are problems with any kind of diagnostic system, but we do need categorisation systems to make sense of the world we live in.
>
> (Female lead psychologist)

The problem is not reductionism or categorisation per se. Rather it is the obfuscation of the social foundations of medical categorisation. Psychiatric diagnosis is presented as if the constructs it relies on are real, rather than socially produced and socially productive. Diagnosis imposes certain formations of disorder that, once named, can shape how individuals view themselves and their actions. Indeed, diagnosis can be understood to have dramatic effects:

> They've been reinforced all their lives to be bad and mad. They're no good and the label actually states that, so they act out. So I suppose if you took the label away maybe their perception of themselves would change, they wouldn't have to live up to [being] the 'bad, mad psychopath'.
>
> (Female nurse therapist)

Yet, diagnosis is presented as being a short-hand marker for what already exists in people, rather than being one of the mechanisms through which disorderly persons are constructed and reality is controlled. Diagnostic practices and diagnostic structures, therefore, can have powerful effects on regulating what counts as the real world. Yet, such means of control go, for the most part, unseen and unnoticed. So their effects may be visible, but the operations of power implicated in such mechanisms of control remain hidden (see Swan, 1999). Indeed, as Foucault (1981: 86) argues, power is tolerable only on 'condition that it masks a substantial part of itself. Its success is proportional to its ability to hide its own mechanisms.' The medical model maintains its centrality to the social management of so-called mentally disordered individuals by concealing the ways it structures psychiatric realities to maintain medical hegemony. The medical model is (re)presented as *the* means through which mental (ill)health can be deciphered and, as such, psychiatry represents *the* discipline most able to do this deciphering. Diagnosis, therefore, not only specifies the ways in which misery can be articulated, but is also implicated in reifying particular formations of expertise. As Madigan argues:

> The process of being inscribed into the DSM IV text always requires a trained – that is to say, highly specialised – professional whose expertise affords him or her the opportunity and privilege to unlock the secrets of the disordered body.
>
> (1999: 152)

The act of diagnosis, therefore, regulates both patients and professionals, and functionally determines not only who is abnormal but also who has legitimate rights to speak about abnormality. The practice of diagnosis requires experts, and expertise is conferred through the act of diagnosis. By contrast, as Shotter (1993: 38) notes, 'those who are considered "abnormal" are not afforded legitimate speaking rights because they are perceived as not acquiring the "proper rational inquiry".' Hence, women's attempts to fashion their own life narratives will be discredited. As one female nurse therapist observed:

> What often happens is that, especially for women, other people tend to define the problem according to how they see the problem manifesting itself. It isn't always the person themselves who have got a voice to define it for themselves. This is because if it isn't a voice that suits the prevailing ideology, it will be because the women 'can't think about it', because they're 'so damaged'. It will be interpreted, I guess, in a way that suits the prevailing orthodoxy.

Whilst any regulation invites resistance, any challenges to the prevailing orthodoxy will themselves invoke greater attempts to control the social space. Hence, those members of staff that challenge medical hegemony may themselves be made liable to derogation and isolation:

> I haven't been impressed in the teaching case conferences I've gone to. It was all medics with very few other professionals there, and I felt like I was a lone voice when I was trying to put the patient's behaviour into some sort of social context. I can remember standing there and feeling like an alien. They were trying to make medical sense of it, and sometimes you can't. They've just got to have a label, the diagnosis at the end.
>
> (Female social worker)

Diagnostic practices, then, may tell us more about prevailing ideologies and social hierarchical structures than about the 'disorders' of which they ostensibly speak. Indeed, far from being rooted in objective empiricism it may be that, as one female nurse therapist said, diagnosis is built on 'shifting sands'. Borderline personality disorder is one such example of this that has increasing relevance for women detained in special hospitals.

Constructing borderline personality disorder: child sexual abuse and the gendering of 'effects'

Borderline personality disorder is an increasingly popular diagnostic category (Warner, 1996a, b) that has undergone various definitional revisions over time. Over the past forty years descriptions of the 'borderline syndrome' have moved away from an emphasis on its 'schizophrenic-like' features (Becker, 1997), towards an affective symptomatology that stresses emotional lability, self-destructiveness, depression, rage and feelings of emptiness (American Psychiatric Association, 1994). Such emotions are frequently associated with normative femininity (Warner, 2001). It is little wonder, then, that women in special hospitals are significantly more likely than men to meet the criteria for borderline personality disorder (WISH, 1999). Indeed, women generally outnumber men within this category at a rate of anywhere from 2:1 to 9:1 – depending upon the sample under investigation (Becker, 1997).

Concomitantly, over the past two decades there has been an increasing acknowledgement that a high percentage of patients who qualify for a borderline personality disorder diagnosis have also been traumatised through childhood abuse (Barnard and Hirsch, 1985; Coons *et al.*, 1989; Brown and Anderson, 1991; Earl, 1991). Child abuse, like borderline personality disorder, is a gender-saturated narrative in which women are more likely than men to be seen as victims rather than perpetrators. This is especially the case with respect to child sexual abuse (Warner, 1996c, 2000d). It is unsurprising, then, that women in special hospitals are not only more likely to receive a diagnosis of borderline personality disorder but are also significantly more likely to report histories of sexual and physical abuse than male patients (WISH, 1999). So, borderline personality disorder and child abuse have a correlative relationship, if not a 'causative' one. The relationship between borderline personality disorder and child abuse becomes even more enmeshed when childhood *sexual* abuse is considered. This may be expected given that many of the 'symptoms' associated with child sexual abuse (such as deliberate self-harm) are interchangeable with the 'symptoms' associated with borderline personality disorder (Warner, 1996a). Indeed, borderline personality disorder can be understood as the social embodiment of childhood sexual abuse, as well as (already pathologised) femininity. It is unsurprising, therefore, that in a study conducted by Westen *et al.* (1990) a history of sexual abuse was found to be a distinguishing feature of so-called borderline patients (rates of physical abuse were found to be high in most psychiatric research samples of other diagnostic categories).

Because child sexual abuse is seen to co-vary with the diagnosis of borderline personality disorder, it can then be used to support the existence of personality disorder. The 'effects' of child (sexual) abuse can be raised as causing changes in personality structure by interfering with normal personality development. For example, Herman (1992) argues that when chronic child abuse occurs the personality is organised around the central principle of fragmentation because fragmentation serves to keep the trauma out of conscious awareness. Fragmentation as a strategy of survival then becomes fixed as a characteristic of personality, through taken-for-granted stories of 'development', that may then be used to confirm the disordered personality diagnosis. As a female nurse therapist stated:

> It's definitely significant trauma: trauma through their upbringing – neglect, physical abuse, verbal abuse, emotional abuse. It definitely has a major impact on the development of their personality, it's so fragmented. It feels like they can't hold themselves together anymore.

It may be that understanding the relationship between so-called borderline symptoms and women's histories is useful because, through socially located women's actions, it normalises their behaviour (Wile, 1984). Yet the recognition of the social foundations of individualised narratives of misery has not necessarily led to a more social model of secure psychiatric care. Indeed, the process of diagnosis acts to keep the social aspects of traumatisation hidden. This is because borderline personality disorder is defined in emotional terms and not with respect to abuse (see American Psychiatric Association, 1995). Hence, the practice of diagnosis does not invite clinicians to focus on the underlying causes of distress. Diagnosis, therefore, acts as a barrier to understanding the impact earlier experiences of abuse may have. As a female nurse consultant noted:

> I think borderline personality disorder describes mostly a form of chronic traumatisation which has occurred or commenced throughout much of their first decade of life. I think that's the kind of personality that's produced as a result of that, but the criteria for diagnosing borderline personality disorder doesn't include any kind of traumatisation, and I think that the link is then missed. So it's then that this person is 'just like this' for some reason that we don't know.

Histories of childhood sexual abuse, then, may be drawn on to confirm borderline personality disorder, but remain largely unexplored:

Most of the female patients who I work with, who have come in under the label of PD or borderline, have that label purely because they've been abused and they self harm, and that's the main reason why they're classified as that.

(Female social worker)

Diagnosis, then, focuses attention on identifying which symptoms are present rather than exploring what functions so-called symptomatic behaviour serves. Women's meaningful coping strategies, once decontextualised in this way, simply become pathological indicators of (personality) disorder:

What might often be good survival methods in terms of letting people know you're in distress – no matter how unhealthy that might be in the long term they probably kept someone alive. But that's not often going to be seen, particularly in a diagnostic criteria.

(Female nurse therapist)

Hence, rather than being perceived as coping with extreme circumstances, women are depicted as being made ill by, or damaged through, their experiences:

I think that most of the people that come into this kind of service [are here] due to maladaptive parenting, losses, separations, abuse. I think the personality develops in very damaging circumstances that lends itself to a damaged personality.

(Female consultant nurse)

In medical terms early childhood trauma is conceptualised as resulting in permanent damage to the personality. Inculcation into the personality disordered identity invites women to view themselves as being the cause of any future social difficulties. It may also be that women, generally, are still all too ready to internalise fault, blame and responsibility in respect of relationships (Becker, 1997). It is unsurprising, therefore, that women in special hospitals may come to view themselves as being pathological and, hence, unable to change: 'I definitely have seen women who at some level take on board that issue. All behaviour then would be defined as ill, for themselves, which is quite powerless thinking' (female nurse therapist).

Narratives associated with child sexual abuse are embedded within current definitions of borderline personality disorder, but are closed down through repeated abstraction effected through the practice of diagnosis. It is little wonder, then, that the diagnosis does not function as a window into a detailed description of a particular form of disorder. Rather, the diagnosis of (borderline) personality disorder, in practice, may function to obscure specificity acting, in effect, as a general marker of abnormality. When diagnosis functions as a general marker for abnormality, unacknowledged assumptions about gender may then be (re)invoked and gender saturated definitions of so-called abnormal personality structures give rise to very different interventions into the lives of men and women so defined.

Implementing the Mental Health Act: borderline personality disorder and the gendering of exclusion

As already noted, women are far more likely to be given the label of having borderline personality disorder than are men. Despite this, gender is not raised as an explicit marker for this diagnosis, yet assumptions about gender are imbricated into its construction. This is the case for the range of personality disorders (Warner, 1999). And, as Becker argues:

[T]o ignore ... the impact of the differential evaluation of masculine and feminine characteristics and behaviour upon the development of personality disorder – or, more accurately, upon the process that eventuates in the labelling of an individual as having a personality disorder – is to seal off the possibility of developing a more complete understanding of how so-called disorder develops.

(1997: xxiii)

Women have long needed to do less than men to acquire the label of personality disorder (see Allen, 1987) and they will be judged more harshly for exhibiting the same behaviour as men (Warner, 2001). As one male clinical leader noted:

We know that women that offend are treated differently from men who offend, and if you don't [conform to] female stereotypes you're labelled. So I think some of them get the harsher label [for] relatively minor personality difficulties. We probably admit more borderline disorders because their acting out behaviours, and their ability to inflict harm on themselves is so, so challenging to our own ideas of how women should behave. [It is] probably more about the male notion of how a woman should behave, and the conflict with how some of these patients actually do behave, that leads them into high secure beds, rather than the extent of the disorder or their individual treatability.

Hence, the diagnosis of borderline personality disorder relies on traditional assumptions regarding how women should behave. Women may be labelled as having borderline personality disorder when they are deemed to act outside of the ordinary boundaries of femininity:

> For a lot of women it isn't acceptable for them to not be good parents, not [to be] good mothers, to be angry and express that in a hostile way within their environment or to commit a crime, which is at conflict to women.
>
> (Female nurse therapist)

Behaviour that contravenes gender stereotypes may be used to signal personality disorder. More than this, such behaviour may lead to very different consequences for men and women. A behaviour that is considered 'mad' when presented by women may be considered 'bad' when engaged in by men. Indeed, the courts are more likely to assign women to psychiatric care, whilst men are more likely to be assigned to prison (Warner, 1996a). As a female nurse therapist reflected:

> Women are constructed in society as being carers and nurturers, so if they step outside of those it's quite hard for all of us. To see that as being a choice and positive gain, and women being angry and expressing that in a similar way that men do would be pathologised rather than punished. So I think at some level society finds it hard to tolerate the idea of women being bad.

Even when women go to prison, they may still be medicalised because women who do go to prison are more likely than men to be given psychiatric treatment and prescribed psychotropic medication (Ussher, 1992). However, intersections around race and gender make this process more complex and less predictable. Black women are over-represented in the prison system, yet relatively under-represented in the special hospital system (Warner, 2000b; Warner and Horn, 2000). Indeed, there has been a general reduction over recent years of the number of women in special hospitals (Warner, 2000b). The decrease of women in special hospitals may not reflect a liberalisation of that system, however, but a more punitive attitude (ibid.) that has seen the numbers of women in prison increase dramatically over the last decade (Warner and Horn, 2000). Whilst the number of women in special hospitals has decreased, such institutions remain the final solution for women who, it can be argued, contravene gender stereotypes:

> The women, they can't cope, they smash a window and that's highlighted that she's got a problem, and they don't want to deal with it so they just chuck you in places like this. It's as if people don't want to know, they don't want women like us.
>
> (Female patient)

Hence, women may be excluded from community care services not because they are deemed to be 'mentally ill', but rather because they are viewed as being difficult to manage and, therefore, too challenging for the people who work with them:

> Women who are the most distressed and distressing, the system will not hold and contain, so it excludes them more easily. So I think that's one of the reasons for us taking in women who don't need high security, but need services we're providing because no one else is providing it.
>
> (Female medical consultant)

Through a diagnostic sleight of hand, what is difficult for society is reconstructed as individualised pathology which warrants exclusion and incarceration. This can lead to the somewhat bizarre situation of women being detained within, and yet banned from, services (Perkins and Repper, 1996). Hence, special hospitals may function as a dumping ground for those women who cause too much (gender) trouble (Butler, 1990) elsewhere: 'Women are probably detained more readily because we've not got the appropriate services and we don't know what to do with them when they're troublesome, or possibly because women aren't meant to be troublesome' (female lead psychologist).

At this point, medical narratives converge with legal narratives, in the context of the Mental Health Act (1983), to restrict liberty and direct people so defined into increasing systems of secure provision:

> [borderline personality disorder] is used as a mental health diagnosis which is the means by which you can be incarcerated here. [This] means people are kept here against any clear rationale, but because they've been particularly difficult to manage, we have to put a label on them so we can detain them under the [Mental Health] Act.
>
> (Female lead psychologist)

The Mental Health Act (1983) recognises three legal categories of disorder: mental illness, mental impairment and psychopathic personality disorder. The medical diagnosis of borderline personality disorder, therefore, would be classified within the legal category of psychopathic personality disorder. Populist representations of psychopathy are masculinised and those women defined as being 'borderline' may be rendered unintelligible (Butler, 1990) and invisible within the wider sweep of psychopathic masculinity:

> There's a strong public opinion that women PD patients don't exist, because we all know women are kind and sweet and loving, so they'd

rather just simply deny that it exists at all. Whereas there's a great ability to believe in the notion of the male PD, psychopath, that's been sensationalised and it's quite sexy really.

(Male clinical leader)

Women may be rendered invisible under the cloak of masculinised narratives of psychopathology. Yet women diagnosed as having a borderline personality disorder may still be judged according to these more public, masculine, versions of personality disorder:

In the wider world PD is only heard about in the most extreme and tragic cases. Their associations with it are all the worst things about the way people can treat people and the fear of it is something because people don't understand it at all. So even those people who are not dangerous are seen as those people who are incurable and almost the modern day lepers, people to be separated from society.

(Male senior manager)

'Personality disorder', then, is a label reserved for the patients that mental health systems (as well as society more generally) struggle to contain and that workers want to avoid:

I think what happened to many of them in the health care system is that they were seen as so difficult that services used the personality disorder label to reject them ... that if you couldn't get them better you labelled them as personality disordered and bad, and then you could have contracts that they couldn't keep, and you could reject them with a clean conscience from the service.

(Female senior medical consultant)

Diagnosis, therefore, rather than offering an avenue in which to 'help' or 'treat' the patient, serves as the container in which to segregate those parts that are socially feared. Specifically, borderline personality disorder has long been recognised as being used in situations of 'diagnostic uncertainty' as a wastebasket category (Reiser and Levenson, 1984; Frances and Widiger, 1987; Fernbach et al., 1989). It is little surprise, therefore, that the category of borderline personality disorder has been judged to be one of the most 'misused and abused' of all psychiatric diagnoses (Becker, 1997: 152). It can be, and has been, employed to blame the patient who makes life hard for the therapist or who does not get better (Aronson, 1985). Indeed, Herman (1992: 54) calls it 'little more than a sophisticated insult'. The category of borderline personality disorder stores all that may be wrong with 'the system' within particular problem women and through this maintains normative boundaries around acceptable expressions of femininity. More than this, because borderline personality disorder is viewed as being something that women bring with them, the contributions current practices make to shaping disordered behaviour can be kept out of sight.

Re-enacting abuse and reproducing disorder: the social regulation of past and current 'effects'

When women are diagnosed as having borderline personality disorder their responsibility for all future difficulties may be over determined. This is because any disorder belongs to them rather than the situation. Even when child sexual abuse is raised in psychiatry as a causative factor in the development of borderline personality disorder, women may still be blamed for current difficulties as women's histories are given as the reason for their current unreasonableness. Yet, women may continue to be abused or feel threatened. As Perry *et al.* (1990: 40) argue: 'the characteristic self- destructive and stormy interpersonal behaviours that follow are an attempt to cope with unbearable feelings of rage, shame, guilt, and terror associated with the symbolic re-experiencing of the trauma.' Hence, experiences of child sexual abuse may foundationalise women's symptomatic behaviour, but its maintenance is ensured through successive practices:

> The thing that you find is the unbelievable psychological trauma that they've experienced early in their lives, and to some extent still do. I think it just maintains them in this kind of atrocious system, but it maintains an abusive quality to their lives, and you can't even begin to imagine what it must be like for their lives to be just a tunnel of invalidation, abuse, you know all those things.
>
> (Female nurse consultant)

When mental health delivery systems, as argued here, may be so instrumental in promoting disorder they must act to protect themselves by deflecting the blame away from 'the system' and into specific pathologised individuals. As Parker (1999: 6) notes, 'a pathological system can survive very efficiently if it can persuade one of its members that they are responsible and they themselves contain the problem'. As one female staff nurse stated:

> By the time they arrive into this kind of setting the women have usually been struggling for a long time. They have usually accumulated lots of disastrous relationships which have exposed them to further abuse and trauma as well. So it's almost as if they're just repeating and repeating, recreating the traumatic conditions and it gets worse. The level of abuse that these women have suffered is so unbearable. It's easier to just think well they're a bad apple.

Such understandings underscore the dynamic quality most relationships have (Warner, 2001). They may protect workers by over-determining women's responsibility for pathological relationships, but they offer no way out. This is because self-reflection must be restricted to preserve the fragile sense of self that workers bring with them. Workers may themselves feel hurt, anger and ambivalence in respect of their own lives, as well as the women they work with. However, they may be unable to acknowledge their feelings within the masculine world of special hospitals and even 'good' therapists may struggle to articulate negative feelings towards their clients. If workers cannot address their own emotional needs, then they cannot begin to address the emotional needs of their clients. Diagnosis provides a get-out clause from engaging in emotionally difficult work because diagnosis operates as an emotional checklist, not as a starting point for exploration. Narratives of child sexual abuse can then be ignored in favour of simple, but static, categorisation. As a female lead medical consultant asserted: 'If the women have been abused and are still cutting and still causing people distress, one way of society managing this is to put them in the sick role. If you put them in the sick role then you keep them here.'

When women are depicted as being 'sick', their active attempts to shape their own lives and cope with both past and present concerns remain obscured. Indeed, they may not be deemed to be coping at all. Women may then be judged as needing to be taught coping strategies so that workers may be protected from the horror that sexual abuse engenders which otherwise may break free from women's pasts. As one female nurse therapist noted:

> Everyone wants to give people coping skills because they're frightened, frightened of what it might mean to look into people's histories, look into their pasts, make connections to how they behave now. I think that it's the level of trauma and abuse with our patients. The patients' histories and narratives that they give now are so, I can't think, gross, that I think people can't cope.

This need to *give* people coping skills further invalidates women because of the refusal to acknowledge they are already doing what they can to cope with past abuse and present services. The acknowledgement that trauma interweaves with borderline personality disorder fails to offer a liberatory script because the emphasis is on women's difficulties and women's pathology. Whether victim of social trauma, or victim of biology, in more traditional psychiatric terms, women remain responsible for all that subsequently happens to them. The medicalisation of social misery, therefore, traps workers and clients in relationships they must maintain but can never explore. Yet it is when we explicate the ways in which such relationships are structured and examine the subject positions opened up and closed down in them that we can begin to loosen the grip of the medical model and challenge the reproduction of gender norms in psychiatry.

As argued, borderline personality disorder reifies particular formations of femininity and particular understandings of the effects of child sexual abuse. As such, it is unsurprising that such narratives extend beyond women patients to women workers or that feelings associated with abusive relationships may become institutionalised:

> Lots of the things that contributed to the women themselves having difficulties, in lots of ways we have similar sorts of difficulties about feeling defensive: about feeling criticised, feeling sort of devalued in a sense, low self esteem, the sort of blame culture of the place. How can we give to other people, when you're not valued in this institution yourself, and you feel powerless in this institution?
>
> (Female psychologist)

Yet, because workers recoil from self-reflection, recognition of commonality is resisted and abusive relationships are, therefore, replayed:

> All the ills and the pathology is located just in the patient, but that of course is not true. So it means that people that are looking after the patients don't understand their own psychopathology – where their own damage impacts on the care and treatment that is offered to patients. And that seems to be one reason why this perpetuation of dysfunction and abuse goes on inside the institution.
>
> (Female nurse consultant)

It is vital, therefore, that professionals feel able to reflect on the ways in which their own life narratives and experiences of (institutional) regulation are implicated in the structuring of their clinical practice. If they do not, their practice will be primarily concerned with protecting themselves. As a senior female psychologist reflected:

> All of you need some sort of control, power, sense of self worth and how are you going to do that? By projecting all of that on to the patients, so that you're very controlling over patients, very punitive towards patients. Because we can't direct those feelings anywhere else, we're blocked from doing it anywhere else, so we come down on our relationships with them.

Hence, although special hospitals may provide physical security, they may still engender feelings of powerlessness that militate against healthy relationships: 'I am sure that this setting is not often containing enough for us to be able to tolerate that person's distress' (female lead psychologist).

The use of classificatory systems, and the very status of theory informed by a metaphor of scientific discovery, utilises language that protects workers, by reifying the distinction between the subject (patient) and 'knower' (professional). Yet positions are relative and are only maintained through iteration as they are 'continuously (re)produced in discursive and (other) practices in the course of social activities' (Stenner and Eccleston, 1994: 89). As argued earlier, the behaviours associated with the diagnosis of borderline personality disorder can be seen as an active attempt by both workers and clients to cope with experiences of distress (by respectively diagnosing and/or acting in symptomatic ways). The coping strategies that people use (whether clients or workers), therefore, indicate not only the kinds of relationships they have had, but are having. When we see the problem as belonging to the individual, we fail to see why people adopt these strategies and so workers respond by punishing their clients and protecting themselves. As one nurse therapist reflected:

> Without any insight or understanding of why people perform or act out in a particular way you defend, you avoid to protect yourself, as staff within the hospital. With no clear understanding of why this happens we will respond in a particular way that defends ourselves, and it's usually very harsh.

Some conclusions

Current definitions of borderline personality disorder deny the normality of women's responses to abnormal events (Linehan, 1993). This is achieved through decontextualising the symptoms that define the disorder, which otherwise indicate the real difficulties women experience through their lives. Even when child (sexual) abuse is raised as being a critical experience in the lives of women diagnosed as having a borderline personality disorder, the social world is still marginalised. This is because in making reference to the causative effects of childhood (sexual) abuse, disorder is sedimented as an internal property of women and, hence, obscures the role of current practices in the maintenance of their misery. Pathologising women's responses to abuse in turn acts as warrant for exclusion from society and such women may then act as the unacknowledged containers of all that is overwhelming, unknown or feared within ourselves. More than this, the diagnostic category of borderline personality disorder is foundationalised in unacknowledged assumptions about gender that are, themselves, implicated within the social regulation of normative femininity. As such, we need to do more than simply change the diagnosis of 'borderline personality disorder'. Changing the diagnosis without reflecting on the way social norms are both the foundation for and effect of diagnosis would only continue to produce and reproduce the same stereotypical (gendered) assumptions. What is required is a permanent conceptual revolution (Warner, 2000d) in which the social threads of theory are exposed and the realities they create are situated rather than simply accepted as objective, empirically derived truths. This revolution does not entail the abandonment of knowledge or a refusal of expertise. As Efran and Clarfield argue:

> To act as if all views are equal and that we-as-therapists have not favourites among them undercuts the very sort of frank exchange we want and expect to have with our clients. It patronises them, compromises our own integrity and treats open dialogue as if it was an endangered species needing 'hothouse' protection.
>
> (1992: 207–208)

Rather, our aim is to situate understanding – politically, historically, institutionally – in order that the effects of our perspective taking remain open to challenge and their regulatory moves can be explored. We may then find different ways to understand women who end up in special hospitals that enable exploration, rather than simply regulation, of their life stories. This is about creating opportunities to articulate multiple narratives about misery and abuse that do not always already pathologise clients or valorise workers. We may then be able to share narratives that no longer maintain women in misery but open up other versions of reality in which women are no longer discursively (and actually) imprisoned but are enabled to live in a community that does not now reject them.

References

Allen, H. (1987) *Justice unbalanced: gender, psychiatry and judicial decisions*, Milton Keynes: Open University Press.

American Psychiatric Association (1995) *Diagnostic and statistical manual of mental disorders (DSM-IV)*, 4th edition, Washington, DC: American Psychiatric Association.

Aronson, T.A. (1985) 'Historical perspectives on the borderline concept: a review and critique', *Psychiatry* 48: 209–222.

Barnard, C.P. and Hirsch, C. (1985) 'Borderline personality and victims of incest', *Psychological Reports* 57: 715–718.

Becker, D. (1997) *Through the looking glass: women and borderline personality disorder*, Oxford: Westview Press.

Brown, G.R. and Anderson, B. (1991) 'Psychiatric morbidity in adult inpatients with childhood histories of sexual and physical abuse', *American Journal of Psychiatry* 148, 1: 55–61.

Butler, J. (1990) *Gender trouble: feminism and the subversion of identity*, London: Routledge.

Caplan, P. (1995) *They say you're crazy: how the world's most powerful psychiatrists decide who's normal*, New York: Addison-Wesley Publishing.

Coons, P.M., Bowman, E., Pellow, T.A. and Schneider, P. (1989) 'Post-traumatic aspects of the treatment of victims of sexual abuse and incest', *Psychiatric Clinics of North America* 12, 2: 325–335.

Earl, W.L. (1991) 'Perceived trauma: it's etiology and treatment', *Adolescence* 26, 101: 97–104.

Efran, J.S. and Clarfield, L.E. (1992) 'Constructionist therapy: sense and nonsense', in S. McNamee and K.J. Gergen (eds) *Therapy as social construction*, London, Sage, pp. 201–212.

Fernbach, B.E., Winstead, B.A. and Derlega, V.J. (1989) 'Sex differences in diagnosis and treatment recommendations for antisocial personality disorder and somatization disorders', *Journal of Social and Clinical Psychology* 8, 3: 238–255.

Foucault, M. (1981) *The history of sexuality, Vol. One*, Harmondsworth: Penguin.

Foucault, M. (1992 [1967]) *Madness and civilization: a history of insanity in the age of reason*, London: Routledge.

Frances, A. and Widiger, T.A. (1987) 'A critical review of four DSM-III personality disorders: borderline, avoidant, dependent and passive-aggressive', in G.L. Tischler (ed.) *Diagnosis and classification in psychiatry: a critical appraisal of DSM-III*, New York: Cambridge University Press, pp. 269–289.

Herman, J.L. (1992) *Trauma and recovery*, New York: Basic Books.

Herman, J.L. (1993) *Sequelae of prolonged trauma evidence for a complex post traumatic syndrome: post traumatic stress disorder: DSM-IV and beyond*, Washington: American Psychiatric Association.

Kleinman, A. (1988) *Rethinking psychiatry: from cultural category to personal experience*, New York: Free Press.

Langer, E.J. and Abelson, R.P. (1974) 'A patient by any other name . . .: clinician group difference in labeling bias', *Journal of Consulting and Clinical Psychology* 42, 1: 4–9.

Linehan, M.M. (1993) *Cognitive-behavioral treatment of borderline personality disorder*, New York: Guildford.

Madigan, S. (1999) 'Inscription and deciphering chronic identities', in I. Parker (ed.) *Deconstructing psychotherapy*, London: Sage, pp. 150–163.

Mitchell, S.A. (1988) *Relational concepts in psychoanalysis: an integration*, Cambridge: Harvard University Press.

Parker, I. (ed.) (1999) *Deconstruction and Psychotherapy*, London: Sage.

Perkins, R.E. and Repper, J.M. (1996) *Working alongside people who have long-term mental health problems*, London: Chapman & Hall.

Perry, J.C., Herman, J.L., van der Kolk, B. and Hoke, L.A. (1990) Psychotherapy and psychological trauma in borderline personality disorder, *Psychiatric Annals*, 20, 1: 33–43.

Plummer, K. (1995) *Telling sexual stories: power, change and social worlds*, London: Routledge.

Reiser, D.E. and Levenson, H. (1984) Abuses of the borderline diagnosis: a clinical problem with teaching opportunities, *American Journal of Psychiatry* 141: 1528–1532.

Shotter, J. (1993) 'The social construction of remembering and forgetting', in D. Middleton and D. Edwards (eds) *Collective remembering*, London: Sage, pp. 35–47.

Stenner, P. and Eccleston, C. (1994) On the textuality of being: towards an invigorated social constructionism, *Theory & Psychology* 4, 1: 84–103.

Swan, V. (1999) 'Narrative, Foucault and feminism: implications for therapeutic practice', in I. Parker (ed.) *Deconstructing psychotherapy*, London: Sage, pp. 103–114.

Ussher, J. (1992) *Women's madness: misogyny or mental illness?* Amherst: University of Massachusetts Press.

Warner, S. (1996a) 'Visibly special? Women, child sexual abuse and Special Hospitals', in C. Hemingway (ed.) *Special women? The experience of women in the Special Hospital system*, Hampshire: Avebury, pp. 59–70.

Warner, S. (1996b) 'Special women, special places: women and high security mental hospitals', in E. Burman, G. Aitken, P. Alldred, *et al.* (eds) *Psychology, discourse, practice: from regulation to resistance*, London: Taylor and Francis, pp. 90–113.

Warner, S. (1996c) 'Constructing femininity: models of child sexual abuse and the production of "woman"', in E. Burman, P. Alldred, C. Bewley, *et al.* (eds) *Challenging women: psychology's exclusions, feminist possibilities*, Buckingham: Open University Press, pp. 36–53.

Warner, S. (1999) 'Special stories: women patients, high security mental hospitals and child sexual abuse', Manchester: unpublished PhD thesis, Manchester Metropolitan University.

Warner, S. (2000a) 'The cost of containment: women, high security mental hospitals and child sexual abuse', *Forensic Update* 62: 5–9.

Warner, S. (2000b) 'Women and child sexual abuse: childhood prisons and current custodial practices', in R. Horn and S. Warner (eds) *Positive directions for women in secure environments: issues in criminological and legal psychology*, Leicester: British Psychological Society, pp. 11–16.

Warner, S. (2000c) 'Child sexual abuse: tactics for survival – identifying issues which contribute to good practice', *Clinical Psychology Forum* 139: 6–10.

Warner, S. (2000d) *Understanding child sexual abuse: making the tactics visible*, Gloucester: Handsell Publishing.

Warner, S. (2001) 'Disrupting identity through visible therapy: a feminist post-structuralist approach to working with women who have experienced child sexual abuse', *Feminist Review* 68, summer: 115–139.

Warner, S. and Horn, R. (2000) 'Introduction', in R. Horn and S. Warner (eds) *Positive directions for women in secure environments: issues in criminological and legal psychology*, Leicester: British Psychological Society, pp. 6–10.

Westen, D., Ludolph, P., Misle, B., Ruffins, S. and Block, J. (1990) 'Physical and sexual abuse in adolescent girls with borderline personality disorder', *American Journal of Orthopsychiatry* 60, 1: 55–66.

Wile, D.B. (1984) *After the fight: a night in the life of a couple*, New York: Guild-ford.

WISH (1999) *Defining gender issues – redefining women's services*, London: Women in Secure Hospitals.

Chapter 11

Writing the effects of sexual abuse

Interrogating the possibilities and pitfalls of using clinical psychology expertise for a critical justice agenda

Nicola Gavey

> As feminists, we need to embrace reflexivity, to incorporate a cultural analysis of our practices into those practices. Whether we are therapists, clients, or researchers, we labor to 'get the story right,' but we need to remember that there is no story that is right forever and for all.
>
> (Marecek, 1999: 180)

This conclusion to Jeanne Marecek's analysis of the lexicon of 'trauma talk' in feminist therapy discourse forms an apt beginning for my task here. Inspired by these very same sentiments, I set out in this chapter to reflexively interrogate some of my own previous clinical psychology practice, writing psychological reports to support compensation claims by women who had experienced rape and sexual abuse. Long troubled by my role in this work, which raises so many contradictory issues for a feminist practitioner, I wanted to return to it, to explicate my ambivalences and expose them to each other. By doing this, I hope to explore some questions I have had about the possibilities and pitfalls of using psychology for a feminist critical justice agenda with women who have been sexually abused.

Ian Parker has referred to critical psychology as operating 'in and against psychology' (1999, 2001), and has argued that 'our concern is for how any system of psychology operates for empowerment or oppression' (1999: 7). The kind of work I will describe is a local and particular instantiation of psychology carried out with feminist sensibilities. Depending on your theoretical perspective, it can be argued to be either empowering or oppressive. It is a form of practice that attempts to strategically use the power of psychology in the name of social justice. But is this actually possible, or is it inherently contradictory?[1] Is the power of psychology such that it co-opts the unruly intentions of any particular practitioner to its own ends? On the other hand, what does it mean to abandon psychology in places and times where it may seem possible that it could further social justice? And, what do we risk losing when we criticise psychology's attempts to facilitate 'empowerment' as insufficiently radical? Can this sometimes reveal a forgetting of the (more?) oppressive and harmful social forces against which such empowering strategies are wielded – that is, the widespread and institutionalised denial, minimisation, and victim-blaming that has accompanied rape and sexual abuse in Western societies for centuries, and which arguably continues in various toned down forms today?

Frustratingly, but perhaps not surprisingly, my reflexive journey around these questions has not yielded clarity or certainty – rather it has taken me into a spiralling maze of possibilities, all of which seem limited and contingent. In the rest of this chapter, I will discuss the tensions inherent in attempting to craft such a 'critical feminist clinical psychology' with women who have been raped and sexually abused as children.[2] I shall first describe the nature of the psychological work that I did, and the context in which it was carried out. I then present two separate feminist readings of this work – a 'clinical psychology' reading and a 'post-structuralist' reading. I end with a third feminist reading, a 'critical psychology' reading, which attempts to take into account and weigh up against each other the more clear-cut 'pro' and 'con' interpretations just offered.

The broader context for this work

In New Zealand, the Accident Compensation Act was passed in 1972[3] to provide a state administered comprehensive scheme to compensate people for accidental injury. It was a no-fault system; in return for guaranteed compensation regardless of fault, New Zealanders gave up the right to sue for compensatory damages. While most of the injuries compensated under the scheme arise from accidents in the home, workplace, motor vehicles or during sport, the Act also provided for compensation to those injured by certain criminal acts (see Couper, 1995; in doing so it subsumed earlier legislation directed specifically at compensation for criminal injuries, Tobin, 1994). The Act came into force in 1974, and by the early-to-mid-1980s the Accident Compensation Corporation (ACC) had been successfully lobbied to provide financial assistance for the development of community-based services for victims of rape and sexual assault.[4] ACC paid for counselling costs, medical expenses and earnings-related income loss.

ACC has become the key funder in New Zealand of services for people who have been sexually abused. It has gone through detailed processes to devise criteria for registering counsellors to provide sexual abuse counselling, and to manage the process of allocating this kind of funding. The relationship between people registered as sexual abuse counsellors by ACC (many of whom work in independent practice, and many of whom have feminist analyses of rape and sexual abuse) and the ACC has been tense in various ways. Notwithstanding this, however, most counsellors working in this area have acted as if the ACC funding is a good thing. In the broader context of economic neoliberal contraction of state responsibilities, many are thankful for this somewhat anomalous situation which provides state funding for sexual abuse counselling, in an environment where it would be much more difficult to obtain state funded counselling for problems unrelated to sexual abuse. Practitioners in the field have critiqued some processes, and have contributed to advising developments for managing the system.[5] However, for obvious reasons, there has been little critique from workers in the field of the whole practice of ACC funding of sexual abuse counselling.

There was also a provision within the ACC legislation for 'lump sum compensation' payments, to a maximum of $10,000.[6] This was generally not well publicised, and it was not until around 1986–1987 that the first applications for lump sum compensation were made by women who had been raped or sexually abused. By 1987 the provision for lump sum compensation for rape and sexual abuse started to be publicised in women's magazines (e.g. McCurdy, 1987; Westaway, 1987), and as general awareness about this grew in the community, an increasing number of women,[7] as well as some children and some men, applied for such compensation from the state.[7]

For lump sum compensation applications, ACC could require clients to see a psychiatrist (or, less commonly, a clinical psychologist) who would provide a report for ACC on 'how the injury has affected them psychologically' (pers. comm., ACC client officer, personal notes, 1987).[8] Although not always required, this referral for psychological assessment tended to become standard practice.

The context of my involvement

In 1986, after qualifying as a clinical psychologist, I started working part-time as a counsellor at an independent community-based sexual abuse counselling agency. At the time, it could have been described as a grass-roots feminist organisation. It was devoted to helping women who had been raped and sexually abused, providing crisis support, counselling, education, as well as political lobbying, and so on.

In 1987, a colleague who was a feminist sexual abuse counsellor at this agency approached me about a client of hers who was making an application for ACC lump sum compensation relating to a rape she had experienced a few years earlier. My colleague, wary from stories about the kinds of experiences that some women had suffered in the process of being assessed by psychiatrists appointed by ACC, inquired to ACC about the possibility of a clinical psychologist being acceptable to write these reports, and then talked me into doing it. We knew of women who had been treated in disrespectful and/or pathologising ways by various psychiatrists, who reportedly approached their task in the mode of a detached clinical assessment, seemingly without recognition of the potential for their assessments to cause further distress to women. One woman we knew of, for instance, was labelled with an unwelcome psychiatric diagnosis of a personality disorder in the process of submitting to this bureaucratic requirement.

I ended up doing this work of writing psychologist's reports on a limited and independent basis over a six-year period between 1987 and 1993. I worked on twenty-seven 'cases' related to ACC claims. About two-thirds of these were primary cases referred by ACC where I worked directly with people making the claims, and about one-third were review cases referred by lawyers, where a woman's initial claim had been turned down or where the amount awarded was being contested by the woman – in three of these cases, I only provided written opinions without re-interviewing the woman herself. Overall, just under half of the women I worked with/for were abused as children; the rest were raped or otherwise sexually assaulted as adults.

The grass-roots feminist milieu, from which I came to this work, was supportive of women making lump sum applications from a social justice point of view. We believed that if women could receive some financial compensation for what they had been through, then that was a good thing. I justified my personal involvement in the process with the belief that I would be able to act 'on women's behalf' as an advocate, using my professional credentials to support their applications, in a way that was affirming of them.

My identity as a clinical psychologist has always been ambivalent and uncomfortable – one I rarely claim. Nevertheless, at the time, even from my perspective as a clinical psychologist, I regarded the horror stories about the treatment some women were getting from some psychiatrists as simply cases of 'bad practice'. My focus here, though, is not on those cases where 'something went wrong' in this way, but rather on a critical rethinking of the whole process itself, in terms of the risks associated with even practice that is attentive to issues of equity, power and justice.[9]

The work

The referral form provided by ACC asked the psychologist/psychiatrist to provide a report with information on any 'loss of the amenities to enjoy life' and 'pain and mental suffering' that the person had suffered:

SECTION 79 (1982 ACT)/(SECTION 120 1972 ACT)
Under Section 79 the Corporation must determine its award within two years of the injury,[10] whether or not the patient's condition has

stabilised. This Section does not allow for re-assessment in the future. Hence in deciding its award, the Corporation must take account of possible future deterioration.

Comment regarding quantum for Section 79 is not required in your report. However, any information which you can provide under the following headings would be invaluable:

1 Loss of the amenities or capacity to enjoy life:
   In particular, restrictions in recreational pursuits, sport, home, and family life, work and social activity.
2 Pain and Mental Suffering
   The extent of pain immediately after injury, during recovery and at the time of the examination. Is this likely to improve or deteriorate in the future?

(ACC Request for Medical Report form)

Typically I would have two appointments with the woman. In the initial two-hour session, I would conduct a fairly detailed semi-structured interview to find out some background about the rape and/or sexual abuse she had experienced, any relevant factors in her background, other related factors or stressors (if any), and then to attempt to identify the ways in which the rape and/or sexual abuse had affected her life. The reports themselves soon became quite formulaic, in terms of structure and style. They contained an account of the sexual abuse suffered by the woman, and relevant background or other factors for helping to understand this in a contextualised way. The legislated categories in the ACC referral – 'Loss of the amenities or capacity to enjoy life' and 'Pain and mental suffering' – were used as a somewhat arbitrary framework for writing about the various areas of apparent effect. For example, under the heading of 'Pain and mental suffering', I used subheadings such as the following (as appropriate for any particular woman): Anxiety and fear, Fear-related behaviour, Depression and suicidal gestures, Self-harm, Guilt, Self-esteem and confidence, Health problems, Shame and embarrassment, Flashbacks, Trust, Eating disturbance and body image, Loss and grief, Sleep disturbance. Under the heading of 'Loss of the amenities or capacity to enjoy life' I used subheadings like: Intimate relationships, Sleep disturbance, Relationships with family members, Home and family life, Friendships, Social life, Work, Sexuality, Drug and alcohol abuse, Schooling.

To conclude the report there would also be separate or combined sections under headings like 'Summary' and 'Prognosis'. These sections contained an attempt to present a concise summary of the ways that the rape and/or sexual abuse had negatively impacted on the woman's life, and some opinion about how lasting this may be. (Part of ACC's brief was to consider 'whether or not the patient's condition has stabilised' and 'possible future deterioration', ACC Request for Medical Report form.)

Below are two extracts, which show the nature of these concluding parts of the reports. (Examples of these particular sections are presented because they are less likely to include potentially identifying detail about the client, and they contain more abstract formulations. This both protects client confidentiality[11] and allows for an analytic emphasis on the professional psychology work itself, rather than on the client.)

(1) Extract from 1990 report

Summary:

S has suffered severe sexual abuse and rape by a much trusted family member, which started when she was very young, and which was ongoing for many years. She now appears to be a bright young woman with good interpersonal skills in a one to one situation, and is independent and self-reliant. However, in her everyday life, S tends to be withdrawn and isolates herself from others. She has been deprived of her childhood, and she now seems to assume quite an adult sense of responsibility for others. For many years S has been chronically depressed and desperately unhappy, to the extent that she has been suicidal.

It seems that things might have become worse for S after leaving primary school. A very significant friendship ended at the end of primary school, and S's life perhaps became more empty at this time. Also, her [male relative's] death, while positive in the sense that it signalled the end of the abuse, may have contributed to S's sense of confusion and guilt.

S's life has been affected in many ways by the abuse. On top of the pain and suffering she has experienced, her achievement at school and her relationships with others both appear to have been negatively affected.

Prognosis:

S appears to be coping with life considerably better this year, than she has in previous years. Hopefully this is a sign of an upwards turn in S's life. However, in light of the serious abuse she has suffered, I would predict that it may take many years for her to overcome the pain this has caused her. I would expect that she will have 'ups and downs' for many years to come. It is very encouraging that she has had a very positive and helpful experience of counselling, which will hopefully mean that she is more likely to seek help or support if she feels desperate and suicidal, or otherwise in need of it in the future.

S is still young, and there are ways in which her life will probably continue to be negatively affected by the sexual abuse she has suffered, which are not apparent yet. Various developmental milestones lie ahead of her. For example, sexual relationships, developing intimate and lasting relationships, and the possibility of having children. In these areas, in particular, S may have problems. For example, sexual relationships may remind her of the abuse, and having children of her own may remind her of her own pain and unhappiness as a small child. Furthermore, disruption of her schooling and the development of peer relationships, may restrict her later career and other lifestyle options.

(2) Extract from 1991 report

Summary and prognosis:

The sexual abuse that R has suffered, and the estrangement and isolation from her family that has gone hand in hand with the abuse, have had a severe and pervasive effect on R's life. As she said, 'never a day goes by when I don't think about it'. She has suffered and continues to suffer an enormous amount of emotional pain and suffering which is, I believe, directly attributable to the sexual abuse and associated factors that she has described. Her life, as she describes it, is currently dominated by fears and anxiety, and it would appear that she has experienced ongoing depression for many years. R has been caught in a pattern of self-destructive behaviours, including self-harm, alcohol and drug abuse, eating disturbances, and aggressive behaviour in relationships – all of which are reported consequences of severe child sexual abuse.

In terms of her capacity to enjoy life, all of these emotional factors and self-destructive patterns are important stumbling blocks. Furthermore, it is important that R has been deprived of a supportive and caring family environment, and is currently isolated and estranged from her mother and siblings, who she cares about. Her early schooling and her later educational and career opportunities were narrowed. Her work life has also been seriously negatively affected. Her ability to form an intimate relationship with a caring and supportive person and to enjoy a sexual relationship with that person is currently very limited.

R has a number of strengths. She is fully aware of the numerous psychological difficulties she has and has a good deal of insight about these problems and how they relate to her family background and the abuse she has experienced. She has made attempts to make changes in her life, and has engaged in counselling, although this has unfortunately not been as useful as it could be. She is resourceful and she is a survivor. She can gain pleasure and comfort from very simple things, such as small animals and nature. She loves children and has enjoyed working with them. I think that R has already started to make progress towards establishing a safer life for herself. I think she would benefit from some good support, and probably from therapy with a skilled psychologist to assist her in this path towards gaining more control over her own life. These steps must occur at R's own pace, however, as only she can really know who she can begin to trust and who will be helpful to her, and when she is feeling safe enough to continue her journey of healing from the sexual abuse and its effects.

After the first appointment and writing a full draft of the report, I would meet with the woman for one more session (usually for an hour) to go over the draft report with her. This meeting was used as an opportunity for further information gathering (to fill in any details I'd missed in the first interview, to correct anything I'd got wrong initially), to ensure she was comfortable with what I had written, and also, importantly, for contextualising the report to the woman. To this end, I would explain why I'd written the report in the way that I had. For example, I'd usually talk about how I had written about a lot of ways in which the rape or sexual abuse had had harmful effects on her life, and then try and put that in context of (1) how this was 'normal' considering what she had been through, and (2) how I also saw her as a person with a lot of strengths and resources. In doing this, I aimed to acknowledge that the report was a 'negative' take on her life that was not the full or only story of her life. I tried to impart a hopeful picture to her, while at the same time offering her a framework for making sense of some of her difficulties in relation to what she had experienced. In doing this I had to walk a delicate tightrope between building a strong case on her behalf for her ACC claim – which required some documentation of 'injuries' – at the same time as conveying to her an analysis that was more fluid and open to change.

Reading this work

While it would be interesting to subject these documents to a more conventional discourse analysis, I set my task here as a more global reading of the professional psychology practice, within the wider bureaucratic, economic and socio-cultural context in which it functions (even though the extent to which I can elaborate these contexts is limited in a single chapter). This approach is inspired by an interest in the broader workings of 'governmentality' (Foucault, 1991; Rose and Miller, 1992). From this perspective, the psychological reports are just one (admittedly important) aspect of the multiple modes of producing and administering 'the "know how" that has promised to make government possible' (Rose and Miller, 1992: 178), as are documents such as the referral forms, form letters sent to ACC clients, and so on. Also important are the normative practices in which all of this takes place – the legislative regulations governing how and to whom a claimant gets referred, the legislated criteria upon which assessments of 'injury' are made, the professional frameworks in which such assessments are carried out, and the techniques used to evaluate harm, as well as how all of these things are communicated to the woman who is making the claim.

It seems to me that the possibilities for analysing this sort of professional work are quite complex. At a very simplified level, I am in 'two minds' about how to regard it – one familiar way I can look at it is through a feminist clinical psychology lens and the other is through a feminist poststructuralist lens. The tension between these two ways of thinking about the ethics and politics of this work, leads to a third approach, which I will refer to here as critical psychology. The rather linear format I will use for discussing these different takes on this work is less than totally satisfying because, of course, the different approaches never exist in bounded forms as this layout might suggest. However, it is a compromise solution for attempting to disentangle the complex array of factors that might need to be considered in critically evaluating the potential of this work for a social justice agenda.

Clinical psychology

At the time I was doing this work, I saw my role first and foremost as a feminist advocate who was able to strategically use my clinical psychology qualifications in the service of acting for women who had been raped and sexually abused, and who were seeking some small form of justice in the form of ACC-funded lump sum compensation. But it was my credentials of psychological expertise that allowed me to document the psychosocial impacts of sexual abuse with authority (see Alcoff and Gray, 1993, for a critical discussion of the role of psy-experts in mediating – judging and evaluating – survivor speech within the confessional mode in which it has come to be delivered). In this way, I was working within a clinical psychology paradigm, albeit a politicised one.

In my work, I was clear that my primary ethical obligation was to the women I saw, even though technically, it was ACC who was my client (in the sense that they provided me with the referral, and they paid me). The work was conducted with at least three goals in mind – respect, advocacy and empowerment. I attempted to conduct the process in a respectful way, so that it was not judgemental or pathologising. I believed in sharing information, giving the woman an opportunity to have input and 'final say' on my report, and giving her a copy unless she preferred not to have one. From my advocacy stance, I aimed to produce a report that presented the woman's 'case' for compensation in the strongest possible way. At the same time as acting as an advocate for her claim, I wanted to provide an experience and a report that gave her a helpful but non-imposing framework for understanding the experience of sexual abuse, and how that may have contributed to difficulties in her life, while at the same time 'empowering' her in some small ways to move beyond this and/or not be overwhelmingly constituted by it (if, indeed, that was her experience). To this end, the reports were always written with two intended audiences. For the audience assessing the claim (ACC), there was a focus on documenting the effects of sexual abuse. But the reports were always also written for the women themselves, with the intent of being respectful (by writing about her strengths as well as her difficulties) and having some *small* therapeutic intervention (such as embedding the suggestion of positive change in relation to states of distress, discomfort and/or ongoing difficulties identified by the woman).

The feminist clinical psychologist, then, can view her role as one of advocacy (working for the woman to help her obtain ACC compensation) and also one of empowerment (providing a framework of understanding for the woman that promotes agency). Clearly, though, the goals of advocacy and empowerment are not always easily compatible. In this context, advocacy necessitated emphasising the psychological effects of the rape and/or sexual abuse that the woman had experienced, which requires a focus on psychological, relational, and other *problems*; on distress, and on suffering. Through the process of the interviews and the presentation of the report an authoritative mirror is created of the woman's life that reflects back a rather negative image. Therefore, in attempting to be respectful and empowering, deliberate active attempts had to be made to help counter this slanted reflection with a more positive, encouraging and optimistic analysis. I tried to carefully balance the tension between advocacy and empowerment, in part by explaining to the woman how and why I was putting the particular story of her experiences into the particular framework I did.

The clinical psychology approach assumes the ontological truth of a connection between the trauma of sexual abuse and mental health consequences (see the large body of literature on the psychological effects of childhood sexual abuse). Given an underlying assumption about this general relationship, as something established by both science and a body of clinical experience, the task for the clinical psychologist remains one of establishing how, if at all, this has manifested in the life of any particular client. As it is assumed that the woman has been harmed in various (unknown, but not unpredictable) ways, it seems reasonable to adopt an advocacy role to work for her by documenting these effects, to present a case for her compensation. Although it is understood that the process is likely to be painful and difficult in various ways, the woman's choice to seek compensation in this way is respected. (Clearly, the issues are more complicated for children.)

Simple interventions like 'normalisation' would be considered likely to provide some small but significant therapeutic effect. It would be assumed that if a woman believes that the nature of her distress is similar to other women who have experienced similar abuses, then it may help her feel less 'pathologised', and it may actually mean it is less likely that she will attribute psychological discomfort and interpersonal difficulties (such as fears, avoidances, relational problems) to some inherent inner flaw. Thus, the experience is hopefully one that is less totalising; one that she has more control over. Another small therapeutic move would be to embed 'suggestions' of positive change or recovery, where possible. (Interestingly this notion, guided by intervention techniques used in, for example, forms of brief, strategic and narrative therapy, shares with post-structuralism some sense of the constitutive nature of language.)

Another consideration in the writing of the reports was to explicitly comment on the woman's strengths, and perhaps her courage. Even though this is strictly irrelevant to the primary purpose of the report, it functions to acknowledge respect and admiration, and hopefully to work against a singular portrayal of the woman's life in limited terms whereby her story could be narrated as one only of the damages of sexual abuse. As well as this, the simple legitimation involved in having one's painful story heard, believed, and ultimately 'compensated' by money may in itself have a significant 'healing' component. New Zealand law academic, Rosemary Tobin, has referred to the 'symbolic significance' (1997: 193) of the $10,000 lump sum compensation, and cites a media article in which three sexual abuse survivors discuss its 'therapeutic importance' (ibid.).

Although O'Dell (1997) and others have rightly criticised the excesses of psychological reductionism found in some of the childhood sexual abuse effects literature – which is often clinical psychology research – clinical psychology is arguably not inherently and inevitably culpable on these grounds. Although laden with somewhat off-putting psy-techno-talk, and traces of evolutionary psychology explanations, the modified cognitive-behavioural 'self-trauma model' of John Briere (2002), for example, is an approach that finds favour among many of my feminist colleagues who are therapists and clinical psychologists.[12] In such recent clinical psychology approaches to understanding the traumatic effects of severe childhood sexual abuse, the model is nuanced, sympathetic and arguably not worlds apart from feminist social constructionist therapeutic models of understanding women's strategies for surviving sexual abuse (e.g. Warner, 2000). Although the broader gender politics of sexual abuse are more prominently foregrounded in approaches such as Warner's (2000) model of 'visible therapy' (see also Warner, this volume), the 'chains of meaning' (Reavey and Warner, 2001: 56) that establish the links between what has happened to a sexual abuse survivor and her current behaviour are certainly retained and emphasised in both approaches. Both the clinical psychology of Briere and the social constructionist therapy of Warner see people's 'coping strategies' (Warner, 2000) or their 'posttraumatic responses' (Briere, 2002: 182), not as signs of 'disorder' (Warner, 2000; see Warner and Wilkins, this volume) or as 'merely symptoms of dysfunction' (Briere, 2002: 182), but as 'survival strategies' (Warner, 2000: 53) or as 'inborn recovery algorithms', 'the survivor's adaptive attempts to maintain internal stability in the face of potentially overwhelming abuse-related pain' (Briere, 2002: 200). While it would be disingenuous to deny the significant differences between these approaches (for instance, Briere makes ample use of an unproblematised notion of posttraumatic stress disorder; Warner introduces more epistemological uncertainty from social constructionism), both approaches clearly formulate the causes of a sexual abuse survivor's distress in their socio-cultural environments.

Post-structuralist

When contemporary anxieties about the difficult imperatives of freedom are installed in the regulatory forces of the state in the form of increasingly specified codes of injury and protection, do we unwittingly increase the power of the state and its various regulatory discourses at the expense of political freedom?

(Brown, 1995: 28)[13]

Wendy Brown's comments here are more specifically directed at legal remedies to protect against discrimination against various 'socially marked groups – people of colour, Jews, homosexuals, and women' (ibid.: 21). Nevertheless, her argument and her notion of an 'injury-identity' (ibid.) are extremely relevant to considering the costs to women who have been sexually abused of seeking justice through the codified avenues of state-funded compensation.

In their emphasis on the constitutive nature of language and discourse, Foucauldian post-structuralist theories argue that, as social beings, we are produced through discourse and culture (e.g. Foucault, 1981; Weedon, 1987). Teresa deLauretis (1987) has, for instance, outlined simple everyday processes by which the social technologies of gender produce us as gendered subjects. Drawing on Foucault, and using the Althusserian notion of interpellation, she describes, for example, how every time we mark the 'female' box on a form we are once again propelled into an identification with the social requirements for our sex. Through reiteration of these processes of interpellation, particular kinds of identities are produced (Butler, 1997; see also Butler, 1993). Not only our minds, but our whole beings, including our bodies, are constructed through this discursive power. As Judith Butler suggests, discourses 'actually live in bodies. They lodge in bodies, bodies in fact carry discourses as part of their own lifeblood' (Meijer and Prins, 1998: 282).

These Foucauldian-inspired understandings about the constitutive relationship between discourse and subjectivity (e.g. Foucault, 1981) pose a difficult challenge for the kind of professional psychology I am discussing. What if, as Nikolas Rose (2000a: 4) argues, 'psychology constitutes its object in the process of knowing it'? What might this mean for women who have been raped and sexually abused, given the ascendancy of psychological ways of understanding the impact of sexual abuse? This social constructionist position begs the question: what is the impact of the professional psychological gaze on the woman who is subjected to it?

From these perspectives, the bogey might not be just the sexual abuse and rape that a woman has experienced, but also, potentially, psychology itself. This is because psychology, as a set of discourses and practices that have considerable currency as frameworks for sense-making in contemporary Western societies, has the power to shape not only how we see the world, but also – according to post-structuralist theories – how we actually experience ourselves in the world. Psychology might not be the transparent window to understanding that many practitioners think of it as, but rather a cultural filter that, in the process of seeking to do good, actually provides ways of understanding and being that shape the world. From this point of view, psychology might need to be carefully monitored to ensure, at least, (1) that it does no further harm to women, and (2) that it does not take up all the privileged (expert) speaking space about sexual abuse, and de-politicise it in the process (see Alcoff and Gray, 1993).

The form of writing that is required in the psychologist's reports uses psychological expertise – obtained from normative scientific data and clinical literature and experience – to write a *particular* kind of account of someone's life. The framework of trauma portrays selves who are not merely hurt, but *damaged*, by the abuse or rape they have experienced. As I baldly wrote about one woman (in a report *not* quoted above): 'There is no doubt that the abuse/assault has left B with permanent emotional/psychological scars.' This writing explicitly imposes a kind of 'fixedness' on someone's experience – it diagnoses a permanency to their states of experience. In the 1990 report that I wrote for 'S', I verge on adopting an ominous time bomb metaphor when I wrote that: 'there are ways in which her life will probably continue to be negatively affected by the sexual abuse she has suffered, *which are not apparent yet*' (emphasis added). If nothing else, this proclamation gives this woman a lens through which she may come to read all manner of future events in her life. Whether this is helpful, unhelpful, or a bit of both, is impossible for the practitioner to predict or control.

The tacit requirements of professional authority – to be able to say something definite and authoritative – possibly helps to impose these predictions. Arguably, as any woman's name is written into such reports, the certainty of these particular renditions of their experience is reinforced. Although not for the first time, she is interpellated into the category of sexual abuse victim – who is represented as a particular kind of person with predictable kinds of psychological damages (see also Hacking, 1995; Rose, 2000b; Reavey and Warner, 2001). How does this impact on the woman reading such a report about herself? Does she accept such assessments with resignation or with relief, or possibly even with rage? Is the process of being subjectified in this way helpful or unhelpful, or is it mixed? Is it something she is equally able to reject as embrace, accordingly?

As Jeanne Marecek (1999: 171) has cautioned about therapists' uses of trauma stories to interpret clients' lives: 'Life histories do not merely tell about the past; they create possibilities for the present and future.' While, from within the framework of clinical psychology, it might be thought to be simply stating the truth about the impact of particular acts on psychological wellbeing, outside of this framework employing this particular interpretive lens might be regarded as a less innocent construction of the truth. Although such claims are made on the understanding they are true, and for the purposes of advocacy on the woman's behalf, post-structuralism is inherently suspicious of all truth claims and is likely to see the potentially problematic side of such statements. For instance, it might lead one to ask how the particular professional constructions presented in the psychologist's report take on a life of their own to become new constitutive forces in shaping the reality of that woman's experience and identity in the future.

The psychology work itself does not exist in a vacuum of course. The whole practice takes part in a socio-cultural context in which the harmful ways that sexual abuse might have impacted on a woman had to be read in a legislative framework that was designed to apply to physical injuries resulting from accidents. So, for example, there were a myriad of trivial and more substantive ways that the processes for administering and deciding upon claims set up a medicalised, mechanistic, pessimistic framework for understanding the effects of rape and sexual abuse. For example, the body of a (presumably standard) letter sent to a woman who had made a claim stated, 'The Corporation is pleased to advise that we have now accepted your claim, and this has been passed to our *Permanent Disability Unit* for processing. If you have any queries please do not hesitate to contact me' (my files, 1993, my emphasis).

Although psychiatric labels were stringently avoided in my feminist approach, several specific forms of psychological disorder are attributed to women – anxiety, depression, self-destructive behaviours, low self-esteem, and so on.[14] These reports were written before a 'trauma model' had become as institutionalised and formalised as it now is as a framework for conceptualising the psychological impact of sexual abuse (although it existed as an implicit framework). As Marecek has argued, the trauma model shares much of the same logic of the medical model, despite the vehement critiques of the medical model by feminist adherents to a trauma model:

> [Trauma talk] subsumes the particularities of a woman's experience into abstractions (e.g. 'trauma', 'abuse') and reduces experience into discrete, encapsulated symptoms (flashbacks; revictimization). It offers cause-and-effect explanations that are linear, mechanistic, and mono-causal. It sets aside a client's understanding of her own experience in favor of a uniform narrative; a single cause reliably (even invariably) produces a fixed set of symptoms.
>
> (1999: 165; see also Lamb's, 1999, critique of PTSD – posttraumatic stress disorder)

Indeed, the specific form of clinical practice under discussion here *requires* a reductive, linear causal narrative of exactly this kind (in a way that therapy arguably does not). Like any organisation under fiscal accounting pressure, ACC has strict criteria for awarding compensation. It will only agree to pay out money when it can be assured by the professional expert that not only does the woman suffer some sort of injury (psychological distress or difficulty),[15] but that it was caused by the sexual abuse she experienced.

According to Rose, it is simply a fact of contemporary life that 'a psy ontology has come to inhabit us' (1988: 190). Perhaps consistent with this characterisation of our times, it is interesting that Georges Vigarello's recent history of rape suggests that it was not until the 1970s that we started to publicly discuss rape in terms of it causing an 'inner trauma ... the shattering of a consciousness, a psychological suffering whose intensity was measured by its duration, even its irreversibility' (Vigarello, 2001: 209). Prior to this time, according to Vigarello, the seriousness of rape was formulated in terms of its moral or social impact, or as an insult or degradation. It is only relatively recently that attention has turned to the 'inner "ravages" caused to the victim by the crime', to its mental health effects (ibid.). To a psychologist, it is difficult, if not impossible, to get a handle on these historicising suggestions, and what they might mean for understanding the impact of rape and sexual abuse. To the feminist clinical psychologist, it is almost impossible to think about rape without seeing it as the kind of act that impacts on a woman's thoughts and feelings about herself, other people, and the world around her, and on her behaviours (or ways of acting) in many areas of her life. That is, it would be virtually impossible not to see it as an act that has (real, direct) psychological effects, and to suggest otherwise would be seen as outrageous and insensitive. To psychologists who work in this area, the effects of severe traumas are seen as *serious*, and the therapeutic work is *delicate*. More widespread recognition of this in recent decades would be assumed to be a progressive clarification of what rape and sexual abuse has always done to children and others – a victory of science, reason, and liberal social change in uncovering the foundational truth of abuse.

While I might quibble that such recognition, and possibly the effects themselves, are only possible because of our particular cultural and historical location (bringing as it does the humanist values of modernity, such as individual rights, autonomy, equality and justice), I, too, am largely convinced by this narrative of progress. Yet I don't see it as the whole story or the only story, and I suggest that it would be helpful to examine the consequences of acting as if it were. It might, for instance, blind us to considering the disempowering effects of imposing expectations about the inevitability of psychological harm for all people who have been sexually abused as children. To cite just one example, I would refer to legal discourse about sexual abuse and its effects in New Zealand. In the context of advocating for the legal rights of sexual abuse survivors, to make room for their claims in courts of law where barriers to entry, such as statutes of limitation, count against the interests of women who have been sexually abused as children, I have been dismayed to find accounts such as the following:

> But the question must be asked: how sensible is the notion of a reasonable sexually-abused person?
>
> It seems to me that the notion is incongruous. To postulate a woman who has been sexually abused as a child and then suppose her to be reasonable in respect of matters relating to that abuse is almost a contradiction in terms. The contradiction would be plain if one were to speak of a 'reasonable abnormal person' or an 'abnormal person acting reasonably'. Yet, the sexually-abused woman will not behave 'normally'. The vice in the construction of a hypothetical reasonable sexually-abused person lies in the tension between the way in which the courts assume such a person will behave and the way in which a real victim, psychologically damaged and disadvantaged, will actually behave. I suspect that in the fullness of time the notion of the reasonable sexually-abused person will be perceived as a grotesque invention of the law.
>
> (Thomas J., cited in New Zealand Law Commission, 2000: 13)

Although the notion of 'reasonable' may well have a specific meaning in the context of law, such paternalistic constructions readily translate outside of the legal arena in ways that function undesirably to deny agency to the woman who has experienced sexual abuse.

It is understandable that psy-professionals who work with women and children who have experienced sexual abuse, and other advocates, will be impatient with the kinds of critiques that could be launched in the name of post-structuralism. To the feminist, in particular, they could also be seen as dangerously invoking antiquated 'rape myths' (Burt, 1980), thereby betraying an allegiance with patriarchal trivialisations of rape. However, I would counter that these constructionist arguments do *not* imply that the suffering caused by sexual abuse is not real; but they do suggest that the particular shape of this suffering, and the form of its ongoing incorporation into any person's identity is also shaped by the cultural frameworks available for making sense of the impact of sexual abuse. And, given the sort of legal commentary quoted above, it might be necessary to soften our rhetoric – in the interests of women who have experienced sexual abuse.

A critical psychology rejoinder

Both clinical psychology and post-structuralism provide clear paths for thinking about this kind of professional psychology work with women who have been raped and sexually abused. Neither are singular models, and both are complex in their own ways, but they nevertheless each provide easy ways to script a response to the work. These responses are almost completely orthogonal; they work at different levels, they prioritise different concerns and they are willing to live with completely different ontological and epistemological assumptions. Both, though, particularly in their feminist guises, are ostensibly ultimately concerned about the welfare of those who have suffered rape and sexual abuse. What I endeavour to do in this section of the chapter, is to move beyond the comfort zones enabled by these approaches on their own; and to begin to interrogate them against each other.

While it is possible to sit back in the academy and deliver a compelling theorised critique of 'real world' practices, there is something naggingly unsatisfying about critiques that demolish practices that attempt to be liberatory on the grounds that they aren't really. It's not that these critiques aren't valuable or essential, even, but they can't be the last word when there are ongoing pragmatic decisions that have to be made about social action. The personal and very practical question I have been grappling with, in the process of writing this chapter, is whether or not I/we (as feminists and critical psychologists) should be doing the kind of professional clinical psychology work that I have outlined here. My feminist clinical psychology voice says, 'Yes, possibly', and my feminist post-structuralist voice says, 'No, probably not'.

How does this kind of work stand in relation to feminist and critical psychology concerns about the power of psychology, and the psy-professions more generally, to work as a conservative social force? And, in more immediate ways, what are the risks that we might pose directly to the women we work with? Are they too great? And, finally, what are the costs of withdrawing?

The potential risk for individual women we work with occurs when psychological practice contributes to an unhelpful and limiting 'fixing' of a particular narrative or framework for her understanding of the experience of sexual abuse (see also Reavey and Warner, 2001). The problem for psychologists is that we can never really know ahead of time how specific interventions[16] and analyses put to our clients are going to impact on them. In our work, we always inevitably call women into a particular discourse of rape and/or sexual abuse. This process of interpellation occurs without a woman's consent. It is, in many cases, beyond the control of the psychologist, and it is too subtle to be accessible to a concept like informed consent. While the dominant feminist and psychological discourse for understanding the impact of rape and sexual abuse is a sympathetic one, and an improvement on the dominant victim-blaming discourses from our recent past, it may still be too limiting. We can never really know ahead of time whether or not the way that we position a 'client' within the discourse of rape and sexual abuse trauma will be helpful or not. (And, indeed, the whole notion of what it means to be 'helpful' isn't always clear.) For instance, how, if at all, is it possible to talk about pain, hurt, and even damage within the psy-complex, without fixing such renditions of injury into stable identities where such pain and hurt might be permanently locked?

It is for these reasons especially,[17] that this kind of practice seems inherently double-edged at best, and potentially capable of causing harm, even against the explicit good intentions of any individual practitioner. The source of this anxiety is based on a belief in the productive (in the sense of constitutive) power of psychology and psychological practice; and also the belief that this power exceeds the control of the individual psychologist. The power is not in our hands, we might say. But for the very same reasons, to do with the productive power of psychological practice, it may also be possible for it to work constructively in a positive sense for the women who are clients in this kind of process.

Reminded of 'Foucault's challenge that because nothing is innocent and "everything is dangerous ... we always have something to do"' (Lather, 2001: 219), the moral and political high ground does not necessarily rest with a refusal to take part as 'the expert' in such psychology work (see Foucault, 1984[18]). As actors faced with the limitations and opportunities provided by systems not of our own making, political action is inevitably fraught with compromise. For one thing, we have to be mindful of what the alternatives are. While the framework of trauma, for instance, might be limiting and problematic in many ways, from a feminist point of view, it has to be seen and judged alongside the other cultural resources that are readily available to children and women for making sense of sexual abuse.

That is, the victim-blaming, shame-inducing, trivialising, silencing, and threatening discourses through which abuse is perpetrated and ignored. With this in mind, a psychologising ontology of the traumatic effects of sexual abuse might in some cases be extremely liberating. Moreover, feminists such as Judith Butler (1993) have emphasised there is potential for refusal and/or rupture in processes of interpellation. No discourses are totalising, and it is possible that I am overstating the power of psychology and psychological practice.

On the other hand, it is not enough for one to engage in such work with good intentions, but without ongoing reflexive engagement and, as Marecek has argued, 'incorporat[ing] a cultural analysis of our practices into those practices' (1999: 180). Clinical psychology is not inherently and necessarily bad, but it requires this kind of active corrective to protect against its colonising tendencies. If, as feminists and critical psychologists, we are to practise within this paradigm, we must offer the women we work with more than a complacent 'trust me' attitude, because the power of psychology always exceeds the intentions of its practitioners. As a starting point we may need to recognise that our frameworks for sense-making – such as understanding the effects of sexual abuse in terms of psychological trauma – *are* points of interpellation. That is, these particular discourses will always offer strong positions through which women can come to understand and shape their experience of the effects of rape or sexual abuse. While, as feminists, we use frameworks we believe will be helpful for women, my point is that we don't necessarily know whether these frameworks will be helpful or not for any particular woman at a particular time. In our efforts for advocacy, empowerment or healing, I think the least we can do is be acutely aware that our own professional work with women is always a process of subjectification. And sometimes our helping hand may actually work to reinforce limiting constructions of subjectivity.

Acknowledgements

A previous version of this chapter was presented at the Millennium World Conference in Critical Psychology, Sydney, Australia in 1999. I thank all those women who have talked to me about their experiences of rape and sexual abuse, and hope that I have been able to learn from their stories. I also thank members of the Gender and Critical Psychology Group in the Department of Psychology, University of Auckland, and members of the Centre for Psychosocial Studies, Birkbeck College, University of London for helpful discussions in relation to work-in-progress presentations of this material. Ginny Braun, Kim McGregor, Tim McCreanor, and Kay Mitchell read a draft of this chapter, and I am grateful for their feedback. This work has been supported in part by a University of Auckland Research Committee grant and a Royal Society of New Zealand Marsden grant.

Notes

1 While such questions are bound to be perennial dilemmas brought about by the kinds of epistemological confrontation arguably important to the vitality of critical psychology, they are certainly not new. In many ways they mirror the kinds of debate within feminist groups during the 1980s, over the uncertain possibilities for working on feminist political projects 'within the system'.

2 I did see one man (abused as an adult) when I was doing this work, but by far the majority of my work, and the work of others I knew, was with women. While the arguments developed in this chapter also apply in various ways to professional work with men raped and sexually abused, I tend to refer to women here to acknowledge the gendered pattern of sexual abuse.

3 The Act has been amended many times, and has since been replaced by the Accident Rehabilitation and Compensation Insurance Act 1992 (ARCIA).

4 File AACT ACC W3912, 102/1 Compensation: PIBA Sexual Violence 1983–85, Archives New Zealand, Wellington, New Zealand.

5 For example, a booklet recently published by ACC detailing therapy guidelines for working with adult survivors of childhood sexual abuse, was written by an independent counsellor/researcher (McGregor, 2001).

6 Although the amount is less than publicised awards from different systems in some other countries (e.g. see Sheehy, 1994; Tobin, 1994), New Zealand society does not have a strong tradition of litigation, and $10,000 (NZD) was a reasonably substantial amount of money at the time – in 1991, the median annual income for females of fifteen years and over in the full-time labour force was $20,202 (NZD New Zealand Official Yearbook, 1993). By 1993, when legislation was changed, the provision for lump sum compensation for people suffering injuries of any kind, was removed. This change was one of a number of measures taken to reduce costs, by what has been described as the New Right thrust of the 1992 bill (e.g. Couper, 1995). In the meantime, some feminist lawyers have advocated civil suits where women can directly sue those who have sexually abused them for punitive damages. This is arguably an even more complicated and messy area because of the direct confrontation with the abuser (although see Sheehy, 1994, for a sensitive feminist analysis of the pros and cons of such action, from a legal point of view). With new changes to ACC legislation being introduced this year, lump sum payments are being reintroduced with different levels of entitlement and different criteria.

7 I have had considerable difficulty locating trustworthy data on the number of claims made and paid out, despite searching published ACC Injury Statistics and consulting directly with ACC (a statistician, a media adviser, and a general inquiry). Currently, however, there has been some public controversy in the media over the proposed reintroduction of lump sum claims. One newspaper reported that 13,000 claims were made for lump sum compensation relating to rape and sexual abuse in 1993 (the final year in which they were available) (Editorial, *Sunday Star Times*, 13 January 2002: A8).

8 I think there was also some tacit understanding that the psychiatrist/ psychologist's report would act as validation of the person's claim to have been sexually abused (given there were no formal requirements for 'corroboration', and that it was not required for the abuse to have been reported to the police).

9 For related critiques of therapy that share some of my discomfort, see, for example, Masson (1988) and Kitzinger and Perkins (1993).

10 In practice this requirement was not upheld for 'sensitive claims' (the term ACC uses to refer to claims relating to sexual abuse).

11 See Gavey and Braun (1997) regarding the ethics of using clinical case material in published work.

12 This is perhaps not surprising given, as Marecek (1999) has pointed out in her study of US feminist therapists' talk, their frameworks for practice are themselves heavily saturated with psychological models of trauma.

13 The significance of this quote might be more clearly conveyed by Kathy Ferguson's summary of the main point in Brown's book: 'emancipatory politics pursued within depoliticizing and regulatory environments will come to resemble the arenas they intend to subvert' (1997: 1037).

14 Policy regarding the cover of 'sensitive claims' is currently under revision. Ironically, and sadly, ACC has proposed that DSM-IV diagnoses will be required when considering claims for funding ongoing counselling (pers. comm., Team Manager, Sensitive Claims, ACC, 6 November 2001); although this is being contested by counsellors (pers. comm., Kim McGregor, January 2002) and mental health advocates (pers. comm., Senior Analyst, Mental Health Commission, December 2001). When I raised concern about the potentially negative impact on people of being given psychiatric diagnoses (for bureaucratic accounting purposes), the Sensitive Claims Team Manager noted that '90 per cent of people would never see the reports written about them' and, as a concession to protecting claimants' feelings, he said that it was 'fine with me if people don't know that they've had their cover accepted because they are deemed to have a mental injury' (pers. comm., 6 November 2001).

15 In the revisions currently being proposed, it may soon have to be established that a person has 'mental injury', that is either a 'cognitive impairment' or a 'behavioural impairment' before counselling will be paid for (pers. comm., Team Manager, Sensitive Claims, ACC, 6 November 2001).

16 And I am coming from a perspective that regards everything the psychologist or therapist says as an intervention; the metaphors we use and the questions we ask all offer an expert framework in which the client is invited to be positioned in various ways – sometimes these will be deliberate, but often they will not.

17 I also have concerns at the broader social level, about the implications of basing campaigns against sexual abuse around emphases on the psychological harm that it causes. For instance, if our moral judgements against sexual abuse become too tightly rooted in evidence of its mental health costs, then what does this mean for women who don't show signs of psychological harm, and where do we stand if prevention strategies that attempt to dilute the injurious effects of rape and sexual abuse are successful, but sexual abuse continues anyway?

18 For related interest, see Young (1994) for a constructive attempt to integrate Foucauldian ideas about disciplinary power and suspicions of the confessional mode, with practical suggestions for more empowering service provision.

References

Alcoff, L. and Gray, L. (1993) 'Survivor discourse: transgression or recuperation?', *Signs: Journal of Women in Culture and Society* 18, 2: 260–290.

Briere, J. (2002) 'Treating adult survivors of severe childhood abuse and neglect: further development of an integrative model', in John E.B. Myers, Lucy Berliner, John Briere, C. Terry Hendrix, Carole Jenny and Theresa A. Reid (eds) *The APSAC handbook on child maltreatment*, Second Edition, Thousand Oaks: Sage Publications, pp. 175–203.

Brown, W. (1995) *States of injury: power and freedom in late modernity*, Princeton: Princeton University Press.

Burt, M. (1980) 'Cultural myths and supports for rape', *Journal of Personality and Social Psychology* 38: 217–230.

Butler, J. (1993) *Bodies that matter: on the discursive limits of 'sex'*, New York and London: Routledge.

Butler, J. (1997) *Excitable speech: a politics of the performative*, New York and London: Routledge.

Couper, F.M. (1995) '*A feminist critique of the Accident Compensation Corporation*', unpublished dissertation for a Bachelor of Laws (Honours) degree, University of Auckland.

deLauretis, T. (1987) *Technologies of gender: essays on theory, film, and fiction*, Bloomington and Indianapolis: Indiana University Press.

Ferguson, K.E. (1997) Review article of Wendy Brown, *States of inquiry: power and freedom in late modernity. Signs: Journal of Women in Culture and Society* 22, 4: 1037–1040.

Foucault, M. (1981) *The history of sexuality, vol. 1: An Introduction*, (Trans. R. Hurley), Harmondsworth, Middlesex: Penguin.

Foucault, M. (1984) 'On the genealogy of ethics: an overview of work in progress', in P. Rabinow (ed.) *The Foucault reader*, London: Penguin.

Foucault, M. (1991) '*Governmentality*', in G. Burchell., C. Gordon and P. Miller (eds) *The Foucault effect: studies in governmentality*, Chicago: The University of Chicago Press, pp. 87–104.

Gavey, N. and Braun, V. (1997) 'Ethics and the publication of clinical case material', *Professional Psychology: Research and Practice*, 28: 399–404.

Hacking, I. (1995) *Rewriting the soul: multiple personality and the sciences of memory*, Princeton: Princeton University Press.

Kitzinger, C. and Perkins, R. (1993) *Changing our minds: lesbian feminism and psychology*, New York and London: New York University Press.

Lamb, S. (1999) 'Constructing the victim: popular images and lasting labels', in S. Lamb (ed.) *New versions of victims: feminist struggles with the concept*, New York and London: New York University Press, pp. 108–138.

Lather, P. (2001) 'Postbook: working the ruins of feminist ethnography', *Signs: Journal of Women in Culture and Society* 27, 1: 199–227.

McCurdy, C. (1987) 'Broadcast: accident compensation for sexual assault', *Broadsheet* 153: 8–10.

McGregor, K. (2001) *Therapy guidelines: adult survivors of child sexual abuse*, (ACC 293), Wellington, NZ: Accident Compensation Corporation.

Marecek, J. (1999) 'Trauma talk in feminist clinical practice', in S. Lamb (ed.) *New versions of victims: feminist struggles with the concept*, New York and London: New York University Press, pp. 158–182.

Masson, J. (1988) *Against therapy*, London: Fontana.

Meijer, Irene Costera and Prins, Baukje (1998) 'How bodies come to matter: an interview with Judith Butler', *Signs: Journal of Women in Culture and Society* 23: 275–286.

New Zealand Official Yearbook (1993)/Te Pukapuka Houanga Whaimona o Aotearoa, Ninety-sixth Edition, Department of Statistics/Te Tari Tatau.

New Zealand Law Commission/Te Aka Matua O Te Ture (2000) *Limitation of civil actions: a discussion paper*, Preliminary Paper 39, Wellington, New Zealand: Law Commission.

O'Dell, L. (1997) 'Child sexual abuse and the academic construction of symptomatologies', *Feminism and Psychology* 7: 334–339.

Parker, I. (1999) 'Critical psychology: critical links', *Radical Psychology* 1(1). Available: http://www.yorku.ca/faculty/academic/danaa/Parker.htm (accessed 9 March 1999).

Parker, I. (2001) 'Critical psychology: excitement and danger', *International Journal of Critical Psychology* 1: 125–127.

Reavey, P. and Warner, S. (2001) 'Curing women: child sexual abuse, therapy and the construction of femininity', *International Journal of Critical Psychology, Special Issue on Sex and Sexualities* 3: 49–71.

Rose, N. (1998) *Inventing ourselves: psychology, power, and personhood*, Cambridge: Cambridge University Press.

Rose, N. (2000a) 'Power and subjectivity: critical history and psychology', *Academy for the Study of the Psychoanalytic Arts*. Available: http://www.academyanalyticarts.org/cnrose.html (accessed 18 July 2000).

Rose, N. (2000b) 'Power in therapy: Techne and ethos', *Academy for the Study of the Psychoanalytic Arts*. Available: http://www.academyanalyticarts.org/rose2.html (accessed 12 October 2000).

Rose, N. and Miller, P. (1992) 'Political power beyond the state: problematics of government', *British Journal of Sociology* 43, 2: 173–205.

Sheehy, A. (1994) 'Compensation for women who have been raped', in J.V. Roberts and R.M. Mohr (eds) *Confronting sexual assault: a decade of legal and social change*, Toronto: University of Toronto Press, pp. 205–240.

Tobin, R. (1994) 'Recent developments in accident compensation: the consequences of mental injury', *Legal Update Series* May: 11–23.

Tobin, R. (1997) 'Civil actions for sexual abuse in New Zealand', *The Tort Law Review* 5, 3: 190–205.

Vigarello, G. (2001) *A history of rape: sexual violence in France from the 16th to the 20th Century*, Cambridge: Polity Press.

Warner, S. (2000) *Understanding child sexual abuse: making the tactics visible*, Gloucester: Handsell.

Weedon, C. (1987) *Feminist practice and post-structuralist theory*, Oxford: Basil Blackwell.

Westaway, J. (1987) 'What women don't know about rape', *New Zealand Woman's Weekly*, 17 August, 33.

Young, I.M. (1994) 'Punishment, treatment, empowerment: three approaches to policy for pregnant addicts', *Feminist Studies* 20: 33–57.

Chapter 12

Working at being survivors

Identity, gender and participation in self-help groups

Marcia Worrell

By plotting the commonalities in women's experiences, feminists working across a range of academic, clinical and grass-roots settings over the 1970s and 1980s have been instrumental in securing a voice and new kind of visibility for women who had been sexually abused in childhood. This voice and visibility was based on the double move of depathologising the trauma of child sexual abuse whilst acknowledging the suffering it gives rise to. The result was to create identities for women contingent on 'survival', agency and resilience. Such a move also provided an understanding of women's experiences of abuse as part of wider processes of subordination. The 'survivor' in such incursions came to be seen as the embodied icon of second-wave feminism with women's experiences of abuse central in framing political struggles against heteropatriarchy.

Although coined by feminists, the term 'survivor' has, in more recent times, slipped into the wider vernacular of child sexual abuse. Whilst being largely (re)produced in the privatised settings of self-help and therapeutics (Reavey and Warner, 2001), survivor narratives have been disseminated more widely by way of the mass media, especially in talk shows, made-for-TV movies, and other genres that combine news and entertainment (Plummer, 1995; Best, 1997). At the same time, information, advice and support offered in the form of groups, guides and autobiographical accounts have proliferated. Much of this offers a gender-based analysis that draws explicitly on, or is loosely aligned to, feminism. These resources enjoin women who have been sexually abused in the past with the promise of understanding, support and increased opportunities to take control over their lives and subjectivity.

Across these texts, as well as those produced in clinical and academic settings, survivors are often referred to as a taken-for-granted singularity (see, for example, Liebman, 1994; Waldman, *et al.* 1998). What was initially used by feminists as a means of coalescing a wide range of women who have been sexually abused has now come to denote a unified identity. What is at work here is a set of foundational assumptions that there is something sufficiently stable about women and their experiences of sexual victimisation in childhood. When read through feminist/post-structuralist concerns, such unitary notions of survivor identity and experience are based on a spurious 'ontology of woman' (cf. Warner, 2001, and also this volume; see also O'Dell and Worrell, 1998; Reavey and Courtney, 1998). These unitary notions not only singularise the many meanings and readings that can be given to child sexual abuse, which itself is marked by a profusion of entangled events. They also conceal the discursive work through which such an identity is made intelligible for women who have been sexually abused.

My aim in this chapter is to draw attention to the discursive work going on when a survivor identity is assumed. To do this, I will examine the ways in which survivors come to know themselves, and each other, by sharing their narratives on abuse within the discursive context of a self-help group. I will also examine the way in which these narratives are, in turn, informed and fashioned by wider discourses on surviving child sexual abuse. My reading of this discursive work is informed by a working relationship between feminist and post-structuralist speaking and analytical positions – as well as the spaces in-between them. A central tenet of this approach is that we never encounter or experience the social world unmediated by the meanings that are given to it. These meanings are constructed through language or other forms of representation (see, for example, Curt, 1994). Additionally, as 'the world out there' neither shows itself completely nor speaks to us directly, there will always be, what Parker (1999), drawing on the earlier work of Woolgar (1988), refers to as an 'interpretative gap' between representations of the world (which include all our observations and constructions of behaviour and feelings) and the things themselves. This interpretative gap is *indexical* because words, phrases and complete accounts are never context free and are always-ever glued to the circumstances and contexts in which they are used. They can only be made sense of in relation to the specific, socially situated, occasions of their use and are, furthermore, *inconcludable* because a complete description of a phenomenon is never possible.

Post-structuralists, especially feminist/post-structuralists, additionally highlight the power/knowledges that the researcher brings to bear on the research process. In particular, they point to questions of how to narrate the voices of others and what claims can be made in the process. In relation to this, Condor (1997: 119) argues that 'the genres we use when producing academic texts and research articles are clearly different to those used by the research participants in producing their own accounts'. This process of narrating the 'voices' of others, Squire (1990) argues, inevitably forms a new narrative. The formation of these 'new narratives' (i.e. those formed through the process of research as opposed to those which are un- or dis-covered in any pre- or extra-discursive sense), presents serious problems for those forms of research that claim to capture unmediated examples of 'naturally occurring' talk. These are unmediated in the sense that they existed prior to the operations of the research, or that these examples of naturally occurring talk can be decoded or interpreted in a way that is detached from the operations of the researcher. Far from being a limitation for feminist/post-structuralist-informed styles of research, the notion that researchers themselves form part of the equation is considered axiomatic. These approaches enable a critical scrutiny of the assumptions operating in the social world. At the same time they also recognise that such approaches are never entirely free of the assumptions they claim to disrupt.

I am interested in the broad ways in which survivor discourses operate as a social and cultural resource that shape the accounts that women who have been sexually abused are able to give. As such my analysis is not concerned with the formal organisation and sequential implicativeness of talk (found in conversation analysis). More specifically, my concern is to address the particular modes of speaking about child sexual abuse that are inscribed in an already constituted system of meanings associated with child sexual abuse and its survival. In offering these readings of survivor narratives, my aim is not to 'relentlessly ... interrogate ... every last claim' (Gill, 1995: 172), and to dissolve these claims in post-structuralist critiques. Rather what I aim to show are the ways in which the women in the group arrived at particular modes of understandings in relation to the abuse they had experienced and how these become invested in survivor subject positions.

The specific analytical tool I will adopt in this chapter is that of subject positioning (Davies and Harré, 1990). This approach points to the ways in which 'identities' are actively produced and negotiated through discursive practices. So construed, 'identity' is not fixed, but provisional. It is conceived as an ensemble of identifications through which subjects are constituted and constitute themselves. This approach also strongly conveys the way in which people either take up, or are ascribed, discursive positions contextually through interaction and talk. By using this analytical tool to prise apart some of the meanings and understandings enfolded in survivor discourses, my aim is to neither show nor assume who or what a survivor is. Rather it is to explore how the presumed unity of survivor identity *works* through the particular discursive modality of self-help and the forms of positionality this gives rise to.

Women's narratives on surviving child sexual abuse

The narratives I look at in this chapter were expressed by women who formed a self-help group for survivors of child sexual abuse based in the South East of England. The group comprised ten white British women who attended sessions on a weekly basis. The aims of the group, in common with other self-help groups for survivors of sexual abuse, included breaking down the isolation that many women feel following experiences of abuse through solidarity with other survivors. The group also explicitly aimed to address healing, and personal as well as social transformation. These aims were stitched together by mutual support given by group members and by the informal leadership of the facilitator, Krystal.[1] As facilitator, Krystal would provide a focus for the weekly sessions by asking the other women to read sections from Bass and Davis' best-selling – although not without its critics (see, for example, Haaken, 1999) – guide to surviving sexual abuse, *The Courage to Heal* (1997). This particular aspect of the group's activity, or 'bibliotherapy' as Taylor (1999) puts it, was seen to provide a road map to the goal of 'personal healing' and to create an awareness that the women's 'individual problems' were shared more widely amongst other survivors of child sexual abuse.

The need to heal

Whether deployed in popular, academic or professional settings, discourses on child sexual abuse commonly convey a statement about the severity of the abuse and its long-term psycho-social consequences for women who have experienced it. For Bass and Davis:

> The long-term effects of child sexual abuse ... permeate everything: your sense of self, your intimate relationships, your sexuality, your parenting, your work life, even your sanity. Everywhere you look, you see its effects.
>
> (1997: 33–34)

Bearing witness to the trauma caused by the abuse to a skilled or sympathetic audience is widely seen to both ameliorate the effects of abuse and break the codes of silence surrounding it. In Petronio and Flores' view

> [t]he weight of their secrets leads to painful lives ... being unable to talk about their experiences results in both physical and emotional health problems ... By keeping the secret of abuse, the perpetrator's crime becomes a lifetime sentence for the victim.
>
> (1997: 101)

Similarly, for Bass and Davis (1997: 58), 'telling another human being about what happened ... is a powerful healing force that can dispel the shame of being a victim'. In light of this, it was therefore not surprising that talking about the effects of abuse was something that occupied much of the group's time. The women talked at length about how the abuse had affected them psychologically, emotionally and physically. What was continually stressed, as these narratives were shared, was that survival was contingent not on *how* women survived the abuse, but the fact that they *did* survive. Moreover, when sharing their narratives, members of the group would actively position themselves, and each other, so as to resist what they perceived to be inappropriate subject positions of 'victim' and 'self-blaming'. These were seen to have undesirable connotations, such as powerlessness and being 'stuck in victim mode' (as Anita, another member of the group, put it), which the women in the group wished to retain a strategic distance from. When individual women's narratives strayed into such inappropriate terrains, other group members would actively intervene to navigate the account and reposition it in alignment with preferred survivor subject positions.

The response to Hayley's narrative about the impact that the abuse had on her relationships with men, provides an example of this collective repositioning:

HAYLEY: I always feel as though I'm waiting to fuck-up or to be fucked-over by some fucker or other [...] men don't stick around long enough to care about me [...] I usually feel [...] when I'm gonna have sex [...] I usually feel that I'm sort of giving in to it [...] I just can't get into it, y'know [...] I met this really nice guy called 'Tim' once. Whenever we tried to do it I'd see *his* face [her abuser's] [...] needless to say he was off like a bullet. Can't blame him really [...] it's just that it kept coming back to me all the time and I guess I made it so as Tim couldn't handle it all.

The other members of the group saw the necessity to calibrate Hayley's narrative as she had expressed what for them was her continued powerlessness in relation to the abuse. Hayley was also impelled by the group to adopt an attitude of self-care: one in which she was no longer vulnerable to the sway of others, especially men. Hayley was encouraged to harden her attitude towards men, not in order to turn away from them altogether, but so that she could 'find the right one'.

Gayle too talked about difficulties in maintaining relationships, this time in the broader context of family, friends and even therapists:

GAYLE: I have been trying to deal with the abuse for years and years [...] I've seen off countless therapists [...] burnt-out loads of friends [...] I've lost touch with most of family except mum because they all think I've lost it big time [...] maybe I have I don't know [...] I mean I haven't been through some of the stuff that many of you talk about, so why is it affecting me so badly? [...] what if I was always mad and this has just made it worse? [...] I've been trying, though, trying really hard to deal with all the anxiety [...] panic attacks are the worst [...] claustrophobia, depression, eating disorders, the lot. You name it – I've got it!

In sharing her narrative on how the experience of abuse had affected her, Gayle doubted her status as a 'true survivor' in terms of her own self-defined lack of resilience in relation to the magnitude of what had happened to her. Other members of the group, including Hayley whose discursive positioning had shifted now she was a 'listener' and not a 'speaker', contested this statement. In a double move, the group acknowledged the effects of the abuse of which she spoke, at the same time as interpolating Gayle into a survivor subject position. Krystal exemplified this double move when she asserted that 'you were a child ... how were you supposed to know what was going on? ... he might have been trying to kill you for all you knew ... course you're going to feel like this.' She further commented that Gayle was indeed 'a survivor as [she was] still here to tell the tale', thereby positioning her as a de facto survivor.

How to heal

Retaining a level of identification with the experience of victimisation and the harmfulness of abuse was seen as an important bridge that connected the women's past experiences with their present selves. Across a number of the sessions I observed, Krystal would note that healing (and by implication 'survival') is 'only possible through changes in thinking'. This was evident when the women sought to recast their experiences in more positive terms, by seeking out 'the benefits' of the abuse. Over the course of these discussions, the abuse was likened to something like an epiphany and sovereign in terms of shaping their post-abuse selves. Many of the women talked about the life-altering nature of the abuse and claimed to have found new resources or to have benefited as a result. Group members explored, for example, the ways in which being abused had developed their ability to 'read social situations' and a 'hyperawareness of others', and had heightened their 'powers of intuition'. Many others asserted that they had obtained powers, skills and overall levels of achievement that they would not have otherwise had. The narratives of Sandra and Dawn provide examples of this discursive work:

SANDRA: Now I'm just so sensitive to other people's needs, their moods as well I suppose. I can just feel when there's something going on that someone doesn't want to talk about [...] I reckon being a survivor does that to you [...] it makes you more in touch with other people [...] you get 'vibes' [...] I guess you kind of instinctively know what's really going on.

Many of the women extended Sandra's point by suggesting that they could intuitively sense who other survivors were. One of the perceived benefits of the abuse was being part of a community of women who knew and understood them 'in a way that no one else could' (Hayley). Among the 'benefits' identified by Dawn was her ability to be 'super organised', 'efficient' and the 'best at everything':

DAWN: I'm the kind of person you'd have hated at school [...] I just have to be the best at everything [...] I can't cope otherwise [...] even now, you know, my house is spotless – even in the places no one ever sees! I'm like that with my work as well. [...] although I think it's really helped me out there as I'm so super organised [...] maybe I'm just competitive, I dunno [...] I guess what people don't see is that even the thought of being out of control terrifies me [...] it makes me remember all those times I never had control over anything [...] I really don't let myself feel like that again.

On the one hand, Sandra's account of her heightened intuitive skills, sensitivity and interconnectedness with others conformed to the normative expectations of what survivors should be like. Dawn's narrative, on the other hand, did not. The response from the other women was to urge Dawn to be easier on herself and others. Their argument was that Dawn's approach could be 'alienating for those who are close to [her]' and 'oppressive'. It was also suggested that it might eventually lead to her isolation, even from other survivors. Dawn's (unintended) articulation of difference, and the dissonance it produced amongst other group members, was eventually repaired by an intervention from the facilitator. Krystal absorbed Dawn's difference by imploring the group to re-position her narrative not as 'being controlling', but as a legitimate way of dealing with the aftermath of the abuse, that was in itself preferable to being a victim.

Speaking outside of the group

The social transformatory aims of the group, and its loose alignment to feminist politics, were highlighted when the women addressed, or contemplated, the issue of speaking outside of the privatised setting of the group. Krystal described this process as, in part, another step 'on the path to recovery' from abuse. At the same time Krystal argued that owning the status of survivor publicly would provide a means of educating wider audiences about child sexual abuse and, in so doing, putting a stop to it. She also argued that speaking outside of the group would enable larger numbers of women to locate themselves within survivor networks. Some of the group members also felt that self-help groups for survivors should not be seen only as an occasion for securing individual support and healing. For these women this carried the attendant risk of creating a situation where survivors learn how to 'cope', 'accommodate' and thereby 'contain' the effects of the abuse. In many respects, women sharing their narratives of abuse within the agentic context of self-help can in itself be seen as mode of resisting and transforming the discursive dominance that constitutes survivors as pathologised. For many of the women, however, it was felt that speaking only to each other would 'take the heat off' perpetrators of abuse and the heteropatriarchial systems that enable and shield their actions. Such a situation, particularly so far as Krystal and Anita were concerned, was untenable:

KRYSTAL: I'm really interested in talking to other survivors [...] we can do something [...] [we can] make a difference if we work at it together [...] we must stop other children from going through what we did [...] abusers need to be stopped [...] I can understand why so many survivors want to stay silent about the abuse [...] I can't blame them. There's such a lot of stigma even now [...] the problem is, if we don't speak out about it [...] if we stay silent we become our own worst enemies – we're so much stronger together, we can't be brushed aside so easily. [...] if we don't stand together we cut ourselves off from other survivors [...] we need to stand up and say *you* did this to me [...] we're here alright and we're not going away that's for sure.

Krystal's account here again resonated with Bass and Davis (1997: 95) who are clear that speaking publicly about the abuse is socially as well as personally transformative. They also argue that this enables survivors to 'join a courageous community of women who are no longer willing to suffer in silence' (ibid.). For Anita, Krystal's emphasis on joining with other survivors simply did not go far enough. In Anita's view, when survivors speak only to each other, whether within or outside the privatised space of the self-help groups, the subversive potential of women challenging both the abuse and abusers was undercut. For her, the solution was far more radical:

ANITA: These men are evil bastards [...] cowards [...] they can get away with it because we don't say anything – well not outside of here anyway [...] ... we just take it and take it and take it so that they can just go on from one child to the next [...] it's all very well us being here, but it's still all secret, we meet here at night nobody sees us [...] we use the side door [...] nobody knows why we're here, we could be learning flower arranging for all anyone knows [...] yeah and we might feel better when we go home because we've talked about what's been bothering us – don't get me wrong and that's really helpful and everything – but what really gets to me is whose life is he fucking over now because I couldn't – well still can't – tell anyone apart from you? [...] there are so many of us and we don't tell, we allow them to get away with it time and time again don't we? [...] If we all [survivors] went to the police tomorrow they'd have to bang-up every other bloke in this country, I tell you they would.

The associated subject positions that the women, led by Krystal and Anita, were invited to take up is well illustrated by the writings of the radical feminist Rosaria Champagne, who argues that:

A survivor of incest is someone who has been molested or raped ... who lives through and remembers the experience, and who comes to understand – through therapy or feminism or some combination of the two – how the experience of childhood sexual violence is 'political'.

(1996: 11)

For Champagne, *not* speaking out about abuse provides a hiding place, or *closet* for heteropatriarchical processes to operate unchallenged and unabated. Her argument is that operations within the discursive arena of surviving abuse can be construed not only as a site for dealing with the individualised long-term effects, but also as a launch-pad for feminist-informed interventions into heteropatriarchy. Similarly, for hooks (1989), 'self-recovery' provides the basis for gaining a critical consciousness through the reconstitution of the self. This radically constituted self, in the view of hooks and Champagne, can then be set to work to both identify and change structures of oppression.

My analysis so far has shown some of the discursive work through which women come to know and understand themselves as survivors of child sexual abuse. In the following section I offer a wider reading of this discursive work. I will go on to then explore the ways in which the women's narratives were shaped by wider discourses on child sexual abuse and to consider some of the implications for women.

Working at being survivors

As stated earlier, for the group, talking about the effects of the abuse was held to serve a number of functions. It was used, for example, as a means of promoting solidarity through mutual understanding and exposing commonalities in experience. It also acted to reinforce the view that resilience, courage and resourcefulness were all needed to survive abuse, even if the assorted survival strategies appear 'self-destructive to [those who do] not understand' (Krystal). Talking about the abuse also provided an opportunity for deploying a corrective to the take-up of undesirable subject positions and potential stasis in 'victim mode'. Specifically, women were encouraged to take up subject positions in which their victimisation was acknowledged but through which they came to see themselves as 'victims no longer' (Anita). Further, even if they were no longer victims, this neither obscured nor elided the need to heal. In this way, talking about the effects of the abuse performed the further function of 'revealing' those aspects of the women's lives that were in need of healing. While speaking out pointed to the need to heal, the interactions amongst members of the group *provided* a means through which healing 'could be' achieved. There was thus, an entwinement of the need to heal with how to heal. Speaking outside of the group was further seen to be demonstrative of personal healing. It was also deployed as politicised technology through which survivors could mobilise and transform social power relations.

However, as I have shown, the confessional genre of the group was also infused with power. This power did not take the crude form of a top-down domination (Foucault, 1988). It was sometimes subtle, but always diffuse, and shifted between members of the group. These operations of power steered women along self-shaping paths. This was particularly evident in the way in which the women were encouraged to avow particular modes of understanding their experiences of abuse and the discomfort they felt when this did not occur. By being guided and constrained through the process of interaction, the women actively positioned themselves and each other in accordance with the categories, assumptions and regulatory ideals of wider survivor discourses.

There was, therefore, a process of attunement at work between the women's personal narratives and those of other women in the group, the facilitator's gained experience of running other groups and external forms of textual authority, such as *The Courage to Heal* and other self-help guides. Together these formed a complex weave of discourses, yoked together by power in highly contingent ways, which appeared as well-formed answers to such questions as, '*Who am I?*', '*To whom am I connected?*' and '*Who can I hope to become?*' (Rappaport, 1993). From a feminist/post-structuralist perspective, 'personal narratives' are discursively mediated and always saturated with the experiences and realities of others. In sharing their narratives on abuse, the women I observed were speaking into already-constituted speaking and listening positions and the dicta of self-help and wider discourses on surviving sexual abuse. Moreover, these positions are thoroughly implicated in power relations.

Doing woman?

At the same time as attributing the responsibility for the abuse to heteropatriarchy, many members of the group also tended to also assess their achievements and shortcomings according to associated hegemonic modes of femininity. Alongside speaking about the psychological effects, many of the women also talked about the ways in which their taken-for-granted modes of 'doing woman' had been dislodged by the abuse. This was particularly evident when the women discussed the difficulties they had had, or were having, with their sexual and non-sexual relationships with men (see, for example, Hayley's account described on page 214). It was also evident in the way in which the women over a number of the sessions I observed tended to assess their sense of physical attractiveness in relation to their perceptions of how men see, or what men want, from women. Thus, in many respects, being a survivor co-articulated with 'doing woman', which here involved drawing on, and reproducing, a wider cultural stock of assumptions and ideas about gender, through which women come to know themselves as individuals and participants in relationships (Simonds, 1996).

In discussing the benefits concerned, here too traditional modes of femininity were performed. These iterated around such claims as women's greater capacity to rear and nurture children, or a heightened sense of intuition, which included the ability to recognise and identify with other survivors. A further demonstration of the women's self-surveilling with respect to hegemonic modes of femininity was seen in the group's response to the benefits of abuse identified by Dawn, who was construed as inappropriately taking on board male values. The transformation of the harmfulness of abuse into something positive or beneficial is central to the construction of survivor identity. The value of this approach for many women is undeniable, not least in terms of dealing with the effects of the abuse, securing support, visibility and resources. And yet this rendering of the harmfulness of abuse as central to survivor identity binds women to the operations of heteropatriarchy, through the very means they seek to resist it. Additionally, although speaking out about abuse (either within or outside the context of self-help) does indeed transform power relations, it does not further follow that this is always self-evidently transgressive (Gavey, 1999). This may re-inscribe women in hegemonic structures through and within which gendered subjectivity is reproduced (Alcoff and Gray, 1993).

Differently positioned narratives

I have argued that throughout my observations many of the women ceded their differently positioned narratives on abuse so as to be positioned within the group story and wider survivor discourses on surviving child sexual abuse. The reduction of difference to sameness through appellations to survivor identity simultaneously opened up particular positions for speaking and listening. These, as I have argued, were demonstrative of a mastery of survivor discourse. At the same time, they obscured or foreclosed the alternative readings that some of the women may have wished to give to their experiences. This eclipsing of difference by the deployment of a unified survivor identity is also evident in survivor discourses more generally.

Although claiming to speak for all women who have been sexually abused, survivor discourses (especially those operating in the discursive context of self-help) are largely based on the assumptive, albeit unstated, experiences of certain women that are designated generic (see Wilson, 1994). These 'generic' experiences have, by way of their social salience and expressive dominance, become codified in survivor discourses as the foundation of survivor identity. Furthermore, in as much as these experiences form the basis of survivor identity politics, they also represent the struggles of all women who have been sexually abused as unitary. This pasting together of women's experiences and agendas fails to give a specificity to the interconnected set of concerns of those women who are differently positioned to the 'generic survivor' commonly invoked within survivor discourses. This includes, for example, women multiply positioned in and by discourses on 'race', age, 'class', sexuality and disability. This lack of specificity leaves unexamined within survivor discourses the situated and specific ways in which the discursive locations of these women co-articulates with their experiences of abuse. This sets in place a framework for making sense of abusive experiences into which not all women can, do or want to fit.

To point to the lack of specificity within survivor discourses is not, as Warner (2001: 119) notes, a simplistic call for the inclusion of 'Others' in ways that invest 'understanding within actual persons'. Rather this solipsism is rejected and replaced by a 'focus on situated knowledges that draw on subjugated perspectives' (ibid.). It is equally not to countenance a slide into overly simplified readings of difference, marginality and exclusion. Such a slide would suggest that marginality derives its meaning from the centre. It is also predicated on notions of fixed centres of power and meanings that structure and order the surrounds (Flax, 1993; Pujal i Llombart, 1998). By reifying those at the 'centre' and 'margins', such notions fail to recognise that within sameness there is difference and within difference sameness. At the same time, they are divested of the notion that one's social location necessarily determines opportunities for speaking, hearing, and being heard (Dow, 1997). What is vital then, as Alcoff (1991: 12) notes, is who is speaking to whom; as this 'turns out to be as important for meaning and truth as what is said; in fact what is said turns out to change according to who is speaking and who is listening.' Survivor discourses are therefore not immune to feminist/post-structuralist questions of who is included in the presumed universal category and whose agendas are being served; as well as who gets to speak, what they are able to say, and what legitimacy is afforded to their voices (O'Dell and Worrell, 1998; Reavey and Warner, 2001).

Towards some conclusions

My argument in this chapter has been that when 'survivor' is used to denote a singularity of experience, it becomes inscribed in discourse as a reified, taken-for-granted identity. Once pulled from the mire of foundationalist assumptions, the notion of a unitary survivor identity is exposed as being 'performatively constituted by the very "expressions" that are said to be its results' (Butler, 1990: 25). In this chapter I have used my observations of a self-help group to show that, both within the group and in relation to wider self-help survivor discourses, this unity similarly disguises the discursive work that brings it into being. The survivor identity, which the group used as an imaginary referent, operated as a regulatory ideal as women monitored themselves, and each other, via the technology of mutual support. As I have shown, the regulatory ideal of this identity was not mobilised in a linear or uni-directional fashion. For, at times, women were positioned, and positioned themselves, as de facto survivors. At others, survivor identity was *immanent* and contingent on the successful negotiation towards the preferred subject positions operating in the group.

Mobilising the unitary survivor identity as a means by which *all* women may challenge heteropatriarchy is also problematic in that it is based on the expressive dominance afforded to just some women who have been abused. In claiming to 'soak up' the experiences of all women, only particular voices and ways of speaking about abuse are legitimated within the deployment of a unitary survivor identity. Its regulatory force, thus, simultaneously 'conceals' certain aspects of women's experiences of abuse whilst 'revealing' others. This not only limits the range and type of experiences that can be heard. It also has implications for which women can speak, and to whom, as well as for those experiences which come to typify survivors.

What is at stake here is more than wrangles over epistemology. A feminist/post-structuralist analysis provides the means for showing how the unity of survivor identity works. This critical work is necessary as, without it, regulatory and homogenising effects at work within notions of a unified survivor identity remain unacknowledged and undisturbed (Flax, 1993). These troubling notions cannot be overlooked; as to do so will fall into the trap of only talking about abuse in ways that are sanctioned by these singularised notions. It also points to how we may engage with the issues engendered by abuse in more complex and nuanced ways. Rather than deciding in advance 'who women are' and what sense can be made of their experiences through recourse to immutable survivor essence, this perspective allows for more open and provisional ways of approaching women's experiences of abuse. It opens up possibilities for seeing survivors in specific and situated terms through their identifications with self-help and survivor discourses more generally. For, instead of revealing a foundation that is unquestionably there, they alternatively show the complex, heterogeneous and nuanced ways in which women, in and through such articulations of difference, 'make sense' of their experiences of abuse. An engagement with multiple articulations of difference not only affords a visibility and specificity to those experiences hitherto obscured by unified notions of survivor identity, it also has the potential to disrupt the essentialising tendencies inherent in such discourses. This allows us to (re)conceptualise narratives of survival, and representations of survivor identities, in terms of their being *political* activities that require different *discursive* strategies depending on the context in which they are enacted (Atmore, 1999, Warner, 2001).

Note

1 The names of women have been changed.

References

Alcoff, L. (1991) 'The problem of speaking for others', *Cultural Critique* 18, 20: 5–32.

Alcoff, L. and Gray, L. (1993) 'Survivor discourse: transgression or recuperation? *Signs* 18, 2: 260–290.

Atmore, C. (1999) 'Victims, backlash and radical feminist theory (or, the morning after they stole feminist's fire)', in S. Lamb (ed.) *New versions of victims: feminists struggle with the concept*, New York: New York University Press, pp. 183–211.

Bass, E. and Davis, L. (1997) *The courage to heal: a guide for women survivors of child sexual abuse*, New York: Harper and Row.

Best, J. (1997) 'Victimization and the victim industry', *Society* 34, 4: 9–18.

Butler, J. (1990) *Gender trouble: feminism and the subversion of identity*, London: Routledge.

Champagne, R. (1996) *The politics of survivorship*, London: New York University Press.

Condor, S. (1997) 'And so say all of us?: Some thoughts on "experiential democratization" as an aim for critical social psychologists', in T. Ibanez and L. Iniguez (eds) *Critical social psychology*, London: Sage, pp. 111–146.

Curt, B. (1994) *Textuality and tectonics: troubling social and psychological science*, Buckingham: Open University Press.

Davies, B. and Harré, R. (1990) 'Positioning: the discursive construction of selves', *Journal for the Theory of Social Behaviour* 20, 1: 43–63.

Dow, B. (1997) 'Politicizing voice', *Western Journal of Communication* 61, 2: 243–252.

Flax, J. (1993) *Disputed subjects: essays on psychoanalysis, politics and philosophy*, London: Routledge.

Foucault, M. (1988) 'Technologies of the self', in L. Martin, H. Gutman and P.

Hutton (eds) *Technologies of the self: a seminar with Michel Foucault*, London: Tavistock Publications Ltd, pp. 16–49.

Gavey, N. (1999) '"I wasn't raped but ...": revisiting definitional problems in sexual victimization', in S. Lamb (ed.) *New versions of victims: feminists struggle with the concept*, New York: New York University Press, pp. 57–81.

Gill, R. (1995) 'Relativism, reflexivity and politics: interrogating discourse analysis from a feminist perspective', in S. Wilkinson and C. Kitzinger (eds) *Feminism and discourse: psychological perspectives*, London: Sage, pp. 165–186.

Haaken, J. (1999) 'Heretical texts: the courage to heal and the incest survivor movement', in S. Lamb (ed.) *New versions of victims: feminists struggle with the concept*, New York: New York University Press, pp. 13–41.

hooks, b. (1989) *Feminist theory: from margin to center*, Boston: South End Press.

Liebman, J. (1994) *Victimized daughters: incest and the development of the female self*, London: Taylor and Francis.

O'Dell, L. and Worrell, M. (1998) 'Trajectories of survivorhood: troubling a singularised identity', Paper presented at the British Psychological Society conference: Psychology of Women's Section, Birmingham University, June.

Parker, I. (1999) 'Critical reflexive humanism and critical constructionist psychology', in D. Nightingale and J. Cromby (eds) *Social constructionist psychology: a critical analysis of theory and practice*, Buckingham: Open University Press, pp. 23–36.

Petronio, S. and Flores, L. (1997) 'Locating the voice of logic: disclosure discourse of sexual abuse', *Western Journal of Communication* 61, 1: 101–115.

Plummer, K. (1995) *Telling sexual stories: power, change and social worlds*, London: Routledge.

Pujal i Llombart, M. (1998) 'Feminist psychology or the history of a non-feminist practice', in E. Burman (ed.) *Deconstructing feminist psychology*, London: Sage, pp. 30–46.

Rappaport, J. (1993) 'Narrative studies, personal stories, and identity transformation in the mutual help context', *The Journal of Applied Behavioral Science* 29, 2: 239–256.

Reavey, P. and Courtney, L. (1998) 'Women, sexual health and sexual abuse: an examination of some apparent tensions in individualist approaches to self-help', *Mental Health Care* 1: 10–17.

Reavey, P. and Warner, S. (2001) 'Curing women: child sexual abuse, therapy and the construction of femininity', *International Journal of Critical Psychology, Special Issue on Sex and Sexualities* 3: 49–71.

Simonds, W. (1996) 'All consuming selves: self-help literature and women's identities', in D. Grodin and T. Lindlof (eds) *Constructing the self in a mediated world*, London: Sage.

Squire, C. (1990) 'Crisis what crisis?: Discourses and narratives of the "social" in social psychology', in I. Parker and J. Shotter (eds) *Deconstructing social psychology*, London: Routledge, pp. 33–46.

Taylor, V. (1999) 'Gender and social movements: gender processes in women's self-help movements', *Gender and Society* 13, 1: 8–33.

Waldman, T., Silber, D., Holmstrom, R. and Karp, S. (1998) 'Incest survivors have different personality characteristics than non-assaulted persons', *Journal of Social Behaviour and Personality* 13, 3: 437–442.

Warner, S. (2001) 'Disrupting identity through visible therapy: a feminist post-structuralist approach to working with women who have experienced child sexual abuse', *Feminist Review* 68, 1: 115–139.

Wilson, M. (1994) *Crossing the boundary: Black women survive incest*, London: Virago.

Woolgar, S. (1988) *Science: the very idea*, Chichester: Ellis Horwood.

Chapter 13

Disrupting identity through Visible Therapy

A feminist post-structuralist approach to working with women who have experienced child sexual abuse[1]

Sam Warner

Introduction

Child sexual abuse represents a key site in which unequal and gendered power relations are played out. Hence, child sexual abuse is of particular concern to feminists who have long been involved in providing contexts in which (child) sexual abuse could be recognised, theorised and its effects on women addressed (Warner, 2000a). This chapter builds on this work to develop a narrative framework for therapeutic interventions with women who have experienced child sexual abuse. This approach, termed 'Visible Therapy', weaves ideas from feminism with post-structuralism (Butler, 1990, 1993; Foucault, 1990; Haraway, 1991) to explicate a socially situated framework for engaging with individualised trajectories of distress.

I begin by arguing that feminism and post-structuralism offer incomplete guides to therapy (regarding women and child sexual abuse), but that together they can provide a critical framework for practice. This framework is described and its application explicated. I interrogate the implicit therapeutic assumption that talking (about child sexual abuse) is always beneficial and critically examine the assumed object of therapeutic concern (aspects of the sexually abusive experience). I describe the 'tactics' of abuse in order to challenge individualised narratives of women's responsibility for past abuse and present re-enactment. I argue that absolute understandings of trust, honesty and survival militate against progressive therapeutic intervention and demonstrate the benefits of socially located revisions of these terms. Implications for adopting a post-structuralist approach to training and supervision are then considered. My aim is to deconstruct mainstream approaches to therapy in order to reconstruct therapy as a socially situated, feminist enterprise.

Therapy and child sexual abuse: feminist politics and post-structuralist concerns

Feminism and post-structuralism are highly contested terms, as evidenced throughout this book. As such, it is a misnomer to talk about feminist or post-structuralist theory, per se (cf. Farganis, 1994). Rather, what is presented here are those aspects found within both feminist and post-structuralist theorising that converge to dispute the notion of a natural social order and which, I argue, can provide a critical framework for therapy. Post-structuralism does this by directly challenging the modernist assumption of an objective world, and with this the implication of any singular understanding of, or approach to, therapy regarding, for example, child sexual abuse. Normative values are no longer hidden (as natural), but exposed (as regulatory fictions) and, as such, are made open to dispute (cf. Deleuze and Guattari, 1984).

Social constructionist approaches to therapy (e.g. White and Epston, 1990; Epston, 1993; Larner, 1995), which draw on these ideas, are often termed 'narrative therapy' (Parker, 1992) because of their focus on discursive practices. They are understood as progressive precisely because democratisation is presumed to be promoted through the displacement of an unproblematised understanding of 'truth' (Frosh, 1995). However, the idea that democratisation is necessarily achieved by refusing absolute understanding is naïve. Therapists occupy a very different social location to their clients and the notion that one can 'give up' power by refusing absolute truth is a sleight of hand which denies its own productive relationship with change (Larner, 1995). Therapy is, after all, a deliberate intervention in the life of someone else.

From some feminist perspectives (e.g. Hartsock, 1990; Jackson, 1992; Weissen, 1993; Benhabib, 1995) refusing absolute truth was never understood to be a progressive strategy. Rather, relativist approaches were viewed as regressive because they invalidate women's knowledge and experience. In particular, post-structuralist frameworks seemingly undermine a principled engagement with the 'real problem' of abuse (see Reavey and Warner, 2001). The concern is that if all knowledge is socially constructed and, therefore, has epistemological equivalence, how is perspective to be theorised as having value? Specifically, how can a feminist understanding that the sexual exploitation of children is wrong be sustained? Yet admitting all knowledge has epistemological equivalence does not necessarily preclude operating a practical morality. And the assumption that principles can only ever be rooted in absolute values reinstates the hierarchy of insight and truth (cf. Frosh, 1995) and, de facto, promotes regulation rather than liberation. Whilst all social practices regulate, it is the *unacknowledged* regulation of social space that can act to reproduce dominant values and militate against a partial liberation from those social structures that bind us precisely because we cannot see them.

This requires an examination of how experience becomes known and knowledge is experienced, through situated discursive action. As Grosz (1995: 27) suggests, we need to ask: 'How does this knowledge, this method, this technique, constitute its object?' – in this case, therapy with women regarding experiences of child sexual abuse. This cannot be theorised when knowledge is assumed to be perspectiveless, as objective accounts of the world would suggest. Nor can particular perspectives be valorised when all knowledge is assumed to be of equal value, as some readings of relativist accounts of the world would suggest. As Haraway (1991) argues, both objectivism and relativism are 'god-tricks' which promise, respectively, vision from nowhere and everywhere and thereby deny their responsibility for the things they survey and construct. Conversely, 'being somewhere' means that perspective is socially located, hidden assumptions can be revealed and the effects of our perspective taking can then be theorised. Specifying perspective, therefore, allows greater access to the process(es) whereby interpretations and analyses are made. Hence, this forces the therapist to a greater responsibility for her actions through attending to 'both the forms by which [therapy] is produced, and the relationships in which it is produced' (Banister et al., 1994: 4). As such, the gaze I cast is neither innocent nor naïve, but is rooted in selective concerns (Haraway, 1991). The aim of Visible Therapy is to privilege some understandings over others, as feminism would assert, without arriving at an absolute position, or at an ultimate understanding, as post-structuralism would suggest. It is necessary, therefore, to provide a framework for theorising the privileging of particular perspectives and to demonstrate how feminism and post-structuralism can be applied to conceptualising therapy with women regarding child sexual abuse.

Situating Visible Therapy: provisional perspectives and provisional practices

An attempt, termed 'feminist standpoint theory', was made by Hartsock (1983) to theorise the value of drawing on particular perspectives. The underlying assumption within this theory is that structural privilege precludes clarity of thought because there is no impetus to theorise 'the norm'. By contrast, structural marginalisation increases clarity of thought because such persons not only have access to dominant understandings but also have access to 'abnormal' or subjugated perspectives. Hence, the reasoning is that:

> [I]n societies stratified by race, ethnicity, class, gender, sexuality, or some other such politics shaping the very structure of a society, the

activities of those at the top both organise and set limits on what persons who perform such activities can understand about themselves and the world around them ... In contrast, the activities of those at the bottom of such social hierarchies can provide starting points for thought – for *everyone's* research and scholarship.

(Harding, 1993: 54)

A post-structuralist revision of standpoint theory does not invest understanding within actual persons, but rather focuses on situated knowledges that draw on subjugated perspectives. This non-materialist revision of standpoint theory is crucial because when identity and experience are understood as provisional, then the ways in which identity and experience are socially regulated can be examined. Hence, a simplistic call for 'inclusion' of others' experiences is rejected. The aim is to problematise experience and identity – to theorise how different experiences and identities are constructed and constrained – and not simply reappropriate them (cf. Spivak, 1993).

Thus, I am less concerned with who others are (or who I am) than with how 'they' (or I) come to know and be known (through practices of child sexual abuse and therapy). It is only when we question the authenticity of identity and experience that we can begin to explore how particular versions of reality are produced, promoted and maintained (Warner, 2000b, c). The modernist desire to interpret what 'this person really meant' is resisted and, it can be argued, attendant difficulties circumvented. Hence, whilst I do not presume to speak for others, I do speak about the social production of (myself and) others. The aim of Visible Therapy, therefore, is to problematise the assumption of categorical *identity* in order to make obvious the tactics of taking up particular and strategic *identifications*. This represents a concern with *doing*, rather than *being*, and is an argument for an epistemological concern with identificatory practices, rather than a search for ontological status or meaning. This, then, is therapy *as* epistemology.

A post-structuralist framework, therefore, allows us to challenge the unproblematic acceptance of any identity and a feminist standpoint enables us to recognise the need to privilege particular (marginalised) perspectives in some situations and on some occasions. Hence, given the cultural validation of professional expertise over everyday experience, it has been important, at times, to valorise women's rights to claim a shared identity and to speak for themselves (see also Plumb, 1993). However, from a post-structuralist perspective, this represents a political strategy, rather than an ontological reality: otherwise false and absolute dualisms continue to fictively (re)create and mobilise the division between 'experience' and 'expertise'; and clients and therapists.

The perspective adopted in this chapter, therefore, is informed by feminism, yet remains provisional. I situate my view from somewhere within marginalised perspectives, rather than within 'me' – my essentialised ontological state (as therapist, woman, and/or survivor, etc.). This is because 'speaking from experience' is not only theoretically problematic, but often acts to mute dissent. Hence, authority is located within realms of understanding rather than claims to location within socially valorised (or subjugated) categorical groups. Like Bola *et al.* (1998: 106) I do not accept that all that is needed is to state my 'social location in order to render it unproblematic: as if taking differences seriously simply means listing one's membership of broad social structural categories.' I do not want any identification that I can muster to afford me status that is unwarranted within the text of this chapter or, indeed, my therapy practice. Nor do I want my concern over women/sexual abuse to be rendered anodyne through representational practices which conflate concern with identity to personalise such concern as being 'my problem' (cf. Charles, 1992; Reavey, 1997). Rather, the value of the perspectives drawn on to develop Visible Therapy relates to their ability to promote critical reflection and to theorise a principled, yet provisional, approach to therapy. Thus, whether therapy occurs in any particular service context is a decision which must remain open (Warner, 2000b). As Kitzinger and Perkins (1993) argue, we should not only consider how therapy is conducted (the approach and perspective adopted), but also whether therapy should happen at all. The first step, then, is to interrogate the assumption that speaking out generally, and therapy specifically, is always a good thing, and, in this, integral to 'recovery' from child sexual abuse.

Deciding (not) to speak: child sexual abuse as a provisional and partial object of concern

The lure of the confessional (cf. Foucault, 1992), and the assumption of the cathartic effects of speaking, is written into the West's current infatuation with self-disclosure and child sexual abuse (Plummer, 1995). It has also been part of a feminist strategy for political action (Entwisle and Warner, 1989). The benefits of speaking (about child sexual abuse) are predicated on the assumption that silence equates with passivity (and ongoing abuse) and speaking out brings relief, provides a context for enlightenment, and thereby promotes change and emancipation. Yet silence is not always passive – this is evident when working with so-called 'elective mutes'. And women are not divested of their sexual abuse simply through verbal rehearsal. From a post-structuralist perspective sexual abuse is not something that can simply be added and then subtracted in order to reveal the essence of a pure and prediscursive woman underneath. Rather, sexual abuse is productive of feminine identity, not something that simply sits on top of that which already exists (Warner, 1996a).

Indeed, when therapists assume identity to be foundational rather than provisional, prescription replaces description and can act as the ground on which normative values are reinstalled. This is because therapy, as a humanist endeavour, individualises selfhood, which renders problems private and, in so doing, obscures their social production. When the social is veiled, the assumption of heterosexuality can then be reinstated, as the assumed, but unspecified goal of normative therapy. This is self-evident in those (traditional) approaches to therapy which privilege the need to trust and (sexually) reintegrate with men (see Jehu *et al.*, 1994) and which, therefore, can pathologise those women who exist outside of the hetero-sexual ideal. Moreover, humanist therapies are also saturated with Western ideals of personhood. Recovery from abuse, then, is a process of inculcation into a racialised sex/gender matrix which is achieved through 'technologies of the self' (Rose, 1990). As McNay argues, applying a Fou-cauldian analysis:

Under the illusion of leading to greater self-knowledge, the disclosure of one's inner self and unconscious desires leads to a more efficient regulation and normalisation of sexuality through the production of self-policing subjects. The confessing subject is both the instrument and effect of domination.

(1992: 87)

The fictive separation between personal and social serves to concretise 'recovered' women as self-disciplining subjects set in opposition to 'unre-covered' women – who are out there, dangerous and unpredictable. The recovered woman is 'open about her problems' and has 'insight'. This woman is no longer 'out of control'. 'Control', in this sense, refers to self-control, rather than ability to control the environment (Plumb, 1993). And personal change is valorised over political transformation (Plummer, 1995). Hence, a feminist conflation of political action with privatised per-sonal needs may be premature, as speaking does not always provide the grounds for emancipation. This is why it is crucial to understand identity as a social construal. To do otherwise is to obscure, and shore up, the gen-dered (re)production of normative femininity and dominant, and singular, versions of reality.

Hence, speaking is an identificatory practice that can engender increased regulation. It may also invoke more punitive responses, particu-larly for already marginalised social groups (Warner, 1996b, c, 2000d; Horn and Warner, 2000), for example, through denial, misrepresentation, and re-enactment (McFarlane, 1989). Moreover, poor and inadequately resourced mental health services reproduce neglect, and women continue to be physically and sexually assaulted within them (Daly, 1997). Speaking out may not, therefore, engender a positive or progressive response, and present practices may amplify the negative emotional sequelea of past experiences (cf. Sedgwick and Frank, 1995).

I argue, therefore, that the assumption that it is always beneficial to talk about abuse should be resisted. Women will have different levels of engagement with their abuse at different times and in different situations and relationships. Indeed, issues concerning present life experiences may be far more pressing than past concerns. Moreover, the implication that it is only through the special conversations that occur in therapy that women gain insight situates women as passive containers. According to such a model, women must pour out the 'badness-which-is-abuse' to be filled up with more beneficial messages provided by the therapist. This divests women of agency and obscures the interactive process of therapy and the multiple relationships women have with the narratives of their lives. It may also be that an emphasis on the productive capacities of therapy subjugates other, 'ordinary', relationships/friendships. Indeed, the assertion that people need friends, not therapists, has also been made by some feminist writers (cf. Kitzinger and Perkins, 1993). However, 'friendship' is an idealised term which requires problematisation as much as any other given relationship.

Nevertheless, it may be important to privilege sexual abuse by asking about it, as has been suggested by a number of authors (e.g. Brown and Anderson, 1991; Lobel, 1992; Palmer *et al.*, 1993). This situates women's distress in relation to the productive constraints of previous (and current) relationships, rather than simply unsituated mental pathology. However, we cannot simply ask *the* questions (as if there is one absolute set which will reveal all that is important), but clarify (and be prepared to explain) our purpose: be it voyeuristic, investigative, diagnostic and/or therapeutic. Thus, whilst sexual abuse represents an intelligible and readily imaginable object of therapeutic concern, it should not be raised as *the* object of concern. Otherwise, this provokes a drift towards diagnosis and specification, realised as dogmatic approaches to treatment.

It is not enough, then, that sexual abuse is asked after, but it is crucial to note who does the speaking, what form the questions take and what institutions and persons are privileged and subjugated through this process (cf. Foucault, 1990). Asking whether someone has been sexually abused invites that person to position herself *as* abused. It may be that women may not recognise themselves in such an identity (and all it seemingly implies), but would recognise themselves as having been hurt or manipulated. Hence, questions which imply absolute identities are less useful than questions which situate specific actions and relationships (Warner, 2000c). This means clarifying what it is about sexually abusive experiences that require articulation and examination and the means through which we manage this actualised concern. In order to clarify the therapeutic focus of concern regarding women and child sexual abuse, it is necessary to return to the original abuse.

Constructing negative versions of experience and identity: child sexual abuse, popular culture and normative prescription

From a post-structuralist perspective, identity is understood as a social practice realised in relationships, rather than as an internal and stable property of individuals. Hence, the experiences we have, and the ways in which we understand our experiences, give rise to particular forms of identity. At the same time our sense of self will shape how we understand the world and our experiences within it. Reality, therefore, is a function of the relationships between understanding, experience and identity (Warner, 2000c). Identity can be understood as a social performance (Butler, 1990) that is given the gloss of stability through reiteration. Child sexual abuse is one context in which negative versions of identity and experience are performed, produced and maintained. Explicating the embedded assumptions produced through abuse can enable women to work out how their own particular sense of self may have been shaped by such relationships.

Abusers set up particular versions of identity and experience that construct themselves as blameless, position children as guilty, and also dissuades others from asking questions and recognising harm. It is through the reitterability of these 'mind-fucks' that the 'body-fuck' is maintained and that (gendered) identity is stabilised. Hence, the focus in Visible Therapy is on the tactics of abuse, rather than the physical act itself. This is because it is the 'mind-fuck', rather than the 'body-fuck', which endures and continues to constitute women. The details that are important, then, are those that connect current feelings about self and others with the psychological tactics of abuse. Problems are not located within individuals – whether as children or adults. Rather, problems are located within the narratives that shape individuals' understandings of past and current relationships but which, through reiteration, obscure their own social production. Thus, as already noted, I am concerned not with who women 'really are' but with how selfhood is constructed through practices of both abuse and therapy. This, then, is about making the tactics of abuse and therapy visible.

The aim of Visible Therapy is to explore how women might invest in particular versions of their past abuse and present adulthood. The task is to contextualise women's identifications (as bad, guilty, etc.) in wider social discourses which enable a personal story to be explored in a situated way (Reavey and Warner, 1998). This requires detailing and exploring the range of psychological, structural and social silencing tactics that support sexually abusive behaviour and which are implicated in the regulation of individual life narratives. For example, Black women and white women have different cultural constraints operating through their multiple experiences of child sexual abuse. My aim is not to obscure the dynamic aspects of women's experiences and identifications, but to recognise the wider social narratives that frame these.

It is necessary, therefore, to look beyond the specific tactics of child sexual abuse to more general accounts of childhood, sex and gender that provide the narrative context in which children, and particularly female children, are interpellated as passive (yet guilty). A common cultural belief is that childhood is a distinct social state typified by innocence, dependence and immaturity. A differentiation is, therefore, effected between the agentic subject of adulthood and the (socially) incomplete, and therefore, objectified child (Lee, 1998). Children's assumed innocence and lack of agency renders them, de facto, unable to consent to sex. Any sexual experience must, therefore, be traumatic as sex is the route out of the 'Garden of Eden' (which is childhood) through knowledge into terrible awareness (which is adulthood). Yet children have complex and varying relationships around sex, and a blanket avowal that childhood necessarily precludes (agentic) consent may have the aim of protecting children, but ultimately fails. Innocence is a powerful narrative which serves as warrant to deny children information, which might offset (some) vulnerability (Dominelli, 1989).

Moreover, the assumption of innocence brings guilt into being. Not only is a differentiation instigated between so-called innocent and guilty victims but, through popular accounts of romantic love, (feminine) innocence and passivity are installed as always already corrupting. Drawing on the metaphor of 'Sleeping Beauty' all girls, like Sleeping Beauty, de facto, cannot consent because they are somnolent in their innocence. They, like her, can only be wakened by the violation of imposed sexualisation. Their innocence is destroyed and their maturation complete. But the innocence lost was always guilty. It was the beauty, not yet awakened, that enslaved the prince (abusers) and forced the kiss (abuse). Innocence is, therefore, always already corrupted by incipient (but unknowing) sexuality which precedes and dictates the subsequent violation. Such stories reify the notion of female passivity *and* culpability, whilst at the same time denying male responsibility: men simply act on invitation and instinct (Warner, 2000c). It is only when individual stories of guilt are socially situated that normative understandings of responsibility may be disrupted.

The limits of innocence: socially situating individual trajectories of responsibility

Narratives of guilt cleave to women through socially dislocated stories of sex and abuse. Women may be depicted as being both globally passive (unable to change), yet globally toxic (in the sense that they corrupt all they come into contact with). The aim of Visible Therapy is to disrupt the operations of power that, through repetition, immobilise such identifications as internalised personality structure or pathology. Visible Therapy, therefore, locates women's beliefs and feelings in terms of externalised tactics of abuse rather than viewing them as symptoms of internalised disorder. The aim is to enable women to understand how guilt is produced and maintained through the social practices of sex and abuse, and to challenge implicit humanist assumptions which individualise choice and autonomy in respect of these.

A tactic of Visible Therapy, therefore, is to actively inform women how children are silenced and produced as powerless, and how 'choice' is a loaded term that cannot be fully achieved. 'Choice' is no longer individualised but is situated within structural (social, economic and cultural) inequalities regarding, for example, abuse, poverty and discrimination (Pollack, 1997). As Pollack (ibid.) argues women (and children) may 'know' what they want but are marginalised through structural oppression and only the socially advantaged have ready access to 'self' determination. Moreover, the valorisation of 'personal choice' over communal values is dangerous for marginalised groups – isolating oneself does not create boundaries against harm; rather, connection does (ibid.). Indeed, isolation within families, from friends, relations and larger communities are the conditions in which abuse may be sustained.

When individualistic narratives of choice and responsibility in respect of past abuse are disrupted, normative therapeutic assumptions regarding present re-enactments may also be challenged. Normative psychological theories of human behaviour, such as cognitive and psychoanalytically derived ones, suggest that childhood experiences act as templates for future relationships (Briere, 1992) and that people recreate past (unresolved) relationships in adulthood. The construction of the compulsion to repeat past experiences is internalised, through the fictions of 'faulty cognitions' or 'unconscious desires' (e.g. Clarke and Llewelyn, 1994). Whilst 'the mind' and 'the unconscious' may be useful metaphors in which to narrativise relationship histories and expectations, they become regulatory when their own cultural production and productive capacities are denied. When 'the social' is separated from 'the personal' the unconscious/mind can then be deployed to account for the propulsion of women into abusive relationships. Such narratives over-determine women's active participation in the re-enactment of abuse and hence, obscure the role of abusers who may target vulnerable women (Warner, 1997).

However, whilst narratives of guilt should be interrogated, it is not enough for therapists simply to say, 'It was not your fault'. Such statements deny agency and seldom accord with women's feelings and beliefs. 'Guilt' is a productive fiction that cannot simply be installed by nefarious abusers and removed by benevolent therapists. Not only does this situate women as empty vessels, it also paradoxically confirms their 'badness' by positioning them as 'wrong'. Women remain guilty – for getting it wrong and, worse than that, resisting their therapists' attempts to enlighten them. Such interventions invite women to remain passive or to risk condemnation. So, as Deleuze and Guattari ask: 'How can we ward off, in the practice of the cure, this abject desire that makes us bend our knees, lays us on the couch, and makes us remain there?' (1984: 65).

The aim should be to socially locate and explore these multiple narratives of guilt and responsibility and to resist the desire to provide singular and unsituated truths. There are 'good' reasons why children feel guilty and why such feelings are resistant to mediation. In order to make sense of women's residual feelings, and to challenge the reproduction of these in therapy relationships, we need to understand, and make visible, the tactics of abuse. For example, we might say, 'I do not think children (or women) choose to be abused, but I do know children (and women) often feel guilty because guilty feelings ensure children do not tell (and women do not leave).' The aim is to enable women to make specific connections between their beliefs and feelings and the tactics utilised to ensure their particular silence and acquiescence within both past and present abusive relationships. Detailing and exploring the contradictions within these personal, yet widely available, (gendered) narratives of responsibility diffuses the reitterability of the 'mind-fuck' through situating its operations.

Verbalising and examining such narratives is one way of disrupting negative versions of identity. The negative effects of past relationships may also be addressed without making any direct reference to the abuse. Rather, therapy relationships which are rooted in negotiation offer a lived experience of relating which is not predicated on someone being *the* victim and someone being *the* abuser, or indeed *the* rescuer (cf. Carr, 1989). However, it may still be necessary to problematise and explicate our practices. Good therapists and effective abusers draw on the same skills to encourage children (and adults) to trust them (Warner, 2000b). Hence, we should be mindful that apparently benevolent behaviour on the part of the therapist may be read by the client as a prelude to abuse. As such, it is also important to explicate not simply the content of therapeutic intervention, but the (psychological) processes invoked in that intervention.

Socially situating trust and honesty: rethinking the 'quality' of relationship between therapist and client

The ultimate active ingredient in a therapeutic outcome is often storied as an unsituated and unspecified 'quality' of the relationship. Whilst 'quality' remains a slippery term, it is frequently operationalised in terms of trust. Trust is seen as the central plank on which therapeutic alliances are built and from which therapeutic change is instigated. Hence, it is often asserted that women need to find someone they can trust to talk to. As such, trust is naturalised as the grounds on which therapy proceeds, rather than trust being understood as an (unstable) effect of the therapeutic encounter. By implication honesty is presumed to be the context in which trusting relationships develop. It may be self-evident that relationships built on trust and honesty are better than relationships built on mistrust and deceit. Indeed, betrayal of trust is viewed as a central mechanism for the negative effects of abuse (Warner, 1999b). Yet, from a post-structuralist perspective neither trust nor honesty are absolute once and for all achievements, but are relative social practices. This understanding disrupts the conventional ways in which narratives of trust and honesty regulate the therapeutic relationship and the focus of therapeutic concern.

Under modernism, in order for therapy (whether behavioural, cognitive or psychodynamic) to be effective, clients are required to provide honest and truthful accounts of their experiences of past abuse and present lives. This is so therapeutic interventions can be targeted at the 'real' issues that disable clients. A post-structuralist approach, however, problematises the assumption that it is ever possible to produce a final and ultimately truthful account of experience. From a post-structuralist perspective, making links between the past and the present is always about integrating two current fictions: past acts can only ever be constituted through current concerns. Conversely, when 'the past' is understood to be stable, the disclosure of accurate and detailed descriptions of the abuse experience is centralised within the therapeutic encounter. Memory, or specifically the limits of this active (and therefore suspicious) process becomes another narrative in which to position women as untrustworthy themselves (e.g. Bagley, 1995). Women are guilty, unable as they are to simply reflect the past; they must always (and wilfully?) construct it. 'Recovered' memories (and their opposition, 'false' memories) then become something to be fought over (Haaken, 1998; Warner, 1999a) and belief becomes an undifferentiated move of all acceptance or non-acceptance. From this perspective, the partial objects that constitute identity are conflated to represent the whole. It can then feel invidious for progressive therapists to query any part of women's stories, as this becomes synonymous with attacking the authenticity of that (whole) person. Conversely, when honesty and trust are situated, then 'belief' becomes a multiplicity of narratives that one may, at times, remain agnostic over.

This is also the case for clients who are no longer simply expected to 'trust' their therapists, as trust is local and contingent. Therefore, therapists should be prepared to make that which can be trusted operant (i.e. explicit and actualised). Such 'things' may include time, location and the physical boundaries around therapy. More than this, therapists should be able to explain how they make sense of what they do and why, in order to enable clients to engage critically with their therapists' therapeutic narratives. This is therapy 'long-handed' where the process is described alongside the content and can be understood as 'situated honesty'. The tactics of therapy are made visible, in contrast to the tactics of abuse which are hidden. Therapists may then share with clients epistemological, rather than ontological narratives of (them) selves. So women may 'know me' from how I make sense of, and describe the world, rather than through self-disclosure of personal experience. As argued, there is no direct access to 'experience' and it is the ways in which personal experiences are socially regulated that is of concern in Visible Therapy.

When honesty and trustworthiness are internalised as personal characteristics, then the ability *to* trust also becomes a property of individuals. This ability to trust is often depicted as being negatively effected by betrayal. Hence, learning to trust others (usually men) can become a main goal of therapy regarding child sexual abuse. However, this is a spurious goal (Dominelli, 1989) when we can only ever 'trust' local and specific things. Yet, women who 'cannot trust' may be condemned and met with 'therapeutic pessimism'. And women who trust too readily may also be viewed with concern. Trust which is partial and specific is all and the best that can be hoped for, aligned with a healthy, and partial, scepticism. Women's challenge is to trust themselves to make sense of that which they feel able to rely on. Women should be validated for meeting some situations with suspicion and taking active measures to protect themselves. Yet, when absolute judgements are made regarding the way women feel and the things that women do, women's strategies of self-protection and survival are frequently undermined. The negative versions of identity foundationalised in past abusive relationships are then reinforced through successive interventions. It is crucial, therefore, to reconsider how we theorise women's means of survival.

Deliberate self-preservation: using coping strategies to make sense of past and present concerns

When children are abused they must find ways of surviving not simply the physical act of abuse, but the continual emotional assaults on their sense of self. If people respond negatively to the ways children survive they further invalidate who those children are. When women's survival strategies are pathologised as being inherently self-destructive, women's actual attempts at self-preservation are discredited and their need to utilise such strategies is paradoxically reinforced. Yet 'risk' is located within individuals rather than the relationships, both past and present, that give rise to such behaviour. Indeed, such strategies may be as indicative of current (therapeutic) relationships as they are of past (deliberately abusive) ones. As such, rather than simply attempt to stop women doing what they do (which paradoxically re-enacts the conditions of constraint in which such actions arise) we should enable women to make specific connections around their actions and emotions (cf. Waller, 1996). Hence, we must ask questions and make links regarding not just *what* women survive but *how* they survive. By attending to these strategies we invoke agentic subjects who can actively participate in their own lives.

The three D's (denial, distraction and dissociation) and 'deliberate' self-harm (including self injury, drug and alcohol use, over-eating and starvation) are common methods of coping with the extremely difficult feelings of powerlessness, guilt and anger often associated with experiences of child sexual abuse (Warner, 1998, 2000b, c). Because of widely available cultural representations of feminine passivity, women may be particularly primed to turn their hurt and anger inwards and self-harm. Traditional readings of dissociation and self-harm, however, fail to recognise them as meaningful coping strategies, located within social structural space. Rather, dissociation and self-harm are often perceived as disembodied symptoms of an underlying personality disorder or mental illness. By bracketing out such behaviour as mental disorder its social production is erased. In such a frame the 'effects' of abuse constitute all that women *do*, as being all that women *are*, and ever can be.

Collapsing different strategies of coping into extant and separable disorders prevents a useful therapeutic engagement with such strategies. The feelings that underlie such strategies may also be ignored, as engagement stops as diagnosis begins. Women's legitimate anger, hurt and ambivalence may then be translated into, for example, a decontextualised notion of 'emotional lability' which reiterates precisely those aspects of femininity which foundationalise gender in the first place. Such gendered discourses may then be used as the unacknowledged referents in the construction of psychiatric classifications. Such labelling further confirms women as essentially wrong or flawed and thus compromises appropriate therapeutic action. This has led Hamilton to conclude: 'It is probable that women with a history of childhood sexual abuse are both overserved (handicapped by an inappropriate label) and underserved by mental health delivery systems' (1993: 157).

Yet such feelings and actions are not incomprehensible symptoms of mental illness, but rather meaningful coping strategies (Romme, 1998) located in social space. When such 'symptoms' are understood as meaningful, then women may be helped to understand their 'symptoms' not in terms of evocations of madness, but in terms of comprehensible strategies of survival. For example, when dissociation is understood as a strategy of survival during abuse, it can be used to explain the non-formation of detailed memories later. This provides a relevant site for intervention – not to 'recover' memories but to account for why some memories will remain 'lost'/incomplete. Women may have a limited narrative for detailing the ways in which their early experiences and sense of self have been structured. Their coping strategies can act as an 'intermediary language' (LeFevre, 1996) that connects past and present versions of self. When professionals try to stop self-harm or refuse to engage with people's voices they deny this intermediary language which can delay the progression to finding different versions of self and experience.

The key issue is to stop placing absolute values on women's feelings and actions, and remain open to exploring the range of meanings they might have. Self-harm and dissociation are neither *the* solution nor *the* problem. At times they may be both. Both provide solutions to the problem of limited choices (Warner, 2000c). From a post-structuralist perspective such strategies are given meaning through situating their operations. Suicide is seldom the goal or effect of 'deliberate' self-harm and, in this sense, self-*harm* may be a misnomer. Deliberate self-preservation should be validated. This does not preclude my right to remain concerned about the methods women sometimes use. I also remain mindful that individual coping strategies are regulated within social structural space and that issues such as race, class, culture, gender and ability can also constrain the options and salience of particular strategies. For example, women's use of alcohol, as a coping strategy, has increased in Britain since women's use of alcohol, socially, has become more acceptable. Also, in response to sexually abusive experiences, women may disfigure their bodies in multiple ways, for example, through excessive cleaning rituals. However, because of wide-spread racism, Black women have additional invitations to view their skin and bodies as being pathological and, hence, Black women may be more likely to scrape off their skin and/or use bleach on their bodies than are white women.

Whilst women may have developed their strategies in isolation it is important, therefore, to socially locate our understanding of this, as no coping strategy is universal but is socially specific. For example, 'dissociation' is a specifically modernist project. In order to be able to dissociate and split parts off (for example, hear voices) there has to be a sedimented social understanding of the humanist subject. If there is no 'I' there can be no 'other' (cf. Boyle, 1990); concomitantly without the 'individual' there can be no 'psy-complex' (Rose, 1990). It is unsurprising, therefore, that the growth of self-regulatory technologies of government within Western societies and the attendant elevation of psy-experts is paralleled in the twentieth century' obsession with pathologising (and diagnosing as variously dementia praecox, schizophrenia, psychosis, borderline personality disorder, etc.) those behaviours which directly problematise the humanist subject. Dissociation can only function, therefore, as a coping strategy within societies that rely on a humanist reading of selfhood. Hence, coping strategies are more usefully understood as socially located practices rather than ontological narratives of disorder and distress.

Whilst it is crucial to engage with the multiple ways in which women survive their lives, it is necessary to resist the desire to over-determine survival as a primary construct of identity. When identity is collapsed around *being* a survivor (or a victim) other identifications are necessarily subjugated and, whether survivor or victim, such women are defined primarily by that which hurts them (Kitzinger and Perkins, 1993). Moreover, narratives of survival (or victimhood) are often sedimented within predefined symptomatologies which are imbued with unacknowledged assumptions regarding the normative limits of femininity (Warner, 1996a; O'Dell, 1997). Women may recognise themselves in such abuse check-lists because such lists become part of what we know (rather than what we propose) to be the effects of child sexual abuse, and hence function as 'the real'. From a post-structuralist perspective any identificatory reduction is unhelpful, particularly those which privatise hurt. Yet from a feminist perspective there may still be an argument for locating women within a narrative of survival because survival invokes agency. However, it is crucial to situate behaviour as what is indicative of survival or victimhood, and the values we place on these, are unstable. Moreover, once the productive capacity of these discourses is made visible, women can then make a more deliberate engagement with both survival and victimhood. And when we engage with identity as a social practice, we can promote competing versions of reality which provide the context in which multiple understandings of behaviour and more positive versions of self may emerge and be sustained.

Supporting therapists: situated strategies for training and supervision

Therapists, like their clients, have multiple and provisional identities that are stabilised through reiteration. At different times identifications made by therapists and clients may converge or diverge and these should be examined, rather than simply assumed. For example, the assumption of similarity between therapist and client sharing the identification of 'woman' can act to obscure power differences in the therapeutic relationship and, hence, militate against this reflexivity. This may be one time when otherness provokes a healthy reaction. Conversely, when therapists view their clients as so different from themselves they may feel unable to engage, unable to understand and, hence, unable to take responsibility for the interventions they make. The trauma that surrounds abuse may, then, be compounded by the contributory effects of the client's, and the therapist's, life narratives clashing and melding.

What, then, do therapists do with the trauma they may bring from their own lives and which they experience in therapy relationships? Sexual abuse confounds efficacy and fractures good relationships. Hence, the mutual dance of therapy is about warding off those feelings that confirm therapists', as well as clients', sense of incompetence. It is no wonder that the lure of containment through diagnosis and categorisation is so strong or that strategies of dissociation may be utilised by mental health workers as well. The institutionalisation of such coping strategies can lead to inter-professional conflicts and punitive interventions including sectioning, med-icating, scapegoating and avoidance of change (Davenport, 1997). When this happens, therapy may not function at all.

Hence, clear boundaries around therapy relationships are not simply for the benefit of clients but are also there to protect therapists' sense of self. Therapists require a permanent space for reflection that permits them to explore the benefits, to themselves and their clients, of taking up their own particular and strategic identifications within therapy relationships. If this reflexivity is not entered into, then therapists themselves will act without understanding to protect their own fragile fictions of self. And whilst women may well have survived worse, they will nevertheless con-tinue to be victimised. One aim of training and supervision within Visible Therapy, therefore, is to enable therapists to develop strategies for ques-tioning their, and their service's, contributory relationships with their clients' distress and the maintenance of behaviour they ostensibly wish to change.

Training and supervision, conceived within a feminist post-structuralist framework, does not pathologise therapists, any more than therapy, con-ceived within a feminist post-structuralist framework, pathologises clients. From this perspective, the beliefs and understandings that individual ther-apists hold are socially and temporally situated. As such, therapists are no longer positioned as being beyond change and development. Socially situ-ating therapists' understandings as discursive practices promotes change because changing one's understanding no longer equates with rejecting one's whole being. Moreover, because absolute versions of identity are rejected, then 'expert' as a category is also fractured. This means that ther-apists can engage with training and supervision without necessarily writing themselves into a story of absolute ineptitude and naïvety. Additionally, a post-structuralist approach would (as some forms of psychotherapy) also accord equal status to process as well as content issues. This means that, just as identity is no longer understood to be set in concrete, neither are treatment strategies. The narrative framework of Visible Therapy pro-vides a critical means of deconstructing objects of therapeutic concern, whilst admitting the value of situated knowledges which actively construct those same objects. Training, therefore, is not about defining pre-determined approaches, but about promoting a reflexive climate that pro-vides a framework for questioning dominant versions of reality through engaging with marginalised perspectives. Marginality is not only located within structural difference but with respect to subjugated ways of under-standing and speaking about that understanding. This is about changing our concern (cf. Henriques *et al.*, 1984) from exploring individual narratives of expertise and/or pathology to addressing the ways in which such narratives sustain particular formations of relationship between therapist and client.

Provisional reflections on Visible Therapy

My aim in this chapter has been to demonstrate the potential for non-foundationalist feminist politics to transform mental health practices, specifically in respect of women and child sexual abuse. My objective was to develop a practical and accessible framework for reconstructing thera-peutic interventions through making the tactics and practices of abuse and therapy visible. Problems regarding child sexual abuse are no longer located within individuals as individual pathology. Indeed, behaviour is no longer conflated with identity. Rather 'problems' are located within wider social narratives which situate personal relationships, both past and present, that give rise to notions of fixed identity. The aim was to demon-strate how Westernised notions of 'the self' are secured through the obfus-cation of the structuring effects of social reiteration. The reorientation of 'the problem' of sexual abuse as socially constituted and constitutive of gendered and Westernised formations of identity provides a means through which the maintenance of women *as* (inherently) pathological could be challenged. Such an approach provides the grounds for progres-sive practice because it militates against the instillation of naturalised sub-jects and, hence, absolute and invariant trajectories of recovery. Reorienting the problem of child sexual abuse in this way provides a way of developing more progressive research, training and therapy practices through enabling a more fully social engagement with personal narratives of child sexual abuse. The challenge is to maintain a permanent space in which relationships (both past and present) are continually reassessed and articulated.

Visible Therapy aims to disrupt identity so that narratives of women's pasts no longer foreclose their futures and more positive versions of reality can be imagined and sustained.

Acknowledgements

I thank the many women and children who have shared their stories of sexual abuse with me. I also thank the research department at Ashworth Hospital for supporting the research out of which this chapter (partly) arose.

Note

1 This chapter is a revised version of an article that first appeared in *Feminist Review* 68: 115–139, 2001.

References

Bagley, C. (1995) 'A typology of child sexual abuse: addressing the paradox of interlocking emotional, physical and sexual abuse as causes of adult psychiatric sequels in women', Paper given to Annual Conference of the Canadian Sex Research Forum, Banff, October.

Banister, P., Burman, E., Parker, I. and Tindall, C. (1994) *Qualitative methods in psychology*, Milton Keynes: Open University Press.

Benhabib, S. (1995) 'Feminism and postmodernism', S. Benhabib, J. Butler, D. Cornell and N. Fraser (eds) *Feminist contentions: a philosophical exchange*, London: Routledge, pp. 17–34.

Bola, M., Drew, C., Gill, R., Harding, S., King, E. and Seu, B. (1998) 'I. Representing ourselves and representing others: a response', *Feminism and Psychology* 8, 1: 105–110.

Boyle, M. (1990) *Schizophrenia: a scientific delusion?* London: Routledge.

Briere, J.N. (1992) *Child abuse trauma: theory and treatment of the lasting effects*, London: Sage.

Brown, G.R. and Anderson, B. (1991) 'Psychiatric morbidity in adult inpatients with childhood histories of sexual and physical abuse', *American Journal of Psychiatry* 148, 1: 55–61.

Butler, J. (1990) *Gender trouble: feminism and the subversion of identity*, London: Routledge.

Butler, J. (1993) *Bodies that matter: on the discursive limits of 'sex'*, London: Routledge.

Carr, A. (1989) 'Countertransference to families where child abuse has occurred', *Journal of Family Therapy* 11: 87–97.

Charles, H. (1992) 'Whiteness – the relevance of politically colouring the 'Non', in H. Hinds, A. Phoenix and J. Stacey (eds) *Working out: new directions for women's studies*, London: The Falmer Press, pp. 29–35.

Clark, S. and Llewelyn, S. (1994) 'Personal constructs of survivors of childhood sexual abuse receiving cognitive analytic therapy', *British Journal of Medical Psychology* 67: 273–289.

Daly, M. (1997) 'Therapy or punishment?', *The Big Issue in the North*, December 15–28: 6–7.

Davenport, S. (1997) 'The interaction of the dynamics of abuse in in-patient (institutional) settings', *Group Analysis North, Monday Seminar Programme*, May 19: notes, unpublished.

Deleuze, G. and Guattari, F. (1984) *Anti-Oedipus: capitalism and schizophrenia*, London: The Athlone Press Limited.

Dominelli, L. (1989) 'Betrayal of trust: a feminist analysis of power relationships in incest abuse and its relevance for social work practice', *British Journal of Social Work* 19: 291–307.

Entwisle, J. and Warner, S.J. (1989) *Taboo – Manchester support group for survivors of child sexual abuse: information sheet*, Manchester: Taboo.

Epston, D. (1993) 'Internalizing discourses versus externalizing discourses', in S. Gilligan and R. Price (eds) *Therapeutic conversations*, New York: W.W. Norton, pp. 161–180.

Farganis, S. (1994) *Situating feminism: from thought to action*, London: Sage Publications.

Foucault, M. (1990) *The history of sexuality, vol. one: an introduction*, Middlesex: Penguin.

Foucault, M. (1992) *Madness and civilisation: a history of insanity in the age of reason*, London: Routledge.

Frosh, S. (1995) 'Postmodernism and psychotherapy', *Journal of Family Therapy* 17, 2: 175–190.

Grosz, E. (1995) *Space, time, and perversion*, London: Routledge.

Haaken, J. (1998) *Pillar of salt: gender, memory and the perils of looking back*, London: Free Association Press.

Hamilton, G.J. (1993) 'Further labelling within the category of disability due to chemical dependency: borderline personality disorder', in M.E. Willmuth and L. Holcomb (eds) *Women with disabilities: found voices*, Tennessee: The Haworth Press, Inc, pp. 153–157.

Haraway, D. (1991) *Simians, cyborgs, and women: the reinvention of nature*, New York: Routledge.

Harding, S. (1993) 'Rethinking standpoint epistemology: what is "strong objectivity"?', in L. Alcoll and E. Potter (eds) *Feminist epistemologies*, London: Routledge, pp. 49–82.

Hartsock, N. (1983) 'The feminist standpoint: developing the ground for a specifically feminist historical materialism', in S. Harding and M. Hintikka (eds) *Discovering reality: feminist perspectives on epistemology, metaphysics, methodology, and philosophy of science*, Dordrecht: Reidel, pp. 283–310.

Hartsock, N. (1990) 'Foucault on power: a theory for women?', L. Nicholson (ed.) *Feminism/postmodernism*, London: Routledge, pp. 157–175.

Henriques, J., Hollway, W., Urwin, C., Venn, C. and Walkerdine, V. (1984) *Changing the subject: psychology, social regulation and subjectivity*, London: Methuen.

Horn, R. and Warner, S. (eds) (2000) *Positive directions for women in secure environments: issues in criminological and legal psychology*, Leicester: BPS.

Jackson, S. (1992) 'The amazing deconstructing woman', *Trouble and Strife: The Radical Feminist Magazine* 25: 25–31.

Jehu, D., Gazan, M. and Klassen, C. (1994) *Beyond sexual abuse: therapy with women who were childhood victims*, Chichester: John Wiley and Sons.

Kitzinger, C. and Perkins, R. (1993) *Changing our minds: lesbian feminism and psychology*, London: Onlywomen Press Limited.

Larner, G. (1995) 'The real as illusion: deconstructing power in family therapy', *Journal of Family Therapy* 17, 2: 191–217.

Lee, N. (1998) 'Towards an immature sociology', *The Sociological Review* 46(3): 458–482.

Lefevre, S.J. (1996) *Killing me softly: self harm. Survival not suicide*, Gloucester: Handsell.

Lobel, C. (1992) 'Relationship between childhood sexual abuse and borderline personality disorder in women psychiatric patients', *Journal of Child Sexual Abuse* 1, 1: 75–81.

McFarlane, A.C. (1989) 'The treatment of post-traumatic stress disorder', *British Journal of Medical Psychology* 62: 81–90.

McNay, L. (1992) *Foucault and feminism*, Cambridge: Polity Press.

O'Dell, L. (1997) 'IV. Child sexual abuse and the academic construction of symptomatologies', *Feminism and Psychology* 7, 3: 334–339.

Palmer, R.L., Coleman, L., Chaloner, D., Oppenheimer, R. and Smith, J. (1993) 'Childhood sexual experiences with adults: a comparison of reports by women psychiatric patients and general-practice attenders', *British Journal of Psychiatry* 163: 499–504.

Parker, I. (1992) *Discourse dynamics: critical analysis for social and individual psychology*, London: Routledge.

Plumb, A. (1993) 'The challenge of self-advocacy', *Feminism and Psychology* 3, 2: 169–187.

Plummer, K. (1995) *Telling sexual stories: power, change and social worlds*, London: Routledge.

Pollack, S. (1997) 'The social construction of the female offender: issues of choice, agency and responsibility', Paper presented at Parables of Possibility: An Interdisciplinary Women's Studies Symposium, Toronto, May.

Reavey, P. (1997) 'What do you do for a living then? The political ramifications of research interests within everyday interpersonal contexts', *Feminism and Psychology* 7, 4: 553–559.

Reavey, P. and Warner, S.J. (1998) 'Curing women: child sexual abuse, therapy, embodiment and femininity', Paper presented at The Women and Psychology Conference, Birmingham: July.

Reavey, P. and Warner, S.J. (2001) 'Curing women: child sexual abuse, therapy, and the construction of femininity', *International Journal of Critical Psychology: Special Issue on Sex and Sexualities* 3: 49–71.

Romme, M.A.J. (1998) *Understanding voices: coping with auditory hallucinations and confusing realities*, Cheshire: Handsell Publications.

Rose, N. (1990) 'Psychology as a "social" science', in I. Parker and J. Shotter (eds) *Deconstructing social psychology*, London: Routledge, pp. 103–116.

Sedgwick, E.K. and Frank, A. (1995) 'Shame in the cybernetic fold: reading Silvan Tomkins', *Critical Inquiry* 21: 496–523.

Spivak, G.C. (1993) 'Can the subaltern speak?' in P. Williams and L. Chrisman (eds) *Colonial discourse and post-colonial theory*, London: Harvester Wheatsheaf, pp. 66–111.

Waller, G. (1996) 'Sexual abuse and the eating disorders: understanding the psychological mediators', *Clinical Psychology Forum* 92: 27–32.

Warner, S. (1996a) 'Constructing femininity: models of child sexual abuse and the production of "woman"', in E. Burman, P. Alldred, C. Bewley, *et al.* (eds) *Challenging women: psychology's exclusions, feminist possibilities*, Buckingham: Open University Press, pp. 36–53.

Warner, S. (1996b) 'Special women, special places: women and high security mental hospitals', in E. Burman, G. Aitken, P. Alldred, *et al.* (eds) *Psychology, discourse, practice: from regulation to resistance*, London: Taylor and Francis, pp. 96–113.

Warner, S. (1996c) 'Visibly special? Women, child sexual abuse and Special Hospitals', in C. Hemingway (ed.) *Special women? The experience of women in the Special Hospital system*, Hants: Avebury, pp. 59–76.

Warner, S. (1997) 'Review article on "Childhood sexual abuse and the construction of identity: healing Sylvia" by Michelle Davies; "No right way: the voices of mothers of incest survivors" by Tracy Orriava; "Beyond blame: child abuse tragedies revisited" by Peter Reder, Sylvia Duncan and Moira Gray', *Feminism and Psychology* 7, 3: 377–383.

Warner, S. (1998) 'Emotional aspects of sexual abuse', in A. Garden (ed.) *Paediatric and adolescent gynaecology*, London: Edward Arnold, pp. 66–377.

Warner, S. (1999a) 'Reviews: *Making monsters: false memories and sexual hysteria*', R. Ofshe and E. Watters, *Psychoanalytic Studies* 1, 2: 248–249.

Warner, S. (1999b) *Special stories: women patients, high security mental hospitals and child sexual abuse*, Manchester: unpublished PhD thesis.

Warner, S. (2000a) 'Feminist theory, the Women's Liberation Movement and therapy for women: changing our concerns', *Changes: An International Journal of Psychology and Psychotherapy* 18, 4: 232–243.

Warner, S. (2000b) 'Child sexual abuse: tactics for survival – identifying issues which contribute to good practice', *Clinical Psychology Forum* 139: 6–10.

Warner, S. (2000c) *Understanding child sexual abuse: making the tactics visible*, Gloucester: Handsell Publishing.

Warner, S. (2000d) 'The cost of containment: women, high security mental hospitals and child sexual abuse', *Forensic Update* 62: 5–9.

Weissen, N. (1993) 'Power, resistance and science: a call for a revitalised feminist psychology', *Feminism and Psychology* 3, 2: 239–245.

White, M. and Epston, D. (1990) *Narrative means to therapeutic ends*, London: Norton Books.

Index

Aboriginal people 27–8, 89
abuse: *see* child abuse; child sexual
    abuse
abuse recovery movement 88
Accident Compensation Act 188
Accident Compensation Corporation
    188–92, 206n6, 206n8; assessments
    189–92; criteria 201; examples of
    reports 192–4; referral 190–2
advocacy 11, 190, 195, 196
Africa: child sexual abuse 57–64;
    patriarchy 69; refugees 82, 83; women
    9; *see also* individual countries
ageing process 47
aggression 56, 80, 81, 161; *see also*
    violence
aid organisations 45
AIDS activism 29n2; *see also*
    HIV/AIDS
Alcoff, L. 150, 195, 199, 221
alcohol 240
Alderson, M. 21
Althusser, L. 198
American Psychiatric Association
    172
anger 80
Antigone figure 121, 127n11
anti-political correctness 19
anti-pornography 18, 21
anti-poverty measures 89
apartheid 60, 61, 62
Armstrong, Louise 95, 134, 144, 150
Armstrong, Stephen 45
Asian culture 143
Association of Chief Officers of
    Probation 110
Association of Chief Police Officers
    110

Atmore, Chris 7, 15, 18, 20, 26–7
Australia: Aboriginal people 27–8, 89;
    feminism 7; media coverage of
    feminism 21–3; and New Zealand 16,
    24
Australian Magazine, The 23

babies, protection of 44
Badgley Report 64
Barnardos 45–6
Bass, E. 151, 154, 213, 217
BBC: *Newsnight* 96; *Strange Days* 99,
    101
Beck, Ulrich 112
Becker, D. 170, 174, 175
Bell, Vikki 9, 134
Bennett, T. W. 59–60
betrayal 65, 85
bio-politics 108
black men 61, 88
black women: and black men 88;
    feminism 9, 17, 28; hardship/abuse
    87–8; reparation 79; self-harm 240
blame 46, 87–8, 178–9, 188, 205, 214
Blume, E. 151
Boateng, Paul 115, 118
body-fucks 233
body language 155
Bola, M. 230
borderline personality disorder: child
    sexual abuse 11, 168, 172–5, 182;
    definitions 182; diagnosis 167–8,
    178–9, 182–3; femininity 176–7, 181;
    medicalisation 168; responsibility
    179; self worth 181; stories 173;
    trauma 173–4
Bordo, Susan 20, 22
Boyle, M. 240

boys 58
Briere, John 197–8, 235
British False Memory Society:
daughters of member 103–4; media
96; power relations 95, 96; psychiatric
terminology 97–8; scientific advisory
board 98–9; strategies 97–9
British Heart Foundation 48
British Psychological Society 136
Brown, Wendy 198
Bruner, Jerome 70
Bulger, Jamie 38
Burman, Erica 7–8, 37, 38, 39, 42, 66,
144
Butler, Judith: Antigone figure 127n11;
discourse/body 198–9;
heterosexuality 141, 157; identity 233;
interpellation 205; political action 5;
psychopathy 177; surviving 222

Canada 63–4, 64, 89
Cape Town 60–1
Carroll, Sue 127n9
Champagne, Rosaria 218
Chesler, P. 97
child abuse, women perpetrators 83
child development 7, 43, 48–9;
emotional 137; hierarchy 37, 136; loss
137–8; social construction 132
child labour 47
child sexual abuse 55, 65, 212; Africa
57–64; borderline personality
disorder 11, 168, 172–5, 182; cultural
factors 57, 70, 143; discourse 69–72;
effects 4–5, 10–11, 64–7, 66, 138–9,
140, 213; family 58, 71, 81–2;
feminism 2, 3, 6, 54, 67, 126, 140, 145,
227–8; feminist post-structuralism
222; gender 39–40, 142; Germany 55;
harm story 131–2, 139, 143–4; identity
46, 230, 233; media 9, 100; memory
41–2, 67, 78; prevalence 41–2, 53,
54–6, 64–7, 123; radical feminism 19;
resistance 69, 232; South Africa 6,
52–4, 58–9; stigma 65, 67, 70; stories
34–6, 90, 135, 150, 180; trauma 53–4,
55–6, 167, 241–2; USA 55; victims
120, 140; see also false memory
syndrome; sexually-abused children;
survivors
child sexual offenders: media coverage
109–10; post-release 117;
rehabilitation 127n6; reoffending risk
127n5; see also perpetrators
child soldiers centre 82
childhood 36–9, 46; and children 7–8;
crisis 41–2; development 136;
innocence 1–2, 48, 204; institutions
35; marginalisation 41; naturalness 7,
41, 42, 44–5; originary state 43;
otherness 37; responsibilities 38–9;
social construction 38–9, 136; stories
34–6; subjectivity 36, 40;
textualisation 37; Western society 53,
66
children: childhood 7–8; as developing
subjects 42; gendered 39–40; labour
47; moral guarantors 48; Paulsgrove
estate 117, 121; rights 43–4, 52–4, 64;
sexuality 49n1, 65, 71; silencing of
235; social constructions 46;
socialisation 66; vulnerability 41; and
women 57; see also boys; girls;
sexually-abused children
Children Act 134–5
Chodorow, Nancy 85
Choi, P. 150
choice/sexuality 153–5, 157–60, 162–3,
235
Christianity 77, 86, 90
civil war 82
Clarfield, L. E. 183
clients/therapists 150, 236–8, 242
clinical psychology 150, 189–90, 195–8
Comaskey, Brenda 89
compensation claims 187, 188–92, 197
Condor, S. 211
confessional mode 219, 230
conflicts of interest 48–9
consciousness-raising groups 77–8
consent 234
contextualisation 138, 151
control/sexuality 161–2
coping mechanisms: diagnosis 174;
homosexuality 141;
institutionalisation 242; intermediary
language 240; psychotherapy 239;
self-preservation 238–41; survivors
180, 198
Coward, Ros 120
credibility 101–2
Crenshaw, Kemberlé 17, 25, 26
criminal justice system 53
critical psychology 187–8, 203–5

critical reflection 230
critical social science 132–3
cross-cultural studies 57, 70, 71–2
cultural constructions: family sexuality
    63; femininity 85; race 233–4; and
    religion 142–3; ritual 89; subjectivity
    149; textual analysis 142; transformed
    94–5; Western imperialism 8, 69
customary law, South Africa 59, 60

Daily Mail 99
Daily Telegraph 96, 101
Daly, M. 231
Davenport, S. 242
Davies, Barbara 117
Davis, L. 151, 154, 213, 217
Deleuze, Gilles 227, 236
DeMause, L. 55
Democratic Psychiatry 39
denial 143, 239
descriptions/explanations 149
desire 78
development: childhood 136; discourse
    132, 135; harm story 136–8;
    modernity 42; state welfare 42
deviance 66, 141
diagnosis: borderline personality
    disorder 167–8, 178–9, 182–3; coping
    mechanisms 174; medicalisation
    168–72
discourse: Butler 198–9; child sexual
    abuse 69–72; critical social science
    132–3; development 132, 135;
    Foucault 66; gendered 95, 239;
    psychology 199; reality 37; survivors
    221
discourse analysis 72, 151
discrimination 198
disease 57
dispute resolution 87
dissociation 239, 240
distraction 239
domestic violence centre 29
domesticity cult 86
Dominelli, L. 140, 234, 238
Donzelot, Jacques 112, 126
double standard: emotion 99–100;
    sexuality 84
Dworkin, Andrea 19, 20, 120

economic development 48–9
editors 103–4

education 39
Efran, J. S. 183
emancipatory politics 5
emotion 87, 99–100, 137
empowerment 11, 84, 195–6
Ennew, J. 57
entitlement feeling 61, 157
Entwisle, J. 230
Epstein, Barbara 86
essentialism 20
ethical obligations 195–6
ethnicity 142–3
experience 91, 94, 151, 232
explanations/descriptions 149

False Memory Syndrome Foundation
    96
false memory syndrome 105–6n2;
    gender politics 96, 104, 141; incest 96;
    media coverage 9, 95, 96–7, 100–2;
    source credibility 101; USA 96–7
family: apartheid 61; child sexual abuse
    58, 71, 81–2; feminism 82, 122;
    honour 143; kinship 81–2, 127n11;
    oppressed communities 83; power
    relations 21; sexuality 63; state 70,
    112–13; victimisation 27; violence 21,
    27–8; *see also* home
Father, Law of 77
female desire 78
femininity: borderline personality
    disorder 176–7, 181; cultural
    representations 85; normative
    157–60; sexuality 160; stereotyping
    175; vulnerability 39–40, 159
feminism: advocacy 190; anti-
    pornography 18; Australia 7; black
    women 9, 17, 28; child sexual abuse 2,
    3, 6, 54, 67, 126, 140, 145, 227–8;
    clinical psychology 195–8; cultural
    transformations 94–5; emancipatory
    politics 5; empowerment 11; family
    82, 122; forgiveness 83–4; frameworks
    204, 205; home 26, 28; incest 81,
    89–90; lesbianism 16; media coverage
    21–3; men's suffering 24; paedophiles
    126; patriarchy 86–7; Paulsgrove
    estate mothers 120–1; post-
    structuralism 3, 4–6, 20, 21, 25, 26, 29,
    131, 145; rape 134; second-wave 82,
    134, 145; sexual violence 20, 22;
    sisterhood 18, 22; social justice 190;

third-wave 82; trauma 204–5; victims/power 16, 17; *see also* lesbian feminism; radical feminism

feminist post-structuralism: child sexual abuse 222; compensation claims 195; mental health problems 168; sexuality 149; stories 211–12; survivors 149, 211; truth 151; Visible Therapy 226, 227

feminist standpoint theory 228–30

Finney, L. D. 151, 155

Firestone, Shulamith 19

First Nations organisations 89

Flax, J. 222

Fleck, Ludwig 66

Flores, L. 213

Flux, J. 151

forgiveness 82, 83–4, 85–6, 237

Foucault, Michel: bio-politics 108; confessional mode 230; discourse 66; governmentality 194; innocence 204; institutions 232; knowledge 5; power 5, 170–1, 219; subject 36

fragmentation principle 173

frameworks/feminism 204, 205

Freud, Sigmund 77

Freyd, Jennifer 96

friendship 232

Frosh, S. 227

Fuss, D. 57

Gallop, Jane 23

Gavey, Nicola 11, 131, 154, 157

Geertz, Clifford 70

gender: child sexual abuse 39–40, 142; children 39–40; credibility 101–2; differences 56, 68; discourse 95, 239; education 39; emotion 99–100; equality 3; identity 56; media coverage 102–4, 105; medical treatment 175, 176–7; perpetrators 56, 83; power 5–6, 53, 56, 131, 148, 160–2; race 25, 176; sexuality 123, 133, 140–2, 158, 160; stereotyping 39, 40, 176–7; subjectivity 54, 56–7, 68, 160–2; victimisation 140–1, 148, 172; vulnerability 140; *see also* men; women

gender politics 96, 104, 123, 141

genital fondling 55

genocide 27

Germany 55

Gilligan, Carol 85

girls 59, 63, 68

Gist, M. 105

God the Father 85

Gough, B. 156

governmentality 108, 194

Gray, L. 150, 195, 199

Grosz, E. 228

Guardian: Barnardos 45; housing policy 124; *News of the World* campaign 118, 119, 120; paedophiles 126–7n4; vigilantes 115, 116–17

Guardian Weekend 96

Guattari, Felix 227, 236

guilt: innocence 1–2, 234; responsibility 236; stories 235–6; women 87, 237

Guinea refugee camps 82, 83

Haaken, Jan 8–9, 95, 148, 156, 157

Habermas, Jürgen 113

Hacking, Ian 1, 94, 95, 148, 150

Haggis, J. 144

Hamilton, G. J. 239

Haraway, Donna 27, 228

Harding, S. 229

Hare-Mustin, R. 148

harm 10, 131, 137–8, 143–4

harm story: child sexual abuse 131–2, 139, 143–4; development 136–8; psychological approach 133–4; survivors 135; universalism 142

Hartsock, N. 228

hate 46

Haug, F. 110

Haugaard, J. J. H. 53

healing of survivors 215–16

Henderson, L. 105

Henriques, I. 66

Herman, J. L. 173

heteronormativity 157, 159–60

heteropatriarchy 219, 222

heterosexuality 141, 152, 157, 160–2

HIV/AIDS 58, 63

Hoch, P. H. 172

Hoggart, Simon 102

Holland, J. 160

Hollway, W. 69

home 26, 28, 41–2; *see also* family

homosexuality 90, 141

honesty 237–8

honour 143

hooks, bell 17, 22, 25, 218

housing estates 115–16, 123–4
housing policies 123–4, 126
Howard, G. S. 70
Humourless Feminist 17, 19–21, 22, 23

identification 46, 101–2, 152, 215–16
identity: child sexual abuse 46, 230, 233;
    gender 56; individual 86; modernity
    144; multiple 131, 142; post-
    structuralism 233; psychotherapy 231;
    reification 144–5; sexual 148; social
    change 80; social class 86; survival
    241; survivors 12, 151, 211, 212, 220,
    221, 222–3; Visible Therapy 243
identity politics 19
incest 134; Armstrong 95; definitions
    55; false memory syndrome 96;
    feminism 81, 89–90; memory 78,
    80–1; patriarchy 81; poverty 133;
    protection from 60; rape 55; stories
    87, 89–90; survivors 153, 218; victims
    95
incest industry 70
indexicality 211
infantilisation 47
infants 52, 58, 84
information 112–14, 115, 117
innocence 1–2, 48, 204, 234
institutions 35, 62, 89, 232, 242
intergenerational crisis 81–2
interpellation 198, 200, 204, 205, 234
interpretations 71–2, 211
intervention 44–5, 56, 58, 197, 239–40
isolation 38

Jehu, D. 148, 231
journalists 102, 103–4; see also media
    coverage

Karoo town 63
Katz, C. 49
Kelly, Liz 54
Kelner, Simon 117
Kempe, C. H. 134
Kempe, R. S. 133, 134
King, Martin Luther Jr. 89
Kingsolver, Barbara 72
Kinsey, A. C. 133
kinship/family 81–2, 127n11
Kitzinger, C. 230, 232, 241
Kitzinger, Jenny: feminism/child sexual
    abuse 134; framing 125; journalists

102, 103; media coverage 9, 104;
    survivors 152, 155, 156; women's
    pages 105
Kleinman, A. 169
knowledge: local 70; power 5, 108;
    professional/everyday 150; situated
    16, 28; subjugated 36; women 227
Korbin, J. E. 57
Kosambi, M. 144
Koss, M. J. 56
Kunzman, K. A. 153

Lamb, S. 134–5, 140, 156, 201
Lather, P. 144, 204
de Lauretis, Teresa 25, 26, 198
Law of the Father 77
lecturer/sexual harassment 16, 18–19,
    24
lesbian chic 21
lesbian feminism: otherness 22; radical
    feminism 18, 19–20, 21
lesbian vampire murder case 15–17
lesbianism 15–17
Levett, Ann 8, 64, 65, 72, 140
liberal discourse 111, 152–3
Lison, K. 151, 153, 154, 155
lobola payment 59
local tribunals 88–9
Lombroso, Cesaire 109, 114, 126n3
looping effect 150
loss 84, 137–8
Lumby, C. 23

McGillivray, Anne 89
MacKinnon, Catherine 18, 20, 26
MacLeod, M. 134
McNay, L. 231
Madigan, S. 171
Mail 96
Mail on Sunday 96
Malamuth, N. M. 56
Malcolm X 89
male domination: aggression 161; child
    sexual abuse 55–6; institutionalised
    62; media 103–4; pleasure 123; South
    Africa 60, 63–4
male violence 79, 156–7
Manchester City Council: Ten Things
    Children Need Most 44
Mani, L. 29
Mann, Sally 49n1
Maori women 26

Marecek, Jeanne 148, 149, 187, 200–1, 205
marginalisation 41, 46
masculinity 56, 160–2
meanings, chains of 197
Medea figure 86
media coverage 9, 100; Australia 21–3; British False Memory Society 96; child sexual offenders 109–10; false memory syndrome 9, 95, 96–7, 100–2; feminism 21–3; gender 102–4, 105; lecturer story 18–19; lesbianism 15–17, 18–19; male dominated 103–4; murder 15–16; paedophiles 109–12; radical feminism 22–3; sexual harassment 101; survivors 210; women's pages 104–5
media sources 101–2
medical treatment/gender 175, 176–7
medicalisation: borderline personality disorder 168; child sexual abuse 134; diagnosis 168–72; social problems 71
Meese Commission in Pornography 21
Megan's law 109, 114
Mejiuni, C. O. 59
memory 77, 78, 80; child sexual abuse 41–2, 67, 78; experience 91; incest 78, 80–1; intervention 239–40; recovered 81–2, 90, 237; sexual violence 94; stories 78; see also false memory syndrome
men: denial 143; feelings of entitlement 61, 157; in oppressed communities 83; power 56; sexuality 123, 158; suffering 24; victimisers 148; victims of domestic violence 29; see also male domination; male violence; masculinity
mental disorder 7
Mental Health Act 168, 177
mental health problems: categorisation 169; child sexual abuse 54, 150; feminist post-structuralism 168; rape 201; survivors 167–8
mental health services 179–82, 239; abuse within 231–2; clinicians 54; survivors 231; therapists 150
mental health workers 179–80, 181; see also therapists
mental illness 177
mental impairment 177
Miller, D. 98

Miller, P. 108
Miller, Peggy 80
Millett, K. 53
Miltenburg, R. 152
mind-fucks 233, 236
mind/unconsciousness 235
Mirror: News of the World campaign 114; paedophiles 111, 122, 126–7n4; public opinion 118; vigilantes 110, 116, 117
Mitchell, S. A. 169
Mizen, P. 47
modernity 38, 42, 144
monster imagery 110–11, 122
Moore, Charles 117
moral panic 27, 28
Morgan, Elizabeth 144
Morris, Meaghan 17, 20–1, 22, 23
mothers: betrayal 85; child murder reactions 122; reparation 85; single 60; state 120, 121; vigilantes 9; violence 116
multiple personality disorder 80, 95
murder 15–16, 122

NACRO 110
narrative therapy 227
narratives: see stories
Native Americans 89
naturalness of childhood 7, 41, 42, 44–5
Neb, Andrew 46
neglect 57
Nelson, B. 53
neocolonialism 72
New Zealand 7; Accident Compensation Act 188; Accident Compensation Corporation 188–92; and Australia 16, 24; lesbians/lecturer 16, 18–19; Morgan 144
New Zealand Accident Compensation Corporation 11
News of the World: criticisms of campaign 118–19; information for parents 113, 114, 118; nationalist/racialist factors 121; paedophiles 109, 112, 122–3, 126–7n4; public opinion 118; Wade 118
news production 105; see also media coverage
Newsnight, BBC 96
Nicolson, P. 150
Nigeria 59

norms: discourse analysis 72; femininity
   157–60; sexuality 7, 10; Western
   society 142; whiteness 143
NSPCC 110, 123

objectification 59
Observer 102
O'Dell, Lindsay 10, 140, 144, 197
oppressed communities 83, 85, 88
original sin 37
originary state 43
O'Sullivan, Sue 15, 23
otherness: childhood 37; ethnicity 143;
   lesbian feminism 22; sexually-abused
   children 35, 132, 135, 138; survivors
   152–5; women 160

paedophiles: boys 58; feminism 126;
   liberal discourse 111; media coverage
   109–12; *Mirror* 111, 122, 126–7n4;
   monster imagery 110–11, 122; *News
   of the World* 109, 112, 122–3,
   126–7n4; populist discourse 110–11;
   power/knowledge 108; rehousing 9;
   reoffending 127n5, 127n10; state
   protection 120; stereotyping 122;
   suicide 110, 115, 116
Paglia, Camille 16, 17, 19
parents: information about paedophiles
   113–14; perpetrators 113; risk
   assessment 112–13; state 117, 119–20,
   125; vigilance 111–12, 115
Parents Against Injustice 105–6n2
Parker, Ian 179, 187–8, 211
Parker, J. 66
passivity 159
Patel, D. 143
Pateman, C. 44
paternalism 64
patients 178–80; *see also*
   clients/therapists
patriarchy 9, 54; Africa 69; female
   desire 78; feminism 86–7; incest 81;
   paternalism 64; power 56, 57, 58–9;
   resistance 63, 69, 87; Western society
   52
Paulsgrove estate: children 117, 121;
   feminism 120–1; housing policy
   123–4; protest 113–14, 120–1, 125;
   vigilantes 109–10, 116–17
Payne, Sara and Michael 119
Payne, Sarah 9, 109, 118, 120

Penthouse 19
Perkins, R. 230, 232, 241
perpetrators: entitlement feelings 61,
   157; gender 56, 83; parents 113;
   protection 63; victims 65, 80, 138, 172;
   see also child sexual offenders;
   paedophiles
Perry, J. C. 179
personal/political 4, 91
personal/social 235
personality, damaged 174
Petronio, S. 213
Pettinger, Angela 116
physical beatings 60
Piaget, Jean 39
pleasure 123
Plummer, K. 153, 167, 230, 231
Pole, C. 47
political correctness 15, 23–4
political/personal 4, 91
politics 5, 121, 144; *see also* gender
   politics
Pollack, S. 235
populist discourse 110–11
Posel, D. 63
Poston, C. 151, 153, 154, 155
post-structuralism: feminism 3, 4–6, 20,
   21, 25, 26, 29, 131, 145;
   gender/sexuality/ethnicity 131;
   identity 233; interpellation 198, 200,
   204, 205, 234; psychology 199–203;
   trust 237
poverty 57, 89, 133
power: Foucault 5, 170–1, 219; gender
   5–6, 53, 56, 131, 148, 160–2;
   knowledge 5, 108; men 56; patriarchy
   56, 57, 58–9; sex 24–5; sexuality 22,
   154; victimisation 16, 17, 24; Visible
   Therapy 234–5
power relations: adults/children 57;
   British False Memory Society 95, 96;
   child sexual abuse 68; conflicts of
   interest 48–9; family 21; gender 53;
   men/women 57; mental
   representations 80; South Africa
   59–61
powerlessness 148, 182
pregnancy avoidance 68
pressure groups 97–9
private/public sphere 56, 122
professionalisation 53, 68–9, 135,
   150

progression 132–4, 136–7
prohibitions 77; see also taboo
protection 44, 63, 68; see also
  vigilantes
pseudo-forgiveness 85–6
psychiatric disorders 10–11, 66; see also
  mental health problems
psychoanalytic social theory 57, 78–9
psychological approach 133–4, 148
psychological trauma 53, 55–6
psychology 9, 79, 199–203
psychopathic personality disorder
  177–8
psychotherapy 197, 227, 231, 239
public health 43
public opinion 118

race 25, 176, 233–4
racism 25–6, 61, 125
radical feminism: black feminism 17;
  child sexual abuse 19; domestic
  violence 23; lesbian feminism 18,
  19–20, 21; media coverage 22–3;
  political correctness 15; sexual
  violence 17–18, 28–9; sexuality 19
Rahnema, M. 44–5
RAPCAN 58
rape 203; feminism 134; incest 55;
  infants 52, 58; lobola payment 59;
  mental health effects 201; South
  Africa 61–2; survivors 156, 187;
  victim-blaming 188; Vigarello 201
Rappaport, J. 219
reality 1–2, 37, 183
Reavey, Paula: chains of meaning 197;
  effects of child sexual abuse 1, 10,
  144, 149; post-structuralism 227;
  survivors 156, 210
reconciliation 84
recovered memory 81–2, 90
recovery 82, 197, 218, 230
refugees/forgiveness 82, 83, 237
relationships 25, 85
religion/culture 142–3
remembering 80–1, 82, 90–1; see also
  memory
Renzetti, Claire 29
reparation 79, 85
Reppucci, N. C. 53
representations 26–7, 85, 121
residential care 41–2
resilience 40, 215

resistance: child sexual abuse 69, 232;
  defiance 80; patriarchy 63, 69, 87;
  survivors 214
respect 195, 196
responsibility: borderline personality
  disorder 179; childhood 38–9; guilt
  236; personal 90; social 46; survivors
  180–1
Rich, Adrienne 20, 78
rights: children 43–4, 52–4, 64; victims
  120; women 229
risk assessment 112–13, 115
risk society 112–17
ritual 89
Roberge, L. 136
Roiphe, Katie 16, 17, 19, 25
Romme, M. A. J. 239
Rose, Nikolas 108, 112, 199, 201, 231,
  240
Rubin, G. 19
Russell, D. E. H. 53, 65

Saraga, E. 134
Schecter, M. D. 136
Scott, Jean 151
secrecy 63
Section 28 127n9
Segal, L. 148, 160
self 243; see also identity
self worth 181
self-blaming 214
self-disclosure 230
self-harm 240
self-help groups 11–12, 213–15; social
  transformation 216–17; solidarity
  218–19; survivors 212–13
self-help texts 151, 152, 219
self-preservation 238–41
self-recovery 218
self-reflectivity 83–4, 180, 181
self-trauma model 197–8
sentimentality 46
separation 84
separatism 19
sex/power 24–5
sex wars 24–5
sexual abuse 2–3, 54, 56, 87–8; see also
  child sexual abuse
sexual coercion 22, 65
sexual drives 158
sexual harassment 16, 18–19, 24, 101
sexual penetration 161–2

sexual violence 90; feminism 20, 22; harm 131; Humourless Feminist 20–1; memory 94; radical feminism 17–18, 28–9; relationships 25; representations 26–7; social class 62; South Africa 61–2; stories 133

sexuality: children 49n1, 65, 71; choice 153–5, 157–60, 162–3, 235; consent 234; control 161–2; deviance 141; double standard 84; family 63; femininity 160; feminist post-structuralism 149; gender 123, 133, 140–2, 158, 160; harm 10; liberal ideology 152–3; men 123, 158; norms 7, 10; power 22, 154; psychological discourse 148; radical feminism 19; stories 77; survivors 151, 153, 157–8, 160, 163, 220; taboo 65; women 133, 160; see also sexual violence

sexually-abused children: difference 37; isolation 38; otherness 35, 132, 135, 138; rights of children 52–3; stigma 43, 64, 138; as victims/survivors 46

Shotter, J. 171

sick role 180

Sierra Leone 82, 83

silencing of children 235

Singer, E. 152

single mothers 60

sisterhood 16, 18, 22

Skeggs, S. B. 145

Smith, Barbara 22

Socarides, C. 57

social change 80

social class: anger/aggression 80; identity 86; politics 121; sexual violence 62; vulnerability 41

social constructions: child development 132; childhood 38–9, 136; children 46; psychotherapy 227

social exclusion 115–16

social justice 190

social movements 83–4, 86, 90–1

social/personal 235

social responsibility 46

social transformation 216–17

socialisation 66, 68

socialist feminism 18, 22, 25–6

Sockoskie, R. J. 56

solidarity 218–19

South Africa: apartheid 60, 61, 62; child sexual abuse 6, 52–4, 58–9;

Constitution 59; customary law 59, 60; male domination 60, 63–4; multilingualism 71–2; power relations 59–61; racism 61; rape 61–2; sexual violence 61–2; single mothers 60; women 62–3

South African Human Rights Commission 52–4

Soyland, A. J. 150

Spaccerelli, S. 55, 64

special hospitals 167–8, 176, 182

Spivak, Gayatri 20, 229

Squire, C. 211

Stainton Rogers, R. 40

Stainton Rogers, W. 40

Stanko, Elizabeth 29

state: child sexual abuse 27; family 70, 112–13; family violence 21; housing policies 123–4, 126; information to public 117; mothers 120, 121; paedophiles 120; parents 117, 119–20, 125

state welfare 42

Steedman, Carolyn 40

Stenner, P. 135

stereotyping: femininity 175; gender 39, 40, 176–7; paedophiles 122; victims 26

stigma: child sexual abuse 65, 67, 70; sexually-abused children 43, 64, 138

stories 90; borderline personality disorder 173; causality 79; child sexual abuse 34–6, 90, 135, 150, 180; childhood 34–6; feminist post-structuralism 211–12; guilt 235–6; incest 87, 89–90; memory 78; multiple 183; prohibitions 77; psychology 79; reality 183; sexual violence 133; sexuality 77; stock scripts 81; survivors 148–9, 158, 163, 210, 212, 220–1; trauma 200; see also harm story

Strange Days, BBC 99, 101

stranger danger 58, 127n8

Straw, Jack 115, 119, 120

subject 36

subjectivity: child sexual abuse 149; childhood 36, 40; gendered 54, 56–7, 68, 160–2; heterosexuality 160–2; modernity 38; Western society 40

suicide 110, 115, 116, 240

Sullivan, T. 63–4, 71

Sunday Times 96, 101, 102

survival strategies 238–9, 241

survivors 163; body language 155;
compensation claims 187, 188–92;
coping mechanisms 180, 198; critical
psychology 203–5; discourse 221;
feminist post-structuralism 149, 211;
harm story 135; healing 215–16;
identity 12, 151, 211, 212, 220, 221,
222–3; incest 153, 218; Kitzinger 152,
155, 156; long term effects 65, 192–4;
male violence 156–7; media coverage
210; mental health problems 167–8;
mental health services 231; otherness
152–5; rape 156, 187; recovery 82,
197, 230; resilience 40, 215; resistance
214; responsibility 180–1; self-help
groups 11–12, 212–15; self-recovery
218; sensitivity 215–16; sexuality 151,
153, 157–8, 160, 163, 220; sick role
180; stories 148–9, 158, 163, 210,
212–13, 220–1; victimisation 214;
visibility 210; Visible Therapy 197–8

taboo 65, 67, 133
talking therapy 187, 213–14
Tanaka, J. S. 56
Taylor, V. 213
textual analysis 135–43
textualisation of childhood 37
therapist/client 150, 236–8, 242
Thomas, J. 202
The Times 101
Tobin, Rosemary 197
tormentors 91
trauma: borderline personality disorder
173–4; child sexual abuse 53–4, 55–6,
167, 241–2; damage to personality
174; feminism 204–5; framework
204–5; holding 82; model for 200–1;
stories 200; talking therapy 187
trust 236–8
truth 1–2, 151
Tuchman, G. 104

UN Convention on the Rights of the
Child 38–9, 43
unconscious 78–9, 80, 235
unemployment 89
United States of America: child sexual
abuse 55; false memory syndrome
96–7; Meese Commission in
Pornography 21; Megan's law 109,
114

universalism 53, 72, 142
Ussher, J. 176

vampire imagery 15, 24, 27, 29
Vance, Carole 21
victim-blaming 188, 205
victimisation: family 27; forgiveness 83;
gender 140–1, 148, 172; power 16, 17,
24; survivors 214
victims: advocacy 11; child sexual abuse
120, 140; credibility 102; experience
94; feminism 16, 17; Humourless
Feminist 22; identification 215–16;
incest 95; men 29; perpetrators 65, 80,
138, 172; rights 120; stereotyping 26;
vulnerability 140; women 148
Vigarello, Georges 201
vigilance 111–12, 115
vigilantes: mothers 9; Paulsgrove estate
109–10, 116–17; vigilance 111–12, 115
violence: domestic 23, 88–9; family 21,
27–8; institutions 89; male 79, 156–7;
mothers 116; pre-modern 116; *see
also* sexual violence
Virgin advertisement 47
virginity 142–3
Visible Therapy 12, 197; critical
reflection 230; feminist post-
structuralism 226, 227; feminist
standpoint theory 228–30; identity
243; power 234–5; survivors 197–8;
tactics of child sexual abuse 233;
training/supervision 242
vulnerability: children 41; femininity
39–40, 159; gender 140; social class
41; victims 140

Wade, Rebekah 118
Walkerdine, Valerie 42
Walrond-Skinner, Sue 84–5
Walters, Natasha 120
Warner, Sam 140; borderline
personality disorder 172, 175; chains
of meaning 197; choice of partner
156; conceptual change 5, 183;
identity 232; mental health services
167, 180; mind-fuck 236; post-
structuralism 227; psychiatric
classifications 10–11; reality 1, 2;
sexuality 234; social/personal 235;
survivors 159, 160, 210, 221, 239; trust
237; Visible Therapy 12, 197, 230

Watney, S. 19
Weeks, J. 19
Weir, R. I. 133
West , Traci 88–9
Westen, D. 173
Western society 52; childhood 53, 66;
  children's sexuality 71; cultural
  imperialism 8, 69; family/state 70;
  forgiveness 83; as norm 142;
  patriarchy 52; professionalisation
  68–9; self 243; subjectivity 40;
  universalism 53
White, Evelyn 88
whiteness as norm 143
Wigginton, Tracey 15, 17
Wile, D. B. 173
Wilkins, Tracy 10–11
Wilson, M. 143
Winnicott, D. 46, 48
WISH 167, 172

Wolf, Naomi 16
women 1, 12; Aboriginal 89; Africa 9,
  62–3, 83; agency 232; black 9, 17, 28,
  79, 87–8, 240; children 57; desire 78;
  emotional attachment 87; friendship
  232; guilt 87, 237; knowledge 227;
  objectification 59; otherness 160; as
  perpetrators 83; relationships 85;
  rights 229; sexual abuse 2–3; sexuality
  133, 160; trust 238; victims 148; *see
  also* femininity; feminism; lesbianism;
  mothers
Women's Liberation Movement 3
women's pages 104–5
Woolgar, S. 211
world development 48–9
Worrell, Marcia 11–12

Zita, Jacquelyn 22